TMLR *Management of Coronary Artery Diseases*

Springer
Berlin
Heidelberg
New York
Barcelona
Budapest
Hong Kong
London
Milan
Paris
Santa Clara
Singapore
Tokyo

M. Klein H. D. Schulte E. Gams (Eds.)

TMLR

Management of Coronary Artery Diseases

With 79 Figures

Springer

Priv.-Doz. Dr. med. Michael Klein
Professor Dr. med. H. D. Schulte
Professor Dr. med. E. Gams

Heinrich-Heine-Universität
Klinik für Thorax- und
Kardiovaskuläre Chirurgie
Moorenstraße 5
D-40225 Düsseldorf

ISBN-13:978-3-642-72136-6

Die Deutsche Bibliothek - CIP-Einheitsaufnahme
TMLR: management of coronary artery diseases / M. Klein ... (ed.). - Berlin; Heidelberg; New York; Barcelona; Budapest; Hong Kong; London; Milan; Paris; Santa Clara; Singapore; Tokyo: Springer, 1998
ISBN-13:978-3-642-72136-6 e-ISBN-13:978-3-642-72134-2
DOI: 10.1007/978-3-642-72134-2

Softcover reprint of the hardcover 1st edition 1998

Cover-Design: Design & Production GmbH, Heidelberg

Data conversion: K+V Fotosatz, Beerfelden

SPIN 10650514 18/3137-5 4 3 2 1 0 - Printed on acid-free paper

Preface

At the beginning of this century, the state of surgical technique only provided for concepts with an extracardial approach to therapy of coronary heart diseases. Decreasing the heart activity by means of denervating the heart or thyroidectomy, resulting in a reduction of the heart's oxygen demand, was strived at. Later, the progress of clinical surgery at the closed beating heart allowed for procedures with myocardial access. In this historical stage of indirect revascularisation, a compensation was supposed to be stimulated operatively by providing an adhesion to the surrounding organs or by manipulating the larger heart veins. The simple ligation of the *Arteria thoracica interna* in the middle third of its course – intended to increase the perfusion of pericardial branches – is based on the fundamental ignorance or misunderstanding of the haemodynamic laws. The first intervention to reach temporary popularity was the implantation of the *Arteria thoracica interna* into the left ventricular myocardial wall. This so-called "Vineberg procedure" was not very risky and did show some permanent improvements with respect to the patient's complaints or even the prognosis. However, this procedure has been almost completely abandoned, despite the fact that some positive long-term courses have been documented. Other indirect revascularisation procedures carried out in the fifties, e.g. the drilling of transmyocardial channels by application of various techniques, including the insertion of small tubes, were not established clinically either, although a positive effect of the "ordinary needle puncture" could be demonstrated experimentally by different investigators in the acute ischaemic model. Unfortunately, no further research into these techniques was carried out at that time, possibly because of the era of open heart surgery which began almost simultaneously and allowed direct access to the coronary arteries. So this was the actual introduction of direct revascularisation techniques. In particular, the rapid development of the technology of extracorporeal circulation (ECC) which followed and the procedures of myocardial protection favoured the establishment of direct revascularisation techniques at the non-beating heart. This was the reason why aorto-coronary bypass grafting (CABG) became and still is the golden standard in surgical therapy of coronary artery disease.

As aggressively as the cardiac surgeons turned to the treatment of coronary heart diseases, applying more and more sophisticated and high-tech techniques, the cardiologists have also continuously introduced increasingly effective drug therapies and established the most successful interventional procedures. Therefore, drug therapy, percutaneous transluminal coronary angioplasty and bypass surgery form the basic strategies for treating coronary heart disease today.

Despite or even because of the general success in controlling exertional myocardial ischaemia, the treatment of patients suffering from end-stage coronary artery disease poses, particularly due to the influence of demographic and medical data, a challenge to medical therapy as coronary artery disease is not only the major cause of death in the Western World but also a leading cause of severe disability. Anginal chest pain limits physical activities and degrades the quality of life of millions of people. This clinical problem has given rise to the demand to extend the therapeutic focus, not only to the proximal lesion of the coronary arteries, but also to include disorders of the small and smallest vessels. This requires techniques that allow for revascularisation of the ischaemic myocardium from an area which is not directly connected to the vessel concerned. In this context, the indirect transmyocardial revascularisation, i.e. a technique of the pre-bypass era, re-gains importance. This has only become possible because investigators, such as Mirhoseini, had faith in this kind of approach and introduced LASER (Light Amplification of Stimulated Emission of Radiation) technology to this field. So, the historical technique of indirect revascularisation, which has possibly been less effective due only to the lack of adequate technological and instrumental means, has experienced a renaissance: it is currently the only promising technique in this context.

Transmyocardial laser revascularisation (TMLR) is a relatively new and indirect approach to myocardial revascularisation. Laser-drilled transmyocardial channels should ideally provide for the preconditions not only to connect these channels to an intramyocardial network of developed collaterals, but particularly to ensure that these channels remain open, endothelialise and serve as a long-term vessel replacement in order to reduce the prevailing myocardial ischaemia. However, the principle of function of this revascularisation method is actually not fully understood. With about two thirds of the patients, clinical follow-up examinations show an identical improvement in their angina pectoris symptomatology and endurance. Experimental data referring to TMLR are partly contradictory and have been captured under different experimental conditions. In addition, the introduction of different laser systems, with different operational principles and the resultant response of the tissue, have given rise to further hypotheses on the "best-suited light" for this technique. So, the discussion is currently characterised by various arguments and speculations.

On the other hand, more and more serious investigators publish scientific papers focusing on pathophysiology and pathology of the diseased heart to possibly find a proper indication for this surgical intervention. As it is, the best surgical approach means nothing without the right indication.

Currently, only a hibernating myocardium seems to be preferably eligible to TMLR. However, TMLR does not appear to be an alternative to CABG procedures. Consequently, methods aiming to prove its efficiency, focusing on the perfusion degree of the treated areas, are likewise in the centre of interest. Therefore, not only cardiac surgeons and cardiologists, but also pathologists, physiologists and scientists of other disciplines, such as nuclear medicine, are involved in this research.

The re-gained importance of TMLR on the one hand and the inconsistency of current data and the lack of communication between the disciplines concerned on the other have induced us to initiate an exchange of thoughts on the status of TMLR at Duesseldorf University on May 15th–17th, 1997.

The articles included in this book reflect current knowledge and attitudes towards TMLR. The availability of appropriate assay techniques is provided; the future will tell whether TMLR is really a successful method to provide clinically and surgically efficient life-extending help to patients with end-stage coronary artery disease.

As such comprehensive research can only be carried out with the massive support of the laser industry we would like to acknowledge the United States Surgical Corporation, Norwalk, Conn., particularly, for generously enabling us to take the first step in this direction. The second step will be made in 1998 by holding an international conference on the Status of TMLR in the management of coronary artery disease. In addition, an international multicentre trial will be started at the beginning of 1998. The aim of this study will be to evaluate the effects of TMLR as an adjunct to direct revascularisation in patients with end-stage coronary artery disease.

M. Klein
H. D. Schulte
E. Gams

January 1998

Contents

List of Contributors

ASFOUR, B., Dr. med.
Westfälische Wilhelms-Universität
Münster
Klinik für Thorax-, Herz- und
Gefäßchirurgie
Albert-Schweitzer-Straße 33
D-48149 Münster

BEEK, JOHAN, PhD
Laser Center
Academical Medical Center
Meibergdreef 9
NL-1105 AZ Amsterdam

BEYERSDORF, FRIEDHELM,
Prof. Dr. med.
Chirurgische Universitätsklinik
Freiburg
Abteilung Herz- und Gefäßchirurgie
Hugstetter Straße 55
D-79106 Freiburg

BÜRKLE, MANUELA, Cand. med.
Chirurgische Universitätsklinik
Freiburg
Abteilung Herz- und Gefäßchirurgie
Hugstetter Straße 55
D-79106 Freiburg

CAMPANELLA, CIRO, MD, FRCS
Royal Infirmary of Edinburgh
Department of Cardiothoracic
Surgery
1 Lauriston Place
Edinburgh, EH3 9YW
United Kingdom

CRYER, COLIN W., Prof. Dr. med.
Westfälische Wilhelms-Universität
Münster
Institut für Numerische und
Instrumentelle Mathematik
Fachbereich 15, Mathematik
und Informatik
Einsteinstraße 62
D-48149 Münster

DAUBEN, H.P., Dr. med.
Heinrich-Heine-Universität
Klinik für Thorax-
und Kardiovaskularchirurgie
Moorenstraße 5
D-40225 Düsseldorf

DÖRSCHEL, KLAUS, Dr. rer. nat.
Freie Universität Berlin
Institut für Medizinisch/Technische
Physik und Lasermedizin
Krahmer Straße 6–10
D-12207 Berlin

EICHSTÄDT, HERMANN,
Univ.-Prof. Dr.
Charité, Campus Virchow-Klinikum
der Humboldt-Universität zu Berlin
Strahlenklinik und Poliklinik
Augustenburger Platz 1
D-13353 Berlin

ERBEL, R., Prof. Dr. med.
Universitätsklinikum, GH Essen
Zentrum für Innere Medizin
Abteilung für Kardiologie
Hufelandstraße 55
D-45122 Essen

FISHBEIN, M., M.D.
Cedars-Sinai Medical Center
650 South San Vicente Boulevard
Los Angeles, California 90048
USA

FISHER, JOHN C., Sc.D.
417 Palmtree Drive
Bradenton, Florida, 34210
USA

FÜHRMEYER, FRAUKE
Medizinische Universität zu Lübeck
Klinik für Herzchirurgie
Ratzeburger Allee 160
D-23538 Lübeck

FUNCK, REINHARD, Dr. med.
Philipps-Universität Marburg
Abteilung für Kardiologie
Baldingerstraße
D-35043 Marburg

GÖHRING, STEFAN, Dr. med.
Herzzentrum Frankfurt
Abteilung für Innere Medizin/
Kardiologie
Postfach 10 10 63
D-60010 Frankfurt/Main

GRÜNDEMANN, PAUL, PhD
University Hospital Utrecht
Heart Lung Institute
P.O. Box 85500
NL-3508 GA Utrecht

GRUNDFEST, WARREN, M.D.
Cedars-Sinai Medical Center
650 South San Vicente Boulevard
Los Angeles, California 90048
USA

HERING, PETER, Prof. Dr. rer. nat.
Heinrich-Heine-Universität
Institut für Lasermedizin
Postfach 10 10 07
D-40001 Düsseldorf

HETZER, ROLAND, Prof. Dr. med., PhD
Deutsches Herzzentrum
Klinik für THG-Chirurgie
Augustenburger Platz 1
D-13353 Berlin

HEUSCH, GERD, Prof. Dr. med.
Universitätsklinikum
Gesamthochschule Essen
Zentrum für Innere Medizin
Abteilung für Pathophysiologie
Hufelandstraße 55
D-45122 Essen

HÖFFKEN, HELMUT, PD Dr. med.
Philipps-Universität Marburg
Abteilung für Nuklearmedizin
Baldingerstraße
D-35043 Marburg

HORT, W., Prof. (em.) Dr. med.
Heinrich-Heine-Universität
Medizinische Einrichtungen
Institut für Pathologie
Moorenstraße 5
D-40225 Düsseldorf

IVANENKO, M.M., Dr. rer. nat.
Heinrich-Heine-Universität
Institut für Lasermedizin
Postfach 10 10 07
D-40001 Düsseldorf

IVRON, R., Ph.D.
Medical Division
Opgal, Karmiel
P.O. Box 402
Israel

KOERFER, R., Dr. med., MD, PhD
Universitätsklinik der
Ruhr-Universität Bochum
Klinik für Thorax-
und Kardiovaskularchirurgie
Georgstraße 11
D-32545 Bad Oeynhausen

KONDRUWEIT, M., Dr. med.
Westfälische Wilhelms-Universität
Münster
Klinik für Thorax-, Herz-
und Gefäßchirurgie
Albert-Schweitzer-Straße 33
D-48149 Münster

KÖRNER, MICHAEL M., Dr. med., MD
Universitätsklinik der Ruhr-
Universität Bochum
Klinik für Thorax-
und Kardiovaskularchirurgie
Georgstraße 11
D-32545 Bad Oeynhausen

KRAATZ, ERNST-G., Dr. med.
Medizinische Universität zu Lübeck
Klinik für Herzchirurgie
Ratzeburger Allee 160
D-23538 Lübeck

KRABATSCH, THOMAS, Dr. med.
Deutsches Herzzentrum
Klinik für THG-Chirurgie
Augustenburger Platz 1
D-13353 Berlin

LIEBACK, EVELYN, Dr. med.
Deutsches Herzzentrum
Klinik für THG-Chirurgie
Augustenburger Platz 1
D-13353 Berlin

LUNKENHEIMER, P.P., Prof. Dr. med.
Westfälische Wilhelms-Universität
Münster
Experimentelle Thorax-, Herz-
und Gefäßchirurgie
Domagkstraße 11
D-48129 Münster

LUTTER, GEORG, Dr. med.
Chirurgische Universitätsklinik
Freiburg
Abteilung Herz- und Gefäßchirurgie
Hugstetter Straße 55
D-79106 Freiburg

LUTZ, CHRISTOPH, Dr. med.
Chirurgische Universitätsklinik
Freiburg
Abteilung Herz- und Gefäßchirurgie
Hugstetter Straße 55
D-79106 Freiburg

MAISCH, BERNHARD, Prof. Dr. med.
Philipps-Universität Marburg
Abteilung für Kardiologie
Baldingerstraße
D-35043 Marburg

MARTIN, JÜRGEN, Dr. med.
Chirurgische Universitätsklinik
Freiburg
Abteilung Herz- und Gefäßchirurgie
Hugstetter Straße 55
D-79106 Freiburg

MISFELD, MARTIN, Dr. med.
Medizinische Universität zu Lübeck
Klinik für Herzchirurgie
Ratzeburger Allee 160
D-23538 Lübeck

MOOSDORF, RAINER, Prof. Dr. med.
Philipps-Universität Marburg
Klinik für Herzchirurgie
Baldingerstraße
D-35043 Marburg

MORGAN, IAN S., MB ChB, FRCSEd
Royal Infirmary of Edinburgh
Department of Cardiothoracic
Surgery
1 Lauriston Place
Edinburgh, EH3 9YW
United Kingdom

MÜLLER, GERHARD J.,
Prof. Dr.h.c. Dr.-Ing.
Laser- und Med.-Technologie
gGmbH, Berlin
Krahmerstraße 6–10
D-12207 Berlin

NITZSCHE, EGBERT, PD, Dr. med.
Universitätsklinik Freiburg
Institut für Nuklearmedizin
Hugstetter Straße 55
D-79106 Freiburg

OLDENBURG, OLAF, Dr. med.
Universitätsklinikum, GH Essen
Zentrum für Innere Medizin
Abteilung für Kardiologie
Hufelandstraße 55
D-45122 Essen

PACALA, T.
United States Surgical Corporation
150 Glover Avenue
Norwalk, Connecticut 06856
USA

PAPAIANNOU, T., M.S.
Cedars-Sinai Medical Center
650 South San Vicente Boulevard
Los Angeles, California 90048
USA

REDMANN, KLAUS, Dr. med.
Westfälische Wilhelms-Universität
Münster
Experimentelle Thorax-, Herz-
und Gefäßchirurgie
Domagkstraße 11
D-48129 Münster

REIFART, N., Prof. Dr. med.
Kardiologisches Institut
Kliniken des MTK GmbH
Kronberger Straße 36
D-65812 Bad Soden / Ts.

RUPPE, C.
Cedars-Sinai Medical Center
650 South San Vicente Boulevard
Los Angeles, California 90048
USA

RYBINSKI, LESZEK, Dr. med.
Philipps-Universität Marburg
Klinik für Herzchirurgie
Baldingerstraße
D-35043 Marburg

SACHINOPOULOU, ANNA, MSc
Laser Center
Academical Medical Center
Meibergdreef 9
NL-1105 AZ Amsterdam

SARAI, KOPPANY, Dr. med.
Chirurgische Universitätsklinik
Freiburg
Abteilung Herz- und Gefäßchirurgie
Hugstetter Straße 55
D-79106 Freiburg

SCHALDACH, BRITA, Dr. rer. nat.
Freie Universität Berlin
Institut für Medizinisch/Technische
Physik und Lasermedizin
Krahmer Straße 6–10
D-12207 Berlin

SCHÄPER, FRANK, Dr. med.
Rudolf-Virchow-Klinikum
Institut für Pathologie
Augustenburger Platz 1
D-13353 Berlin

SCHELD, H.H., Prof. Dr. med.
Westfälische Wilhelms-Universität
Münster
Klinik und Poliklinik für Thorax-,
Herz- und Gefäßchirurgie
Albert-Schweitzer-Straße 33
D-48129 Münster

SCHMID, CHRISTOF, Priv.-Doz.,
Dr. med.
Westfälische Wilhelms-Universität
Münster
Klinik für Thorax-, Herz-
und Gefäßchirurgie
Albert-Schweitzer-Straße 33
D-48149 Münster

SCHMIDTKE, CLAUDIA
Medizinische Universität zu Lübeck
Klinik für Herzchirurgie
Ratzeburger Allee 160
D-23538 Lübeck

SCHULZ, RAINER, PD Dr. med.
Universitätsklinikum
Gesamthochschule Essen
Zentrum für Innere Medizin
Abteilung für Pathophysiologie
Hufelandstraße 55
D-45122 Essen

SCHWORTZ, B.
Cedars-Sinai Medical Center
650 South San Vicente Boulevard
Los Angeles, California 90048
USA

SEITELBERGER, RAINALD,
Prof. Dr. med.
Universitätsklinik für Chirurgie
Abteilung für Herz-Thorax-Chirurgie
Währinger Gürtel 18–20
A-1090 Wien

SHEHADA, R., M.S.
Cedars-Sinai Medical Center
650 South San Vicente Boulevard
Los Angeles, California 90048
USA

SHI, W., Ph.D.
Cedars-Sinai Medical Center
650 South San Vicente Boulevard
Los Angeles, California 90048
USA

SIEVERS, HANS H., Prof. Dr. med.
Medizinische Universität zu Lübeck
Klinik für Herzchirurgie
Ratzeburger Allee 160
D-23538 Lübeck

SPECHT, VON, B., Prof. Dr. med.
Chirurgische Universitätsklinik
Freiburg
Abteilung für Chirurgische Forschung
Hugstetter Straße 55
D-79106 Freiburg

STUBBE, HANS-MARTIN, PD Dr. med.
Cardioclinic
Heilwigstraße 39
D-20249 Hamburg

TAKAHASHI, NORIYOKO, Dr. med.
Chirurgische Universitätsklinik
Freiburg
Abteilung Herz- und Gefäßchirurgie
Hugstetter Straße 55
D-79106 Freiburg

TAMBEUR, LUC, Dr. med.
Deutsches Herzzentrum
Klinik für THG-Chirurgie
Augustenburger Platz 1
D-13353 Berlin

TENDERICH, G., Dr. med.
Universitätsklinik der
Ruhr-Universität Bochum
Klinik für Thorax-
und Kardiovaskularchirurgie
Georgstraße 11
D-32545 Bad Oeynhausen

TJAN, T.D.T., Dr. med.
Westfälische Wilhelms-Universität
Münster
Klinik für Thorax-, Herz-
und Gefäßchirurgie
Albert-Schweitzer-Straße 33
D-48149 Münster

VERDAASDONK, RUDOLF M., Ph.D.
University Hospital Utrecht
Department of Clinical Physics and
Biomedical Engineering
P.O. Box 85500
NL-3508 GA Utrecht

VOSBERG, H., Prof. Dr. med.
Heinrich-Heine-Universität
Medizinische Einrichtungen
Nuklearmedizinische Klinik
Moorenstraße 5
D-40225 Düsseldorf

WILD, THOMAS, Dr. med.
Universitätsklinik für Chirurgie
Abteilung für Herz-Thorax-Chirurgie
Währinger Gürtel 18–20
A-1090 Wien

WOLFRAM, JOHANNA, Dr. med.
Universitätsklinik im AKH
Abteilung für Kardiologie
Währinger Gürtel 18–20
A-1090 Wien

YOSHITAKE, MICHIO, Dr. med.
Chirurgische Universitätsklinik
Freiburg
Abteilung Herz- und Gefäßchirurgie
Hugstetter Straße 55
D-79106 Freiburg

ZUCKER, M., Ph.D.
Medical Division
Opgal, Karmiel
P.O. Box 462
Israel

PART I

Pathology and Physiology of Myocardial Ischaemia

CHAPTER 1

Pathologic-Anatomic Aspects of Chronic Myocardial Ischaemia

W. Hort

1.1 Compensational Abilities of Coronary Arteries in Coronary Atherosclerosis

Most often, severe coronary sclerosis is the reason for chronic myocardial ischaemia. However, before resulting in a relevant deterioration of the blood flow in the myocardium, the coronary vascular system disposes of several options for compensation.

Under normal conditions the diameter of coronary arteries is - regardless of the cyclical variations - no invariable factor but depends on regulatory humoral and neural influences, one of them being the vasodilating factor (EDRF) produced by the endothelium and the acetylcholine, which leads - also mediated by the ERDF [30] - to a vasodilation of the normal coronary artery.

This regulatory mechanism can even influence the luminal width in segments with eccentric coronary sclerotic foci (which are more frequent than concentric ones), as the unaffected part of the wall remains mobile. This can be seen, for example, when a coronary spasm occurs.

After a longer period of time, the development of a coronary arteriosclerotic plaque leads to a relevant narrowing of the lumen. At first, the foci develop, so to speak, in an outward direction, as reported by Glagov et al. [11]: coronary arteries fixed post mortem under application of physiologic pressure almost keep their standard luminal width if the cross-section of the lesion does not exceed 40% of the total cross-section limited by the elastica interna.

According to morphological findings, no strict parallelism exists between the degree of narrowing of a coronary artery lumen and the effects to be seen in its myocardiac supply area, e.g. the degree of myocardial fibrosis. This is also seen by clinicians when they compare the exent of the hypokinesia to the coronary angiographic narrowing of the lumen. Here, the collateral can still provide for sufficient perfusion, even over a longer period of time. However, one should bear in mind that even the best collateral is not as good as an intact coronary vessel.

To a limited extent, new branches of the main coronary arteries can be developed even by adult hearts, as shown in a study concerning the left descending branch [25]. This is even more astonishing, as the number of branches is rather fixed, and at birth already as high as in a fully developed heart [28]. This is also true for other mammals, e.g. pigs [27] and cattle [7]. A slight but nevertheless significant increase in the number of branches was found, however, in human hearts with cardiac hypertrophy and severe coronary atherosclerosis. The additional branches had developed mostly in the vi-

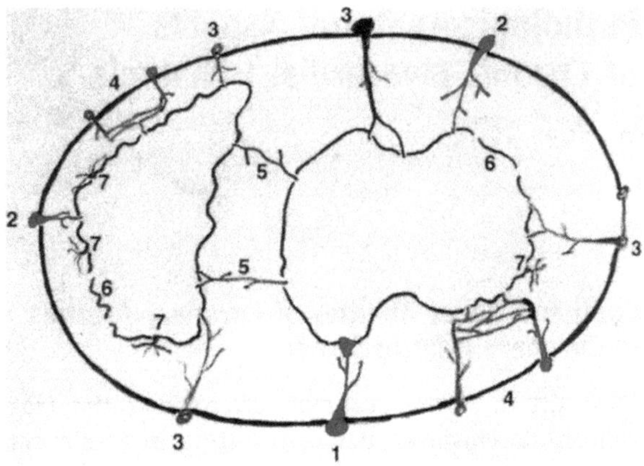

Fig. 1.1. Schematic presentation of the coronary-ventricular and transseptal anastomoses as well as the small Thebesian veins and Lannelonge's channels (from [23], with kind permission). *1*, Arterio-sinusoidal vessel; *2*, arterio-ventricular vessels; *3*, veno-ventricular anastomoses; *4*, capillaro-ventricular anastomoses; *5*, transseptal anastomoses; *6*, Lannelong's channels; *7*, small subendocardial Thebesian veins

cinity of the strongest stenosis, as postmortem coronary angiograms indicated. Whether these were formerly tiny little branches not visible on a traditional angiographic image and were now enlarged or whether they were completely newly developed has not yet been definitely decided.

In some rare cases, patients showing even an old complete occlusion of both coronary ostia survived for quite some time [19]. In this context, we should bear in mind the protective effect of natural anastomoses surrounding the heart, which are in effect a natural equivalent to bypass surgery. These natural anastomoses are found mostly around the ostia of the pulmonary veins, at the pericardial sac near the large vessels and in the adjacent fatty tissue. Furthermore, anastomoses have been reported with neighbouring branches of the a. mammaria interna, and with the anterior mediastinal, pericardial, bronchial, phrenic, intercostal and oesophageal branches of the aorta [15].

Moreover, the question may be raised whether ventricular blood could not be supplied to the myocardium under ischaemic myocardial conditions. The anatomic options have been described in detail in a recently published review [23] (Fig. 1.1).

1.2 Further Routes of Blood Supply to the Myocardium

One of the best-known ways are the Thebesian veins, discovered about 300 years ago. The venous blood of the coronary circulation does not completely flow off via the coronary sinus (in dogs only 60% of the blood flows off in this way [9]). Exterior to the coronary sinus, smaller branch veins open into the right ventricle and the right atrium and quite a number of smaller, often star-shaped subendocardial veins carry the regional venous blood directly into the ventricular lumen.

In addition, direct small coronary arterial branches are sometimes also directly connected to the ventricular lumen. Those with a narrow opening have been named arterioluminal, those with a wide opening have been called arteriosinusoidal vessels by Wearn et al. [31]. With respect to the latter, the inosculation of a small artery into a subendocardial sinus probably begins with embryogenesis. Some direct connections of capillaries with the myocardial cavities have also been reported [18].

In addition, and this is of particular interest for medical historians, the transseptal anastomoses should be mentioned. They were assigned an essential role in ancient times. Galen was of the opinion that the blood was generated in the liver. From there, he assumed, it would flow, enriched with the "spiritus naturalis", into the right heart and partly seep into the left ventricle. Following this assumption, even Leonardo da Vinci depicted the interventricular septum as porous in his early anatomic drawings [3]. These transseptal channels did not correspond with Harvey's concept of a closed circulatory system, however. Nevertheless, a small number of small transseptal connections do exist, and small foramina which are connected to unbranched, blind channels (Lannelonge's channels) are sporadically found in the endocardium.

The fact that anstomoses of the coronary vascular system can actually assist in the supply of blood to the myocardium was shown by Swedenborg [26] in the eighteenth century. The right ventricular wall of an isolated cat heart still contracted for a long time when supplied with blood over a cannula fed through the atrium into the right ventricle.

Whether an influx of blood from the ventricle into the coronary vascular system is relevant under physiological or pathological conditions is so far unknown. Patients suffering from severe coronary sclerosis show an increased number of foramina in the ventricular endocardium, according to Hoffmann et al. [12]; however, Ritter [29] found no evidence for this. Above all, the idea that blood can flow from the left ventricle via the foramina (i.e. also retrograde via Thebesian veins) into the underperfused myocardial areas has not yet been clearly proven.

The numbers of endocardial foramina at the human heart given in the literature vary widely. It is difficult to find them all, as some of them lie deep in the trabecular system and they can be very small. Coronary ventricular anastomoses can be demonstrated postmortem by injecting into the coronary vessels and observing the endocardium or – inversely – with an injection into the foramina. Wearn et al. [31] described eight to ten ventricular connections of the left descending coronary artery; taking the anastomoses of the other coronary arteries and veins into account as well, this is not far from the number of laser channels typically made for therapeutic purposes. Thus, it is unclear so far whether the condition of chronically underperfused areas can be improved by supplying blood from the ventricle via natural coronary venticular anastomoses.

1.3 Myocardial Lesions Under Chronic Ischaemic Conditions

Depending on its severity, underperfusion results in a variety of lesions, from minor functional impairment to a fully developed infarct. Under physiological conditions the myocardium consumes the major part of the energy fed to it for contraction; what remains is then used to maintain its structure.

The myocardium adapts itself to chronic underperfusion by "hibernating". Its function is reduced and all transitional stages from hypokinesia to complete akinesia are found. If the remaining blood flow is no longer sufficient to keep up the entire structure, organelles are degraded, causing increasing vacuolisation of the myocardial cells, until only largely emptied myocytes are left.

Electron microscopically, a reduction of myofilaments, small mitochondria, an increased amount of glycogen [8, 10] and reduced T-tubuli and sarcoplasmic reticulum [1], as well as an increased disorganisation of the cytoskeleton [8] have been detected in the long-term hibernating myocardium. These transformations are also called colliquative myocytolysis. According to Kawano et al. [16], their extent is correlated with the duration of the ischaemia. Whereas Elsässer and Schaper [8] interpret the transformations within the myocardial cells as degeneration, Ausma et al. [1] describe them as dedifferentiation.

Within the interstitium of the hibernating myocardium collagenous connective tissue types I and III is increased; according to Ausma et al. [1], this is responsible for the delayed restoration of contraction after perfusion has normalised.

The hibernating myocardium can be studied best in the surviving subendocardial muscle layer of an infarct, as here all transitional stages from a completely intact structure to necrosis can be found. As an infarct is generally irregularly limited, its periphery can hardly be sufficiently examined by needle biopsy. The periphery usually shows the most varied forms of tissue lesions.

The clearest conditions are found in the subendocardium, where a periphery nearly 0.1 mm wide with several layers of myocytes almost always survives [14]. Normal endocardium being thinner than a myocardial cell, the immediate subendocardial layer of myocardial cells which is fed from the lumen is generally well preserved. In the following layers an increasing number of vacuolisations and some almost completely emptied myocardial cells are found next to necrosis (Fig. 1.2).

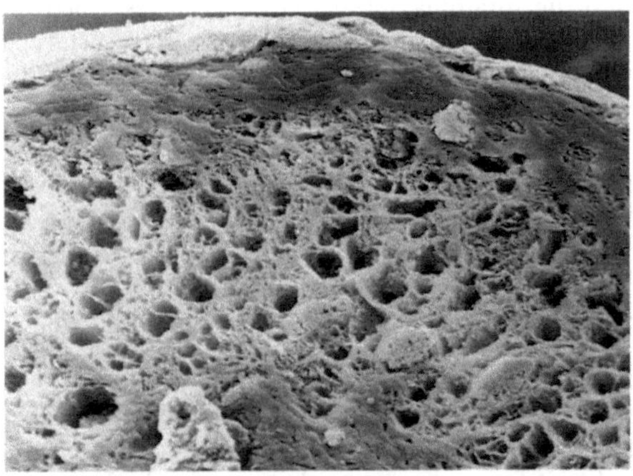

Fig. 1.2. Preserved subendocardial layers at infarct. The myocytes (*above*) directly neighbouring the endocardium are maintained; those more removed include an increasing number of areas without organelles and looking like vacuoles. SEM, ×180

There are good reasons for believing that the myocardial cells can replace the degraded organelles once perfusion has begun again. However, we do not know the minimum extent to which organelles must be preserved in order to allow successful regeneration.

1.4 Morphological Aspects of Transmural Laser Revascularisation

If all interventional and bypass surgical options have been exhausted for patients suffering from the chronic myocardial ischaemia of terminal coronary heart disease and if complaints of pectoral angina and heart insufficiency make life a misery, present-day transmyocardial laser revascularisation often enables us to provide for subjective relief. With this technique, 20–30 channels vertically penetrating the entire left chamber wall are cut by means of laser beams.

The mode of action of this intervention has not yet been sufficiently clarified. The "reptilisation" of the human heart has often been postulated based on the false belief that the entire reptile heart is nourished by diffusion from the lumen. However, this is true only for the very extensive, spongious, elaborately positioned filigree-like inner parts of the ventricular myocardium of reptiles and amphibious animals (Fig. 1.3). Their nutrition is supported by an intensive convection of the surrounding blood [20]. Also with reptiles and amphibious animals the compacta, like those parts of the spongiosa which have exceeded a certain critical size, is nourished by coronary vessels.

A comparison of the surfaces newly created by the laser channels to the immense surface areas of the amphibian and reptile spongiosa is also very weak. A small coat of cardiac muscle situated around the laser channels and

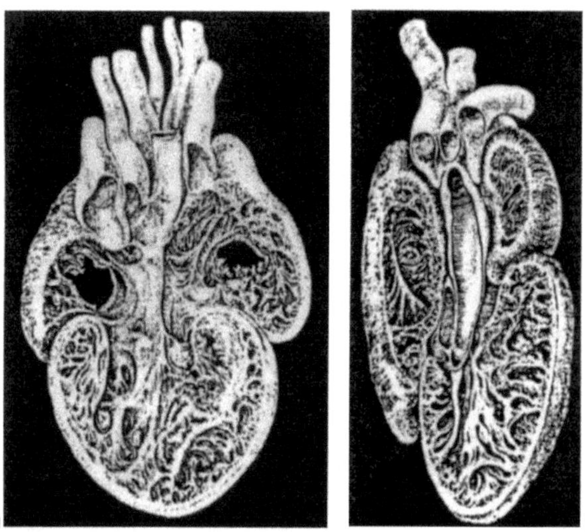

a b

Fig. 1.3 a, b. Frontal section of reptile hearts (**a** lizard, **b** snake). The compacta is narrow, the spongiosa abundantly developed. (From [5])

comparable to the surviving subendocardial muscle layer under infarct conditions could be nourished by means of diffusion. These parts of the myocardium would, however, be smaller than those destroyed when the laser channels are generated [23], so a success of laser therapy could hardly be attributed to this. On the other hand, a connection of the laser channels to the coronary vascular system in the myocardium might really improve blood circulation.

First contrast echocardiographic [2] and colour-coded echocardiographic [24] findings indicating a systolic filling of the channels and a diastolic flow off or a systolic-diastolic flow in the channels have been published. However, it is not easy to distinguish the channels clearly from coronary ventricular anastomoses.

Furthermore, the fate of laser channels has not been indubitably determined. The possibilty of their remaining open has been reported several times [6, 22], and Mirhoseini et al. [21] depicted open, endothelialised channels even years after the actual intervention took place. Other laser channels, however, are quickly occluded. Krabatsch et al. [17] have examined the hearts of seven patients who died within the first 3 weeks following transmural laser revascularisation. Only two of 220 channels were found to be still open. After 2–3 weeks, the clot in the channels had been replaced by a granulation tissue varying in strength and incorporating many macrophages. In addition, a large amount of type IV collagen, which typically is found mostly within the basal membranes of the vessels, was detected. Finally, an increased number of hollow spaces surrounded by basal membranes and lined with endothelium were found in the granulation tissue. Currently, we do not know whether they are connected to the ventricular lumen or not. Theoretically, this is surely possible. Similar processes are found in the organisation of thrombi or emboli, which can almost completely disappear during the rechannelisation of arteries.

In the area of the laser channels the development of the granulation tissue coincides with a neoangiogenesis, which is thought to be furthered by the expression of vascular endothelial growth factor. Brilla et al. [4] assume that - regardless of whether the channels remain durably patent or not - the extent of the vascular neogenesis induced by the transmural laser revascularisation is decisive for its long-term success. If the regional blood supply in a chronically ischaemic myocardium cannot be improved, however, it is difficult to imagine how perfusion should be improved by newly developed capillaries, particularly when the sophisticated pattern of the myocardial capillaries is taken into account. Many questions remain unanswered.

References

1. Ausma J, Cleutjens J, Thoné F, Flameng W, Ramaekers F, Borgers M (1995) Chronic hibernating myocardium: interstitial changes. Mol Cell Biochem 147:35–42
2. Berwing K, Bauer EP, Strasser R, Klövekorn WP, Bertschmann W (1996) Transmurale Laserrevaskularisation: erste Nachweise einer Perfusion offener Laser-Kanäle. Z Kardiol 85 [Suppl 2]:197
3. Boenheim F (1957) Von Huang'ti bis Harvey. Fischer, Leipzig, pp 11–12

4. Brilla CG, Rybinski L, Gehrke D, Rupp H (1997) Transmyokardiale Laserrevaskularisation - ein innovatives pathophysiologisches Konzept. Herz 22:183–189
5. Brücke E (1852) Beiträge zur vergleichenden Anatomie und Physiologie des Gefäß-Systems. Denkschrift Wien Akad Wiss 3:335–367
6. Cooley DA, Frazier OH, Kadipasaoglu KA, Pehlivanoglu S, Shannon RL, Angelini P (1994) Transmyocardial laser revascularization: anatomic evidence of long-term patency. Tex Heart Inst J 21:220–224
7. Dorenbeck U (1997) Quantitative Untersuchungen des Gefäßbaumes der Arteria coronaria sinistra an verschieden großen Säugetierherzen - Untersuchungen an Koronarangiographien und Korrosionspräparaten. Medical dissertation, Düsseldorf
8. Elsässer A, Schaper J (1995) Hibernating myocardium: adaptation or degeneration? Bas Res Cardiol 90:47–48
9. Evans CL, Starling EH (1913) The part played by the lungs in the oxidative processes of the body. J Physiol 46:413–434
10. Flameng W, Suy R, Schwarz F, Borgers M, Piessens J, Thone F, et al (1981) Ultrastructural correlates of left ventricular contraction abnormalities in patients with chronic ischemic heart disease: determinants of reversible segmental asynergy post revascularization surgery. Am Heart J 102:846–857
11. Glagov S, Weisenberg E, Zarins CK, Stankunaviciu R, Kolettois GJ (1987) Compensatory enlargement of human atherosclerotic coronary arteries. N Engl J Med 316:1371–1375
12. Hoffmann E, Ringler W, Gebhardt C (1967) Die Bedeutung ventrikulokoronarer Verbindungen für die Ausgleichsversorgung des Herzmuskels bei Koronarsklerose. Z Kreislaufforschg 56:1218–1226
13. Hoffmann E, Gebhardt Ch, Kisseler B (1971) Morphologie der ventrikulocoronaren Anastomosen bei Herzen mit intaktem und pathologisch verändertem Coronargefäßsystem. Eine injektionstechnische Studie an menschlichen Leichenherzen. Langenbecks Arch Chir 328:180–200
14. Hort W (1968) Capillarisation of the myocardium under normal and pathological conditions. In: Lübbers DW, Luft UC, Thews G, Witzleb E (eds) Oxygen transport in blood and tissue. Thieme, Stuttgart, pp 150–158, 253–254
15. Hudson CL, Moritz AR, Wearn JT (1932) The extracardiac anastomoses of the coronary arteries. J Exp Med 56:919–925
16. Kawano H, Kawano Y, Shirai T, Okada R (1994) Histologic study on adaptation of cardiac myocytes to chronic ischemia. In: Nagano M, Takeda N, Dhalla NS (eds) The adapted heart. Raven, New York, pp 211–219
17. Krabatsch T, Schäper F, Tambeur L, Leder C, Thalmann U, Hetzer R (1997) Histomorphologie nach transmyokardialer Laserrevaskularisation. Herz 22: 205–210
18. Langer L (1880) Die Foramina Thebesii im Herzen des Menschen. Sitzungsbericht der Akademie der Wissenschaften d. math-naturwissenschaftl Klasse III. Abt, vol 82, nos. 1–16, meeting of June 17, 1880, p 25 ff.
19. Leary T, Wearn JT (1930) Two cases of complete occlusion of both coronary orifices. Am Heart J 5:412–423
20. Lübbers D, Barbey KJ (1954) Die Bedeutung der Wandstruktur für die Sauerstoffversorgung des Froschherzens. Pflugers Arch 260:87–103
21. Mirhoseini M, Fisher JC, Cayton MM (1983) Myocardial revascularization by laser: a clinical report. Lasers Surg Med 3:241–245
22. Mirhoseini M, Shelgicar S, Cayton MM (1990) Clinical and histological evaluation of laser myocardial revascularization. J Clin Laser Surg Med 9:73–78
23. Moosdorf R, Schoebel FC, Hort W (1997) Transmyokardiale Laserrevaskularisation - morphologische, pathophysiologische und historische Grundlagen der indirekten Revaskularisation des Herzmuskels. Z Kardiol 86:149–164
24. Nägele H, Kalmar P, Rödiger W, Stubbe HM (1997) Farbdopplerechokardiographischer Nachweis transmyokardialer Kanäle im Langzeitverlauf nach Laserrevaskularisation. Z Kardiol 86 [Suppl 2]:214
25. Oberste-Vorth K (1997) Dissertation in preparation
26. Pratt FH (1932) Emanuel Swedenborg on the thebesian system of the heart. Science 76:488–489
27. Reinecke P, Hort W (1988) Untersuchungen über das Wachstum der Koronararterienäste - morphometrische Untersuchungen an Korrosionspräparaten des R. interventricularis der A. coronaria sinistra bei Schwein und Ferkel. Z Kardiol 77:299–304
28. Reinecke P, Hort W (1992) Untersuchungen über das Wachstum der Koronararterienäste beim Menschen unter physiologischen Bedingungen. Morphologische Untersuchungen an Korrosionspräparaten des R. interventricularis anterior. Z Kardiol 81:110–115

29. Ritter G (1962) Morphologische und quantitative Untersuchungen der Vasa minima des menschlichen Herzens. Dissertation, Göttingen
30. Vanhoutte PM (1986) Could the absence or malfunction of vascular endothelium precipitate the occurrence of vasospasm? J Mol Cell Cardiol 18:679–689
31. Wearn JT, Mettier SR, Klump TG, Zschiesche IJ (1933) The nature of the vascular communications between the coronary arteries and the chambers of the heart. Am Heart J 9:143–164

CHAPTER 2

Hibernating Myocardium: A Review

G. Heusch · R. Schulz

2.1 Summary

Within a few seconds after a sudden reduction of coronary blood flow regional contractile dysfunction ensues. The mechanisms responsible for the rapid reduction in contractile function during acute myocardial ischemia remain unclear, but may involve a rise in inorganic phosphate. When severe ischemia, such as resulting from a sudden and complete coronary artery occlusion, is prolonged for more than 20–40 min, myocardial infarction develops, and there is irreversible loss of contractile function. When myocardial ischemia is less severe but nevertheless prolonged, the myocardium is dysfunctional but can remain viable.

In such ischemic and dysfunctional myocardium, contractile function is reduced in proportion to the reduction in regional myocardial blood flow; i.e. a state of "perfusion-contraction matching" exists. The metabolic status of such myocardium improves over the first few hours, as myocardial lactate production is attenuated and creatine phosphate, after an initial reduction, returns towards control values. Ischemic myocardium, characterized by perfusion-contraction matching, metabolic recovery and lack of necrosis, has been termed "short-term hibernating myocardium". Short-term hibernating myocardium can respond to an inotropic stimulation with increased contractile function, however, at the expense of a renewed worsening of the metabolic status. This situation of an increased regional contractile function at the expense of metabolic recovery during inotropic stimulation can be used to identify short-term hibernating myocardium. When inotropic stimulation is prolonged, the development of short-term hibernation is impaired and myocardial infarction develops. The mechanisms responsible for the development of short-term myocardial hibernation remain unclear at present; a significant involvement of adenosine and of activation of ATP-dependent potassium channels has been excluded.

Whereas short-term hibernation is well characterized in animal experiments, the existence of hibernation over weeks or months (chronic hibernation) can only be inferred from clinical studies. Hibernation, as defined by Rahimtoola, is a state of chronic contractile dysfunction which is fully reversible upon reperfusion. Clinical syndromes consistent with the existence of myocardial hibernation include unstable and stable angina, acute myocardial infarction and left ventricular dysfunction and/or congestive heart failure. In chronic hibernating myocardium morphological alterations occur; the myofibrils are reduced in number and disorganized and myocardial glycogen content as well as the extracellular collagen network are increased. Thus, despite the fact that the myocardium remains viable during persistent ischemia and contractile dysfunction is reversible upon reperfusion, there are severe morphological alterations. Understandably, full functional recovery following reperfusion might therefore require weeks or even months.

2.2 The Concept of Myocardial Hibernation and its Evolution

The term "hibernation" is borrowed from zoology and implies an adaptive reduction of energy expenditure through reduced activity in a situation of reduced energy supply. In the context of coronary artery disease, myocardial hibernation refers to an adaptive reduction of myocardial contractile function in response to a reduction of myocardial blood flow. Thus, in the concept of myocardial hibernation the observed impairment of myocardial contractile function is not regarded as the consequence of an energetic deficit, but instead as a regulatory event which serves to maintain myocardial integrity and viability.

The concept of myocardial hibernation was founded on clinical grounds when Shahbudin Rahimtoola in the early eighties reviewed the results of coronary bypass surgery trials and identified patients with coronary artery disease and chronic left ventricular dysfunction that improved upon revascularization (Rahimtoola, 1982; Rahimtoola, 1985). However, the clinical concept of hibernation quickly merged with a number of experimental observations. Also in the early eighties, several laboratories found that the long held concept of myocardial ischemia as an imbalance between energy supply – as determined by myocardial blood flow – and energy demand – as determined by contractile function – was not correct on the regional myocardial level. In fact, the reduction in regional contractile function was proportionate to the reduction in regional myocardial blood flow (Vatner, 1980; Weintraub *et al.* 1981; Gallagher *et al.* 1983; Canty, 1988) (for review see: (Heusch, 1991)). Gallagher, in that context, coined the term "absolute ischemia" (Gallagher *et al.* 1983) and Ross later the term "perfusion-contraction matching" (Ross Jr. 1991). Such perfusion-contraction matching was observed for a period of 5 hours of moderate ischemia in conscious, chronically instrumented dogs with eventual full recovery of contractile function upon reperfusion and without the occurrence of infarction in the dysfunctional myocardium (Matsuzaki *et al.* 1983). Further experimental evidence for the concept of myocardial hibernation was gained from studies demonstrating the recovery of metabolic markers during ongoing persistent ischemia (Fedele *et al.* 1988; Pantely *et al.* 1990).

The entire concept of myocardial hibernation was popularized by the 1986 editorial by Braunwald and Rutherford (Braunwald & Rutherford, 1986) and has received ever increasing attention and interest, both from clinicians and basic scientists, since then.

2.3 Time Sequence of Events Following Acute Ischemia

Upon acute coronary artery occlusion contractile function in the ischemic region rapidly ceases. Within a few cardiac cycles systolic segment shortening and systolic wall thickening are reduced (hypokinesis), later abolished (akinesis) and within 30 s to 2 min replaced by paradoxic systolic segment lengthening and systolic wall thinning (dyskinesis, bulging) (Theroux *et al.* 1974; Theroux *et al.* 1976). Electrophysiologic changes in the surface ECG occur only after the loss of systolic wall excursion, and changes in the local subendocardial ECG occur even later than those in the surface ECG (Battler *et al.* 1980). During more moderate regional contractile dysfunction distal to a coronary artery stenosis, ischemic changes become apparent in the local ECG, but not in the surface ECG (Battler *et al.* 1980). Thus, loss of regional contractile activity is a rapid, sensitive, and important consequence of regional myocardial ischemia.

2.4 Mechanisms of Acute Ischemic Contractile Dysfunction

ATP is well-accepted to be the ultimate source of energy for the contractile process. Understandably then, the effect of acute myocardial ischemia on the concentration of ATP has been proposed as the mechanism of acute ischemic contractile dysfunction (Hearse, 1979) (Table 2.1). A causal link between the appearance of regional ischemic contractile dysfunction and the loss of regional myocardial ATP, however, has never been proven experimentally. In the inner myocardial layers of anesthetized swine, the ATP concentration is reduced within 15 cardiac cycles following an acute reduction in myocardial blood flow; however, contractile dysfunction occurs prior to changes in myocardial ATP concentration (Arai *et al.* 1992). A compelling argument against reduced concentration of ATP as the mediator of acute ischemic contractile failure is that the result of reduced concentration of ATP should be rigor of the myofibrils rather than the observed loss of wall tension (Katz, 1973). This apparent discrepancy can be at least partially reconciled if the early reduction in ATP concentration acts not as a primary energy depletion, but through a modulatory mechanism which could interfere with excitation-contraction coupling (Kübler & Katz, 1977).

Activation of ATP-dependent potassium channels by an ischemia-induced decrease in the myocardial ATP concentration, an increase in the intracellular proton or lactate concentrations or by activation of adenosine-A_1-receptors could increase potassium efflux, thereby reduce action potential duration and subsequently calcium influx into the myocyte (Noma, 1983). Such decreased intracellular calcium concentration could then reduce contractile function and ATP consumption. Indeed, blockade of ATP-dependent potassium channels abolishes the hypoxia-induced reduction of global left ventricular function in saline-perfused rat hearts (Decking *et al.* 1995). In contrast, in anesthetized swine in situ, blockade of ATP-dependent potassium channels does prevent the ischemic reduction of action potential duration but not al-

Table 2.1. Potential mechanisms of acute ischemic contractile dysfunction (sequence according to appearance in text)

- Reduction in myocardial ATP-concentration
- Reduction of phosphorylation potential or free energy change of ATP-hydrolysis
- Accumulation of protons and lactate
- Disturbance in calcium handling of the sarcoplasmic reticulum
- Collapse of coronary arteries
- Accumulation of inorganic phosphate
- Desensitization of myofibrils for calcium

ter ischemic contractile dysfunction or the myocardial ATP concentration (Schulz *et al.* 1995c).

Apart from changes in the absolute concentration of myocardial ATP, decreases in the phosphorylation potential or the free energy change of ATP-hydrolysis could be responsible for the decrease in contractile function. Indeed the reduction in the phosphorylation potential (Clarke *et al.* 1987) or the free energy change of ATP-hydrolysis (Kammermeier *et al.* 1982) correlates well with the onset of contractile dysfunction in isolated saline perfused hearts.

Other mediators which have been proposed to be involved in the development of early ischemic contractile dysfunction are the accumulation of lactate (Jacobus *et al.* 1982), a decrease in the intracellular pH (Jacobus *et al.* 1982) or a disturbance in the calcium handling of the sarcoplasmic reticulum (Krause & Hess, 1984; Kübler & Katz, 1977). Also, a collapse of the coronary arteries has been suggested to be responsible for the decrease in contractile function early during ischemia (Koretsune *et al.* 1991). The accumulation of inorganic phosphate resulting from the ischemic breakdown of myocardial creatine phosphate and ATP, however, is the most likely candidate responsible for the early ischemic decrease in contractile function (Kusuoka *et al.* 1986). The increase in the concentration of inorganic phosphate could reduce contractile function by direct binding to contractile proteins (Rüegg *et al.* 1971), an uncoupling of the myofibrilar ATP-ase activity (Schmidt-Ott *et al.* 1990) or by desensitization of myofibrils for calcium (Kentish, 1986).

2.5 Transition from an Imbalance between Supply and Demand towards Short-term Myocardial Hibernation

Within the first few seconds following an acute reduction of myocardial blood flow, energy demand of the hypoperfused myocardium clearly exceeds the reduced energy supply. However, this imbalance between energy supply and demand is an inherently unstable condition since ischemia induces mechanisms which reduce contractile function and thus energy demand (Guth *et al.* 1993). In the subsequent steady state condition, the amount of contractile dysfunction is in proportion to the reduction of myocardial blood flow (Vatner, 1980; Weintraub *et al.* 1981; Gallagher *et al.* 1983; Canty, 1988), i.e. a state of perfusion-contraction-matching exists (Ross Jr. 1989; Ross Jr. 1991) (Table 2.2).

Table 2.2. Characterization of short-term hibernating myocardium

- Balance between the reduced regional myocardial blood flow and the reduced contractile function (perfusion-contraction-matching)
- Recovery of contractile function during reperfusion
- Recovery of metabolic parameters (creatine phosphate, lactate) during persistent ischemia
- Recruitable inotropic reserve at the expense of metabolic recovery

In chronically instrumented, conscious dogs, a reduction in myocardial blood flow associated with a decrease in regional contractile function by 40% can be maintained for 5 hours without the development of necrosis within the dysfunctional myocardium. Regional contractile function recovers during reperfusion, but full recovery requires 7 days (Matsuzaki *et al.* 1983).

2.6 Metabolism of Short-term Hibernating Myocardium

Within the first 5 minutes of an acute coronary inflow reduction, coronary venous pH and lactate extraction are reduced and coronary venous pCO_2 increases, but these parameters gradually return towards control values during continued moderate ischemia (Fedele *et al.* 1988). Likewise, during constant moderate ischemia the myocardial creatine phosphate concentration is significantly decreased immediately after the onset of ischemia, but gradually recovers over time towards control values, whereas regional contractile function is persistently reduced (Downing & Chen, 1990; Pantely *et al.* 1990; Arai *et al.* 1991; Downing & Chen, 1992; Schulz *et al.* 1992).

These studies are consistent with the idea that there is only a transient phase of an energetic supply-demand imbalance during early myocardial ischemia. The ensuing reduction in regional myocardial function may induce a downregulation of energy demand and allow stabilization at a new metabolic level characterized again by an energetic balance, as indicated by the recovery of metabolic markers.

2.7 Recruitment of an Inotropic Reserve at the Expense of Metabolic Recovery in Short-term Hibernating Myocardium

Although baseline contractile function is depressed, the hypoperfused myocardium retains its responsiveness to an inotropic challenge (Figure 2.1) (Schulz *et al.* 1992). When, after 85-90 minutes of sustained moderate ischemia in anesthetized pigs, dobutamine is infused selectively into the ischemic region, contractile function increases, although regional blood flow remains reduced. Thus, energy is available in the ischemic myocardium which is not used to maintain baseline function, but permits the increase in contractile function upon an inotropic challenge. These results suggest that the decrease in contractile function secondary to a reduction in myocardial blood flow is not simply the consequence of an energetic deficit, but rather reflects an active adaptive process of the myocardium. Imposition of an inotropic stimulus

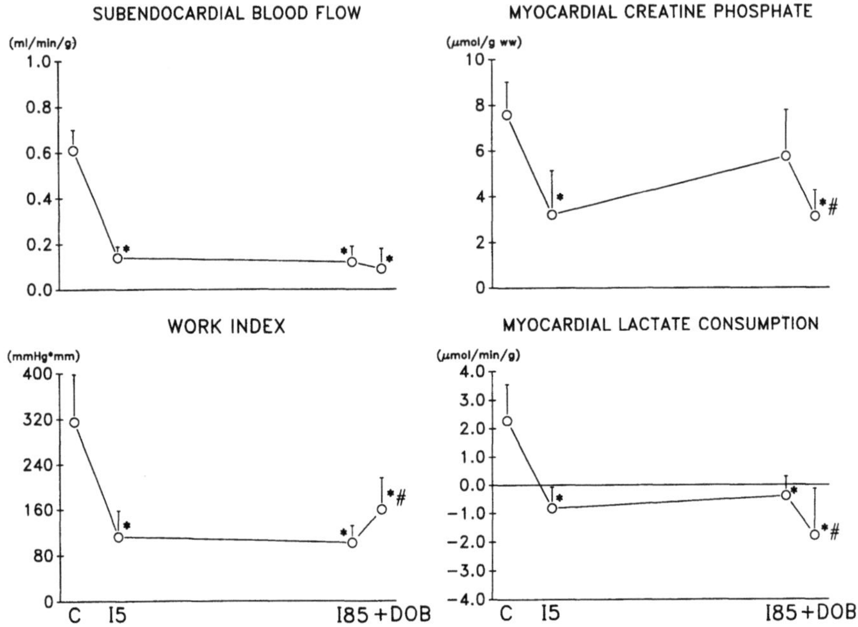

Fig. 2.1. The reduction in subendocardial blood flow of the anterior myocardium at 5 minutes ischemia (I5) is associated with decreased regional contractile function. The creatine phosphate concentration falls and lactate consumption is reversed to net lactate production. With the extension of ischemia to 85 minutes (I85) at a constant subendocardial blood flow, there is a tendency for a further decrease in regional contractile function. In contrast, lactate production is attenuated and the creatine phosphate concentration recovers to a value no longer significantly different from control. Infusion of dobutamine (+DOB) after 90 minutes of ischemia increases regional contractile function at an unchanged subendocardial blood flow. This increase in contractile function, however, is associated once more with increased lactate production and a decreased creatine phosphate concentration. *$p<0.05$ vs CONTROL (C), #$p<0.05$ vs preceding value. (From Schulz & Heusch, 1995)

on the short-term hibernating myocardium disrupts this adaptive process, as indicated by the once more decreased myocardial creatine phosphate concentration and increased lactate production (Figure 2.1).

A similar disruption of the developing metabolic balance after prolonged moderate ischemia is observed upon a chronotropic challenge (Arai *et al.* 1991). Increasing heart rate by atrial pacing in this particular study, however, increased the severity of ischemia and reduced regional myocardial blood flow, function and creatine phosphate concentration and increased lactate production. Since the severity of ischemia was increased, the observed metabolic deterioration during pacing does not conclusively demonstrate active adaptation of energy demand during the preceding more moderate ischemia.

2.8 Limitations of Short-term Hibernation

As already stated, the development of such delicate balance between regional myocardial blood flow and function during early ischemia is disturbed by

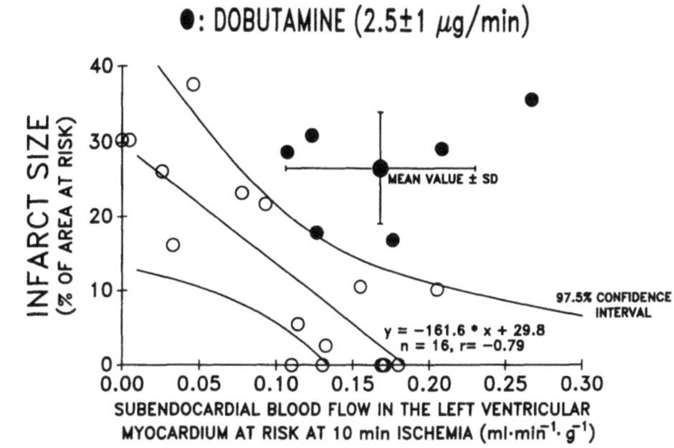

Fig. 2.2. Relationship between subendocardial blood flow in the left ventricular myocardium at risk (x-axis) and infarct size (y-axis). Open circles represent data from control animals undergoing 90 minutes of ischemia of varying severity. With increasing severity of ischemia infarct size is increased. In animals subjected to 90 minutes of ischemia with 85 minutes of dobutamine infusion (closed circles) infarct size is increased above the level expected from the blood flow reduction alone. (From Schulz *et al.* 1993)

unfavourable alterations in supply and demand. When in anesthetized pigs after 5 minutes of ischemia, at a blood flow reduction compatible with the development of myocardial hibernation over 90 minutes, energy supply is further reduced by a further reduction of myocardial blood flow, necrosis develops. The lower limit of myocardial blood flow compatible with the development of short-term myocardial hibernation amounts to approximately 25% of baseline in this experimental setting (Schulz *et al.* 1993).

Also, a further increase in energy demand by continuous inotropic stimulation with dobutamine induces necrosis (Schulz *et al.* 1993) (Figure 2.2). Thus, both the further reduction in energy supply by an increasing severity of ischemia and an enhanced energy expenditure by continuous inotropic stimulation impair the development of short-term myocardial hibernation and precipitate myocardial infarction.

2.9
Experimental Identification of Short-term Hibernating Myocardium

In contrast to dysfunctional, irreversibly damaged myocardium, the short-term hibernating myocardium retains an inotropic reserve. Recruitment of such inotropic reserve is at the expense of metabolic recovery (Figure 2.1) (Schulz *et al.* 1992; Schulz *et al.* 1993). The extent of postsystolic wall thickening in ischemic myocardium also permits to distinguish irreversibly damaged from viable, hibernating myocardium (Rose *et al.* 1993). The extent of postsystolic wall thickening at the end of a 90 minutes ischemic period correlates inversely to the extent of necrosis, and positively to myocardial creatine phosphate concentration, the dobutamine-recruitable inotropic reserve and the functional recovery upon reperfusion. Thus the greater the postsystolic

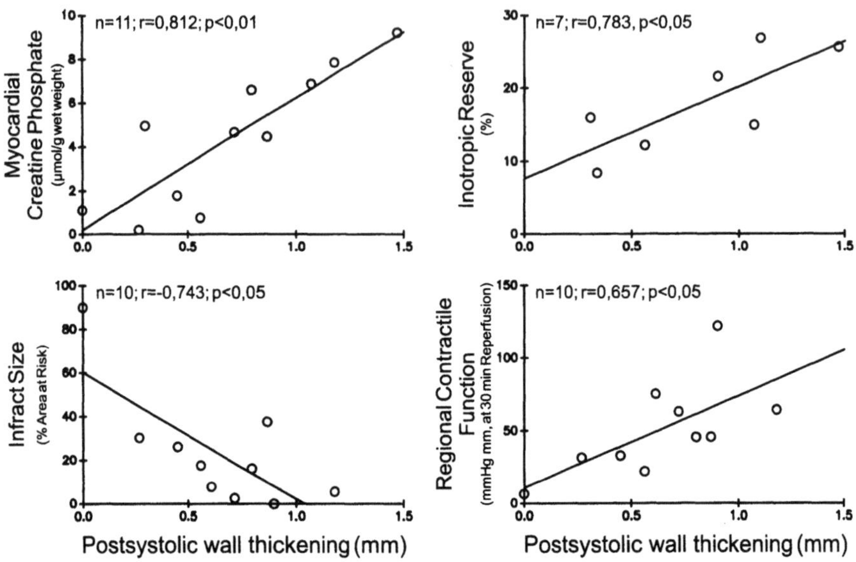

Fig. 2.3. Correlation between the extent of postsystolic wall thickening at the end of a 90 minutes ischemic period and the extent of necrosis, the myocardial creatine phosphate concentration, the dobutamine-recruitable inotropic reserve and the functional recovery upon reperfusion. The extent of postsystolic wall thickening at the end of a 90 minutes ischemic period correlates inversely to the extent of necrosis, and positively to the myocardial creatine phosphate concentration, the dobutamine-recruitable inotropic reserve and the functional recovery upon reperfusion. Thus, the greater the postsystolic wall thickening, the more myocardium is successfully hibernating. (From Rose *et al.* 1993)

wall thickening, the more myocardium is successfully hibernating (Figure 2.3).

2.10 Mechanisms of Short-term Hibernating Myocardium

The mechanisms responsible for the development of short-term myocardial hibernation remain unclear at present. Alterations in the ß-adrenoceptor density or affinity as the underlying mechanism of such adaptive process have been excluded (Schulz *et al.* 1993).

As mentioned earlier, the ischemia-induced activation of ATP-dependent potassium channels might increase potassium efflux, thereby reduce action potential duration and subsequently calcium influx into the cardiomyocyte. Such decreased intracellular calcium concentration could then reduce contractile function and ATP consumption, thus finally allowing the development of myocardial hibernation. Indeed, the monophasic action potential duration shortens during ischemia, and this shortening is prevented by blockade of ATP-dependent potassium channels with glibenclamide. However, complete blockade of ATP-dependent potassium channels does neither alter contractile function nor metabolic parameters nor myocardial viability. Obviously, activation of ATP-dependent potassium channels is therefore not

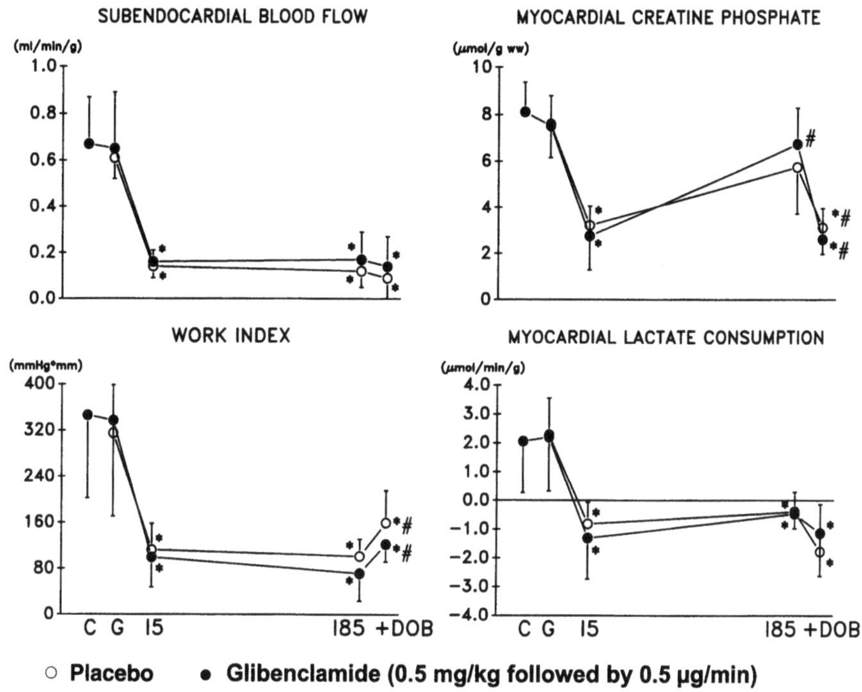

Fig. 2.4. The reduction in subendocardial blood flow of the anterior myocardium at 5 minutes ischemia (I5) is associated with decreased regional contractile function in placebo swine and swine receiving the ATP-dependent potassium channel antagonist glibenclamide (G). Within the first 5 minutes of ischemia, the creatine phosphate concentration decreases and lactate consumption is reversed to net lactate production in both groups of swine. With the extension of ischemia to 85 minutes (I85) at a constant subendocardial blood flow, there is a tendency for a further decrease in regional contractile function in both groups of swine. In contrast, lactate production is attenuated and the creatine phosphate concentration recovers to a value no longer significantly different from the respective control value. Infusion of dobutamine (+DOB) after 90 minutes of ischemia increases regional contractile function at an unchanged subendocardial blood flow to a comparable extent in both groups of swine. This increase in contractile function, however, is associated once more with increased lactate production and a decreased creatine phosphate concentration. *$p<0.05$ vs CONTROL (C), #$p<0.05$ vs preceding value. (From Schulz *et al.* 1995c)

involved in the development of short-term myocardial hibernation (Figure 2.4) (Schulz *et al.* 1995c).

Endogenous adenosine which is released during ischemia might, through a number of secondary mechanisms, such as inhibition of adenylate cyclase activity, inhibition of norepinephrine release from sympathetic nerve endings or inhibition of L-type calcium channels, attenuate the decrease in myocardial energy rich phosphates and the increase in intracellular calcium concentration, thereby preserving myocardial viability during ischemia. However, a role for endogenous adenosine in the development of hibernation has been excluded, since neither contractile function nor metabolic parameters nor viability are altered by increased catabolism of endogenous adenosine by infusion of adenosine deaminase (Figure 2.5) (Schulz *et al.* 1995c).

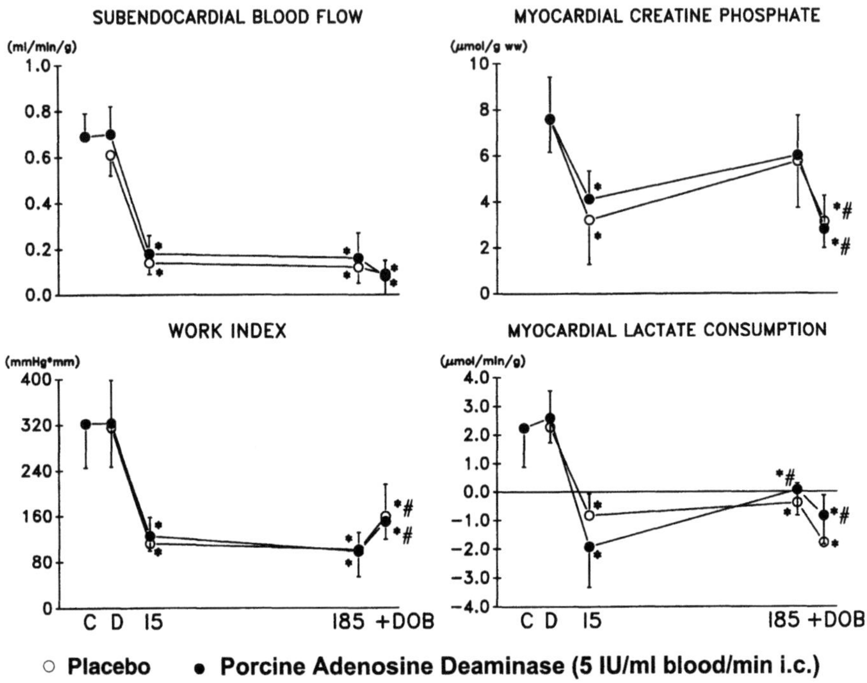

Fig. 2.5. The reduction in subendocardial blood flow of the anterior myocardium at 5 minutes ischemia (I5) is associated with decreased regional contractile function in placebo swine and swine receiving adenosine deaminase (D). Within the first 5 minutes of ischemia, the creatine phosphate concentration decreases and lactate consumption is reversed to net lactate production in both groups of swine. With the extension of ischemia to 85 minutes (I85) at a constant subendocardial blood flow, there is a tendency for a further decrease in regional contractile function in both groups of swine. In contrast, lactate production is attenuated and the creatine phosphate concentration recovers to a value no longer significantly different from the respective control value. Infusion of dobutamine (+DOB) after 90 minutes of ischemia increases regional contractile function at an unchanged subendocardial blood flow to a comparable extent in both groups of swine. This increase in contractile function, however, is associated once more with increased lactate production and a decreased creatine phosphate concentration. * $p<0.05$ vs CONTROL (C), # $p<0.05$ vs preceding value. (From Schulz *et al.* 1995c)

In short-term hibernating myocardium, regional contractile function is decreased without apparent alterations in the calcium sensitivity. In anesthetized pigs after 90 minutes of ischemia, at a time when lactate production is attenuated and the creatine phosphate concentration is restored to a value no longer significantly different from the respective control value, the maximal responses to graded intracoronary calcium infusion and postextrasystolic potentiation are decreased. However, the relationships between the fractional increases in regional contractile function and dose of added intracoronary calcium and the postextrasystolic time interval, respectively, are not different. Thus, overall calcium responsiveness of short-term hibernating myocardium is substantially reduced. The reduction of calcium responsiveness is, however, attributable to a decrease in maximal developed force and not to a decrease in calcium sensitivity (Heusch *et al.* 1996).

2.11 Short-term Hibernation vs. Ischemic Preconditioning

Ischemic preconditioning, i.e. the delay of infarct size development resulting from prolonged and severe myocardial ischemia by one or more preceding short episodes of ischemia and reperfusion, is the most powerful endogenous cardioprotective effect observed so far. Myocardial ATP and creatine phosphate concentrations remain somewhat higher in preconditioned hearts than in hearts subjected to prolonged ischemia without ischemic preconditioning (Murry *et al.* 1990; Kida *et al.* 1991). Also, glycolysis and lactate production have been reported to be attenuated in ischemic preconditioned hearts (Asimakis *et al.* 1992; Wolfe *et al.* 1993), though this remains controversial (Janier *et al.* 1994).

Thus, both hibernating and ischemic preconditioned myocardium are characterized not only by preserved myocardial viability, but also by attenuation of metabolic alterations during prolonged ischemia. Recent data from Ferrari and associates point to a further link between hibernating and ischemic preconditioned myocardium in isolated buffer-perfused rabbit hearts. Myocardial ATP concentration recovered and lactate production was reversed towards lactate consumption after prolonged low-flow ischemia when hearts underwent a preceding short period of no-flow ischemia. During reperfusion following the sustained ischemia, only a transient creatine kinase release occurred and contractile function rapidly recovered towards preischemic values. Thus, the authors proposed that the development of myocardial hibernation requires an initial period of no-flow ischemia, in which the rapid decrease in pH initiating the decrease in contractile function allowed for a renewed balance between energy supply and energy demand (Ferrari *et al.* 1996). Also in anesthetized swine in situ, infarct size caused by sustained low-flow ischemia was reduced by a preceding short period of no-flow ischemia (Schulz *et al.* 1995a). Activation of ATP-dependent potassium channels and endogenous adenosine are involved in the infarct size reducing effect of ischemic preconditioning (Schulz *et al.* 1994; Schulz *et al.* 1995b), but not in short-term myocardial hibernation (Schulz *et al.* 1995c). The observed reduction in infarct size by the initial period of no-flow ischemia, like in classical ischemic preconditioning (Schulz *et al.* 1994), was abolished by blockade of ATP-dependent potassium channels with glibenclamide (Schulz *et al.* 1995a).

Thus, a brief episode of no-flow myocardial ischemia without intermittent reperfusion increases the tolerance to sustained low-flow ischemia. This cardioprotective effect is mediated by activation of ATP-dependent potassium channels, and therefore relates to ischemic preconditioning rather than to myocardial hibernation. Thus, despite certain similarities between ischemic preconditioning and myocardial hibernation, those two cardioprotective phenomena are different in nature.

2.12 Short-term Hibernation vs. Stunning

Both the short-term hibernating and the stunned myocardium are characterized by reversibly reduced contractile function. In short-term hibernating myocardium ischemia is still ongoing, whereas in stunned myocardium blood flow is fully or almost fully restored. In contrast to dysfunctional, irreversibly damaged myocardium, both short-term hibernating and stunned myocardium retain an inotropic reserve. To further distinguish short-term hibernating from stunned myocardium, either regional myocardial blood flow must be measured (Bolli, 1992) or the metabolic changes associated with an inotropic challenge be analyzed. The recruitment of an inotropic reserve in short-term hibernating myocardium is at the expense of metabolic recovery (Schulz *et al.* 1992; Schulz *et al.* 1993) (Figure 2.1), while in stunned myocardium no metabolic deterioration occurs during inotropic stimulation (Ambrosio *et al.* 1987; Arnold *et al.* 1985; Görge *et al.* 1990). Also, whereas prolonged inotropic stimulation causes infarction in short-term hibernating myocardium (Schulz *et al.* 1993), it does not cause necrosis in stunned myocardium (Bolli *et al.* 1985).

2.13 Transition from Short-term Hibernation to Chronic Hibernation

There are a few experimental studies which tried to investigate the transition process from short-term hibernation to chronic hibernation by subjecting swine to either a prolonged partial coronary artery stenosis for a duration ranging from 1 day to 32 weeks (Bolukoglu *et al.* 1992; Liedtke *et al.* 1994; Mills *et al.* 1994; Chen *et al.* 1995; Liedtke *et al.* 1995) or a progressive narrowing of the coronary artery until complete occlusion by use of an ameroid constrictor (Shen & Vatner, 1995; Fallafollita *et al.* 1997). These studies, however, failed to continuously monitor myocardial blood flow and contractile function over the entire time period of coronary hypoperfusion. When resting regional myocardial blood flow was measured (Shen & Vatner, 1995; Chen *et al.* 1995; Liedtke *et al.* 1995; Mills *et al.* 1994; Fallafollita *et al.* 1997), it was either found to be reduced at the beginning (Chen *et al.* 1995; Mills *et al.* 1994) and the end of the stenosis protocol (Chen *et al.* 1995; Mills *et al.* 1994; Fallafollita *et al.* 1997) or was normal (Shen & Vatner, 1995) or almost normal at the beginning and the end of the stenosis protocol (Liedtke *et al.* 1995). At normal or almost normal resting blood flow, however, coronary reserve was impaired (Shen & Vatner, 1995; Liedtke *et al.* 1995; Mills *et al.* 1994; Fallafollita *et al.* 1997). With impaired coronary reserve there could be repetitive episodes of exercise-induced ischemia and reperfusion inducing stunning, offering an alternative explanation for the observed chronic reduction of contractile function during persistent coronary stenosis. Indeed, in one study episodes of apparent stunning were documented (Shen & Vatner, 1995). However, since myocardial blood flow and contractile function were not measured continously, these studies do not prove or disprove the existence of true "myocardial hibernation".

2.14 Morphology of Chronic Hibernating Myocardium

In chronic hibernating myocardium morphological alterations occur. In myocardial biopsies from patients with prolonged contractile dysfunction which was reversible after bypass surgery, the thin filament complex and titin are reduced and the remaining myofibrils as well as the sarcoplasmic reticulum are disorganized (Flameng *et al.* 1981; Elsässer & Schaper, 1995). The intracellular glycogen content is increased and extracellular matrix proteins such as desmin, tubulin and vinculin accumulate (Flameng *et al.* 1981; Elsässer & Schaper, 1995). Up to a certain degree of severity these degenerative alterations are reversible (Elsässer & Schaper, 1995). Apart from such degenerative alterations, the distribution of titin and cardiotin, which reflects an embryonic phenotype pattern, and the expression of alpha-smooth muscle actin suggest a dedifferentiation of cardiomyocytes (Borgers & Ausma, 1995). Thus, despite the fact that the myocardium remains viable during persistent ischemia and contractile dysfunction is reversible upon reperfusion (Rahimtoola, 1985), there are severe morphological alterations. Understandably, full functional recovery following reperfusion might therefore require weeks or even months (Rahimtoola, 1985).

2.15 Hibernation in the Clinical Setting

Hibernation over weeks or months (chronic hibernation), as defined by Rahimtoola, is a state of chronic reduction of contractile function which is fully reversible upon reperfusion (Rahimtoola, 1985), and can only be inferred from clinical studies. Clinical syndromes consistent with the existence of myocardial hibernation include unstable and stable angina (Rahimtoola, 1989; Carlson *et al.* 1989; Bonow *et al.* 1991; Ferrari *et al.* 1992; Sambuceti *et al.* 1993), acute myocardial infarction (Chatterjee *et al.* 1973; Rahimtoola, 1989; Montalescot *et al.* 1992) and left ventricular dysfunction and/or congestive heart failure (Akins *et al.* 1980; Louie *et al.* 1991) (Table 2.3).

It is still under debate whether chronic reduction of contractile function observed in patients with coronary artery disease occurs during persistent ischemia, i.e. true "hibernation", or is the result of repetitive episodes of ischemia and reperfusion, i.e. "stunning". In patients with a complete occlusion of a major coronary artery but an extensive collateral circulation, chronic contractile dysfunction is observed at somewhat reduced resting myocardial blood flows (van Overschelde *et al.* 1993), although given the small number of patients included in this study the decrease in myocardial

Table 2.3. Clinical conditions of myocardial hibernation

- Unstable and stable angina
- Acute myocardial infarction
- Congestive heart failure and/or LV dysfunction

blood flow was not significant when compared to normal values from a different group of individuals. Since, however, coronary reserve was significantly diminished in these patients, there could indeed be repetitive episodes of exercise-induced ischemia and reperfusion inducing stunning, which then result in chronic reduction of contractile function. Nevertheless, this study does not rule out the existence of true myocardial "hibernation", i.e. a situation of chronic reduction of contractile function during persistent ischemia, in the clinical setting.

2.16 Diagnosis of Hibernating Myocardium

In nuclear cardiology, the approach for detection of myocardial hibernation depends on demonstrating a match between reduced contractile function and reduced blood flow or a mismatch between perfusion and metabolism. Segmental contractile dysfunction is determined by echocardiography, contrast ventriculography or gated tomography of labelled agents, perfusion is assessed with ^{201}TI or ^{99m}Tc-Sestamibi using scintigraphy or with $^{13}NH_3$ or $H_2{}^{15}O$ using positron emission tomography, and metabolism is assessed with ^{18}F2-deoxyglucose using positron emission tomography (Table 2.4).

Positron emission tomography techniques (Schelbert, 1991; Marwick *et al.* 1992) may help not only to identify viable, dysfunctional myocardium, but also to distinguish hibernating from stunned myocardium and predict the success of reperfusion procedures (Conversano *et al.* 1992; Dilsizian & Bonow, 1993; Erdmann & Kirsch, 1993).

2.17 Therapy of Hibernating Myocardium

Hibernating myocardium, although exhibiting a number of cardioprotective features, is nevertheless at least intermittently ischemic and therefore a pathological condition. Thus, the only causal therapy of hibernating myocardium is to restore adequate blood flow to the hypoperfused tissue by revascularization.

2.18 Open Questions Related to Myocardial Hibernation

1. How long can the ischemic myocardium maintain its metabolic integrity? It is possible that the metabolic status of short-term hibernating myocardium once again deteriorates over time. In this scenario, the decrease in contractile function during persistent moderate ischemia is only a temporary mechanism to prolong myocardial viability but is inherently time-limited. On the other hand, it is possible that the successfully adapted myocardium can maintain such a state indefinitely and will proceed into chronic hibernation.
2. What are the mechanisms responsible for the transition from an initial supply-demand imbalance to a state of perfusion-contraction matching?

Table 2.4. Diagnosis of myocardial hibernation

Demonstration of a perfusion-contraction match
• Positron emission tomography (^{13}N ^{15}O) • ^{201}Tl scintigraphy, in particular with redistribution or reinjection • ^{99m}Tc-Sestamibi scintigraphy, in particular with redistribution or reinjection (Techniques requiring concurrent assessment of function by other methods: e.g. ventriculography, echocardiography)
Demonstration of a perfusion-metabolism mismatch
Positron emission tomography (^{18}FDG ^{13}N, ^{15}O)
Demonstration of an inotropic reserve at the expense of worsening of myocardial metabolism
• Dobutamine echocardiography • Postextrasystolic potentiation during contrast ventriculography or echocardiography (Techniques requiring concurrent assessment of myocardial metabolism by other methods: e.g. positron emission tomography, coronary sinus lactate)

3. How long can the ischemic myocardium respond to an inotropic stimulation? A progressive loss of myofibrils in ischemic myocardium may result in a reduction and finally loss of response to an inotropic challenge. Thus, the identification of viable, chronic hibernating myocardium by an inotropic challenge may eventually be lost.
4. Does chronic contractile dysfunction in patients reflect true hibernation; i.e. a situation of chronic contractile dysfunction during persistent ischemia, or repetitive episodes of ischemia and reperfusion; i.e. repetitive stunning?
5. Can myocardial hibernation be induced or reinforced? This is a challenging therapeutic goal, as it would extend the time frame for reperfusion interventions in patients with acute ischemic syndromes. In this respect, short-term myocardial hibernation, i.e. an endogenous cardioprotective mechanism during acute ischemic syndromes, may be a much more common and important phenomenon than chronic myocardial hibernation (Schulz & Heusch, 1995).

References

1. Akins CW, Pohost GM, Desanctis RW, Block PC (1980) Selection of angina-free patients with severe left ventricular dysfunction for myocardial revascularization. Am J Cardiol 46:695–700
2. Ambrosio G, Jacobus WE, Bergmann CA, Weisman HF, Becker LC (1987) Preserved high energy phosphate metabolic reserve in globally stunned hearts despite reduction of basal ATP content and contractility. J Mol Cell Cardiol 19:953–964
3. Arai AE, Pantely GA, Anselone CG, Bristow J, Bristow JD (1991) Active downregulation of myocardial energy requirements during prolonged moderate ischemia in swine. Circ Res 69:1458–1469
4. Arai AE, Pantely GA, Thoma WJ, Anselone CG, Bristow JD (1992) Energy metabolism and contractile function after 15 beats of moderate myocardial ischemia. Circ Res 70:1137–1145

5. Arnold JMO, Braunwald E, Sandor T, Kloner RA (1985) Inotropic stimulation of reperfused myocardium with dopamine: effects on infarct size and myocardial function. J Am Coll Cardiol 6:1036–1044
6. Asimakis GK, Inners-McBride K, Medellin G, Conti VR (1992) Ischemic preconditioning attenuates acidosis and postischemic dysfunction in isolated rat heart. Am J Physiol 263:H887–H894
7. Battler A, Froelicher VF, Gallagher KP, Kemper WS, Ross Jr. J (1980) Dissociation between regional myocardial dysfunction and ECG changes during ischemia in the conscious dog. Circulation 62:735–744
8. Bolli R, Zhu W-X, Myers ML, Hartley CJ, Roberts R (1985) Beta-adrenergic stimulation reverses postischemic myocardial dysfunction without producing subsequent deterioration. Am J Cardiol 56:964–968
9. Bolli R (1992) Myocardial "Stunning" in man. Circulation 86:1671–1691
10. Bolukoglu H, Liedtke AJ, Nellis SH, Eggleston AM, Subramanian R, Renstrom B (1992) An animal model of chronic coronary stenosis resulting in hibernating myocardium. Am J Physiol 263:H20–H29
11. Bonow RO, Dilsizian V, Cuocolo A, Bacharach SL (1991) Identification of viable myocardium in patients with chronic coronary artery disease and left ventricular dysfunction. Circulation 83:26–37
12. Borgers M and Ausma J (1995) Structural aspects of the chronic hibernating myocardium in man. Basic Res Cardiol 90:44–46
13. Braunwald E and Rutherford JD (1986) Reversible ischemic left ventricular dysfunction: evidence for the "hibernating myocardium". J Am Coll Cardiol 8:1467–1470
14. Canty JM (1988) Coronary pressure-function and steady-state pressure-flow relations during autoregulation in the unanesthetized dog. Circ Res 63:821–836
15. Carlson EB, Cowley MJ, Wolfgang TC, Vetrovec GW (1989) Acute changes in global and regional rest left ventricular function after coronary angioplasty: comparative results in stable and unstable angina. J Am Coll Cardiol 13:1262–1269
16. Chatterjee K, Swan HJC, Parmley WW, Sustaita H, Marcus HS, Matloff J (1973) Influence of direct myocardial revascularization on left ventricular asynergy and function in patients with coronary heart disease With and without previous myocardial infarction. Circulation 47:276–286
17. Chen C, Li L, Chen LL, Prada JV, Chen MH, Fallon JT, Weyman AE, Waters D, Gillam L (1995) Incremental dosis of dobutamine induce a biphasic response in dysfunctional left ventricular regions subtending coronary stenoses. Circulation 92:756–766
18. Clarke K, O'Connor JA, Willis RJ (1987) Temporal relation between energy metabolism and myocardial function during ischemia and reperfusion. Am J Physiol 253:H412–H421
19. Conversano A, Herrero P, Geltman EM, Pérez JE, Bergmann SR, Gropler RJ (1992) Differentiation of stunned from hibernating myocardium by positron emission tomography. Circulation 86 (Suppl.I):I–107 (abstract)
20. Decking UKM, Reffelmann T, Schrader J, Kammermeier H (1995) Hypoxia-induced activation of KATP channels limits energy depletion in the guinea pig heart. Am J Physiol 269:H734–H742
21. Dilsizian V and Bonow RO (1993) Current diagnostic techniques of assessing myocardial viability in patients with hibernating and stunned myocardium. Circulation 87:1–20
22. Downing SE and Chen V (1990) Myocardial hibernation in the ischemic neonatal heart. Circ Res 66:763–772
23. Downing SE and Chen V (1992) Acute hibernation and reperfusion of the ischemic heart. Circulation 85:699–707
24. Elsässer A and Schaper J (1995) Hibernating myocardium: adaptation or degeneration? Basic Res Cardiol 90:47–48
25. Erdmann E and Kirsch C-M (1993) "Stunned" und "Hibernating Myocardium"-Diagnostik und klinische Implikationen. Z Kardiol 82 (Suppl. 5):143–147
26. Fallafollita JA, Perry BJ, Canty JM (1997) 18F-2-deoxyglucose deposition and regional flow in pigs with chronically dysfunctional myocardium. Evidence for transmural variations in chronic hibernating myocardium. Circulation 95:1900–1909
27. Fedele FA, Gewirtz H, Capone RJ, Sharaf B, Most AS (1988) Metabolic response to prolonged reduction of myocardial blood flow distal to a severe coronary artery stenosis. Circulation 78:729–735
28. Ferrari R, La Canna G, Giubbini R, Visioli O (1992) Stunned and hibernating myocardium: possibility of intervention. J Cardiovasc Pharmacol 20 (Suppl.):S5–S13

29. Ferrari R, Cargnoni A, Bernocchi P, Pasini E, Curello S, Ceconi C, Ruigrok TJC (1996) Metabolic adaptation during a sequence of no-flow and low-flow ischemia: a possible trigger for hibernation. Circulation 94:2587–2596
30. Flameng W, Suy R, Schwarz F, Borgers M, Piessens J, Thone F, van Ermen H, de Geest H (1981) Ultrastructural correlates of left ventricular contraction abnormalities in patients with chronic ischemic heart disease: Determinants of reversible segmental asynergy postrevascularization surgery. Am Heart J 102:846–857
31. Gallagher KP, Matsuzaki M, Osakada G, Kemper WS, Ross Jr. J (1983) Effect of exercise on the relationship between myocardial blood flow and systolic wall thickening in dogs with acute coronary stenosis. Circ Res 52:716–729
32. Görge G, Papageorgiou I, Lerch R (1990) Epinephrine-stimulated contractile and metabolic reserve in postischemic rat myocardium. Basic Res Cardiol 85:595–605
33. Guth BD, Schulz R, Heusch G (1993) Time course and mechanisms of contractile dysfunction during acute myocardial ischemia. Circulation 87 (Suppl. IV):IV-35–IV-42
34. Hearse DJ (1979) Oxygen deprivation and early myocardial contractile failure: a reassessment of the possible role of adenosine triphosphate. Am J Cardiol 44:1115–1121
35. Heusch G (1991) The relationship between regional blood flow and contractile function in normal, ischemic, and reperfused myocardium. Basic Res Cardiol 86:197–218
36. Heusch G, Rose J, Skyschally A, Post H, Schulz R (1996) Calcium responsiveness in regional myocardial short-term hibernation and stunning in the in situ porcine heart – inotropic responses to postextrasystolic potentiation and intracoronary calcium. Circulation 93:1556–1566
37. Jacobus WE, Pores IH, Lucas SK, Weisfeldt ML, Flaherty JT (1982) Intracellular acidosis and contractility in normal and ischemic hearts examined by 31P NMR. J Mol Cell Cardiol 14:13–20
38. Janier MF, Vanoverschelde J-LJ, Bergmann SR (1994) Ischemic preconditioning stimulates anaerobic glycolysis in the isolated rabbit heart. Am J Physiol 267:H1353–H1360
39. Kammermeier H, Schmidt P, Jüngling E (1982) Free energy change of ATP-hydrolysis: a causal factor of early hypoxic failure of the myocardium? J Mol Cell Cardiol 14:267–277
40. Katz AM (1973) Effects of ischemia on the contractile processes of heart muscle. Am J Cardiol 32:456–460
41. Kentish JC (1986) The effects of inorganic phosphate and creatine phosphate on the force production in skinned muscle from rat vesicle. J Physiol 370:585–604
42. Kida M, Fujiwara H, Ishida M, Kawai C, Ohura M, Miura I, Yabuuchi Y (1991) Ischemic preconditioning preserves creatine phosphate and intracellular pH. Circulation 84:2495–2503
43. Koretsune Y, Corretti MC, Kusuoka H, Marban E (1991) Mechanism of early ischemic contractile failure. Circ Res 68:255–262
44. Krause S and Hess ML (1984) Characterization of cardiac sarcoplasmic reticulum dysfunction during short-term, normothermic, global ischemia. Circ Res 55:176–184
45. Kusuoka H, Weisfeldt ML, Zweier JL, Jacobus WE, Marban E (1986) Mechanism of early contractile failure during hypoxia in intact ferret heart: Evidence for modulation of maximal Ca-activated force by inorganic phosphate. Circ Res 59:270–282
46. Kübler W and Katz AM (1977) Mechanism of early "pump" failure of the ischemic heart: possible role of adenosine triphosphate depletion and inorganic phosphate accumulation. Am J Cardiol 40:467–471
47. Liedtke AJ, Renstrom B, Nellis SH, Subramanian R (1994) Myocardial function and metabolism in pig hearts after relief from chronic partial coronary stenosis. Am J Physiol 267:H1312–H1319
48. Liedtke AJ, Renstrom B, Nellis SH, Hall JL, Stanley WC (1995) Mechanical and metabolic functions in pig hearts after 4 days of chronic coronary stenosis. J Am Coll Cardiol 26:815–828
49. Louie HW, Laks H, Milgalter E, Drinkwater Jr. DC, Hamilton MA, Brunken RC, Stevenson LW (1991) Ischemic Cardiomyopathy Criteria for coronary revascularization and cardiac transplantation. Circulation 84 (Suppl.III):III-290–III-295
50. Marwick TH, MacIntyre WJ, Lafont A, Nemec JJ, Salcedo EE (1992) Metabolic response of hibernating and infarcted myocardium to revascularization. A follow-up study of regional perfusion, function, and metabolism. Circulation 85:1347–1353
51. Matsuzaki M, Gallagher KP, Kemper WS, White F, Ross Jr. J (1983) Sustained regional dysfunction produced by prolonged coronary stenosis: gradual recovery after reperfusion. Circulation 68:170–182

52. Mills I, Fallon JT, Wrenn D, Sasken H, Gray W, Bier J, Levine D, Berman S, Gilson M, Gewirtz H (1994) Adaptive responses of coronary circulation and myocardium to chronic reduction in perfusion pressure and flow. Am J Physiol 266:H447–H457
53. Montalescot G, Faraggi M, Drobinski G, Messian O, Evans J, Grosgogeat Y, Thomas D (1992) Myocardial viability in patients with Q wave myocardial infarction and no residual ischemia. Circulation 86:47–55
54. Murry CE, Richard VJ, Reimer KA, Jennings RB (1990) Ischemic preconditioning slows energy metabolism and delays ultrastructural damage during a sustained ischemic episode. Circ Res 66:913–931
55. Noma A (1983) ATP- regulated K+ channels in cardiac muscle. Nature 305:147–148
56. Pantely GA, Malone SA, Rhen WS, Anselone CG, Arai A, Bristow J, Bristow JD (1990) Regeneration of myocardial phosphocreatine in pigs despite continued moderate ischemia. Circ Res 67:1481–1493
57. Rahimtoola SH (1982) Coronary bypass surgery for chronic angina – 1981. Circulation 65:225-241
58. Rahimtoola SH (1985) A perspective on the three large multicenter randomized clinical trials of coronary bypass surgery for chronic stable angina. Circulation 72 Suppl.V:V-123–V-135
59. Rahimtoola SH (1989) The hibernating myocardium. Am Heart J 117:211–221
60. Rose J, Schulz R, Martin C, Heusch G (1993) Post-ejection wall thickening as a marker of successful short term hibernation. Cardiovasc Res 27:1306–1311
61. Ross Jr. J (1989) Mechanisms of regional ischemia and antianginal drug action during exercise. Prog Cardiovasc Dis 31:455–466
62. Ross Jr. J (1991) Myocardial perfusion-contraction matching. Implications for coronary heart disease and hibernation. Circulation 83:1076–1083
63. Rüegg JC, Schädler M, Steiger GJ, Müller G (1971) Effect of inorganic phosphate on the contractile mechanism. Pflügers Arch 325:359–364
64. Sambuceti G, Parodi O, Marzullo P, Giorgetti A, Fusani L, Puccini G, Salvadori P, L'Abbate A (1993) Regional myocardial blood flow in stable angina pectoris associated with isolated significant narrowing of either the left anterior descending or left circumflex coronary artery. Am J Cardiol 72:990–994
65. Schelbert HR (1991) Positron emission tomography for the assessment of myocardial viability. Circulation 84 (Suppl I):I-122–I-131
66. Schmidt-Ott SC, Bletz C, Vahl C, Saggau W, Hagl S, Rüegg JC (1990) Inorganic phosphate inhibits contractility and ATPase activity in skinned fibers from human myocardium. Basic Res Cardiol 85:358–366
67. Schulz R, Guth BD, Pieper K, Martin C, Heusch G (1992) Recruitment of an inotropic reserve in moderately ischemic myocardium at the expense of metabolic recovery: a model of short-term hibernation. Circ Res 70:1282–1295
68. Schulz R, Rose J, Martin C, Brodde OE, Heusch G (1993) Development of short-term myocardial hibernation: its limitation by the severity of ischemia and inotropic stimulation. Circulation 88:684–695
69. Schulz R, Post H, Sakka S, Wallbridge DR, Heusch G (1995a) Intraischemic preconditioning. Increase tolerance to sustained low-flow ischemia by a brief episode of no-flow ischemia without intermittent reperfusion. Circ Res 76:942–950
70. Schulz R, Rose J, Post H, Heusch G (1995b) Involvement of endogenous adenosine in ischemic preconditioning in swine. Pflügers Archiv 430:273–282
71. Schulz R, Rose J, Post H, Heusch G (1995c) Regional short-term hibernation in swine does not involve endogenous adenosine or KATP channels. Am J Physiol 268:H2294–H2301
72. Schulz R and Heusch G (1995) Acute adaptation to ischemia: short-term myocardial hibernation. Basic Res Cardiol 90:29–31
73. Schulz R, Rose J, Heusch G (1994) Involvement of activation of ATP-dependent potassium channels in ischemic preconditioning in swine. Am J Physiol 267:H1341–H1352
74. Shen Y-T and Vatner SF (1995) Mechanism of impaired myocardial function during progressive coronary stenosis in conscious pigs. Hibernation versus stunning. Circ Res 76:479–488
75. Theroux P, Franklin D, Ross Jr. J, Kemper WS (1974) Regional myocardial function during acute coronary artery occlusion and its modification by pharmacological agents in the dog. Circ Res 35:896–908
76. Theroux P, Ross Jr. J, Franklin D, Kemper WS, Sasayama S (1976) Regional myocardial function in the conscious dog during acute coronary occlusion and responses to morphine, propranolol, nitroglycerin, and lidocaine. Circulation 53:302–314

77. vanOverschelde JLJ, Wijns W, Depré C, Essamri B, Heyndrickx GR, Borgers M, Bol A, Melin JA (1993) Mechanisms of chronic regional postischemic dysfunction in humans. New insights from the study of noninfarcted collateral-dependent myocardium. Circulation 87:1513–1523
78. Vatner SF (1980) Correlation between acute reductions in myocardial blood flow and function in conscious dogs. Circ Res 47:201–207
79. Weintraub WS, Hattori S, Agarwal JB, Bodenheimer MM, Banka VS, Helfant RH (1981) The relationship between myocardial blood flow and contraction by myocardial layer in the canine left ventricle during ischemia. Circ Res 48:430–438
80. Wolfe CL, Sievers RE, Visseren FLJ, Donnelly TJ (1993) Loss of myocardial protection after preconditioning correlates with the time course of glycogen recovery within the preconditioned segment. Circulation 87:881–892

CHAPTER 3

Indicators of a Dualistic Organisation of Heart Muscle Structure and Function

P. P. LUNKENHEIMER · K. REDMANN · H. H. SCHELD · C. W. CRYER

3.1 Introduction

Among cardiologists, morphology is held in low esteem. One main reason is the lack of preparation techniques which make it possible to gain access to the intricate weave of the heart muscle. Tissue analysis has remained at a mainly cellular level. A common morphological substrate of myocardial failure has not been identified [57]. Morphology will not succeed in yielding a comprehensive understanding of the wide palette of adaptive heart diseases until tissue analysis is also applied to the mesh texture of the heart. In fact, until recently there were no appropriate methods available for analysing spatial myocardial and connective tissue weave, either post mortem or in vivo. However, new advances in imaging techniques indicate that in the near future pathomorphology will be obliged to broaden its analytical spectrum to keep abreast with clinical diagnostics.

With the following suggestion, Frank shattered the results of more than a century of research [24] and discussion: "So little is known about the orientation of the myocardial fibres that any determination of tension in individual fibres seems to be impossible... The longitudinal direction of the myocardial fibres must generally be tangential with respect to the ventricular surface. If these fibres were in a normal direction to the wall surface, their shortening would induce ventricular dilatation rather than a reduction in ventricular volume..."

More than two centuries prior to Frank's attempt, Lower [38] had delineated the helical continuum of a myocardial band that he supposed to be coiled around both ventricles. This concept implied oblique transmural trajectories.

However, noninvasive imaging methods still tacitly assume that in any individual heart there is a geometrically predictable transmission of myocardial force to ventricular pressure. Points of concern are (a) that all myocardial fibres are assumed to be aligned in parallel to the epicardial and/or endocardial surfaces, and hence, it is taken for granted that all forces generated are acting in the direction of ventricular emptying; (b) histologically determined main myocardial fibre alignment has been unconditionally taken as the sole alignment of stress transmission pathways.

3.2 Pathomorphology Underinterpreted

Clinicians are not used to examining the functional implications of structural myocardial remodeling. Thus, pathomorphological diagnostics remains focused on myocellular or global ventricular observations. Alterations in fibre orientation have not shared in diagnostic evaluations.

The recent arbitrary amalgamation of diverse pathomorphologies, subsumed under the term "cardiomyopathies", reflects the clinician's uncompromising preference for purely global haemodynamic descriptions rather than primary pathomorphological definitions. However, inhomogeneities in ventricular wall function and any putative dualistic organisation of functional anatomy remain hidden behind any contractility index derived from global ventricular pressure. This is a restrictive condition, as there is growing evidence that inhomogeneities in wall motion and stress distribution increase in the diseased heart [56].

Our concept implies the interaction of tangential forces promoting ventricular ejection and radial forces mediating active wall thinning, and hence, sustaining ventricular dilatation. Ventricular constrictive forces should prevail, but permanently active dilating forces are also supposed to exist, in addition to the intracavitary filling pressure [41, 44]. So a *dualistic organisation* of the myocardial structure and function was conceived. In the case of myocardial fibre disarray, in fibre rearrangement related to ventricular hypertrophy, in myocardial fibrosis and in some storage diseases, we speculate that the equilibrium between the constricting and dilating forces becomes unbalanced. Intramural performance, i.e. hidden work, may be excessive, and myocardial hypertrophy therefore ensues without apparent haemodynamic stimulus [41, 44].

During the late nineteenth century and the beginning of the twentieth century dilating forces affecting ventricular wall motion were widely discussed [22]. Following this historical line [6, 7, 22, 23, 27, 29, 50, 53], our intention was linked essentially to the search for the driving forces involved in ventricular diastolic unfolding: In 1965 the morphologists Puff and Feneis coined the expression "garden hose effect" [53]. In 1968, Lochner et al. [37] rediscovered the phenomenon and again called it "the garden hose phenomenon". In the American literature the impact of coronary perfusion on ventricular dimension had long been documented as "the Gregg effect" [27]. Historically, it is worth mentioning that the Austrian physiologist Brücke [8] described the ventricular dilating effect mediated by the coronary perfusion pressure as long ago as 1856. Between the early 1960s and the late 1980s, the most extensively investigated approach to ventricular dilatation was the contribution of an intramural hydraulic driving mechanism [16, 12, 42].

In favour of a hydraulic mechanism involved in ventricular mechanics seemed to us to be the existence of wide intercapillary sinusoids, which were supposed to serve as a compliant intramural blood reservoir [43]. However, the rare incidence of sinusoids in the human heart tempered belief in the importance of coronary perfusion dynamics on intramural hydraulics. Recently, Djavakhisvili presented data demonstrating that in coronary heart disease there is an enormous proliferation of sinusoids [19]. They are understood as an emergency blood supply system. Modern laser revascularisation attempts to duplicate this channel system. In the search for mechanisms mediating ventricular diastolic unfolding, however, it seems to be of minor importance.

In the early 1970s we postulated an oblique transmural contractile element to be involved in actively reducing wall thickness and supporting early diastolic ventricular unfolding [42, 44]. The concept implied the interaction of (a) a fibre component more or less obliquely aligned in an endoepicardial direction, yielding a permanently active dilating force, and (b) a hydraulic function of intramural fluids including blood, lymph and the myocardial mass itself [54, 56]. This concept called for direct measurements of intramural mechanics, namely local fibre stress measurements.

We used needle force probes, small in dimension and shaped to be applicable to any measuring site within the beating heart in situ [39–41]. What we found, by intermittent and long-term measurements and by systematic mapping of the left ventricular free wall [56], is not completely covered by Streeter's morphology [59] or by Ingels' harmonic layered fibre activity, either in the normal or in the hypertrophied heart [32]. Therefore, we conclude that results obtained by intramyocardial measuring approaches, whether pressures [2, 35, 54, 55], forces [30, 33, 39–42, 44–46, 55, 60] or shortening distances, emphasize that a renewed study of morphology is definitely mandatory.

3.3 Back to Ventricular Morphology

The study of left ventricular structure has a history stretching back to Vesalius (1514–1564). Lower's standard unwinding preparation [38], i.e. the blunt preparation technique of the heat-denatured heart muscle (BUT), lent support to the idea that the ventricles were made up of discrete, overlapping muscle bands, each band being consistently identifiable.

The myocardial fibre strand peel-off technique (SPOT) which we used [46] on the heat-denatured or enzymatically decollagenised heart allows for fibre digitising, giving access to even small directional changes in myocardial fibre alignment including those in an oblique transmural, i.e. endoepicardial direction. This procedure, which ultimately reveals the three-dimensional myocardial weave architecture in all areas of the heart, is definitely less time consuming and more efficient and appears more reliable than any histomorphological analysis.

Peeling off fibre strands from the surface by pulling on a randomly selected fibre population exposes deeply perforating, i.e. oblique, transmurally aligned grooved surfaces. The three-dimensional myocardial meshwork thus exhibited displays a pronounced oblique transmural netting component.

We refer to the striated, i.e. fibrous surface structures displayed by SPOT in terms of the *contractile pathway alignment (CP)*. What one recognises on the exposed surfaces after having peeled off superjacent fibre strands is the mainly longitudinal alignment of myocardial cell bundles, called CPs in the following. We keep in mind that in any case we are dealing with randomly selected fragments of the three-dimensional mesh continuum.

3.4 Material and Methods

Adult cow hearts in rigor mortis and dilated (early post mortem) adult pig hearts were procured from a local slaughterhouse. The atria were trimmed

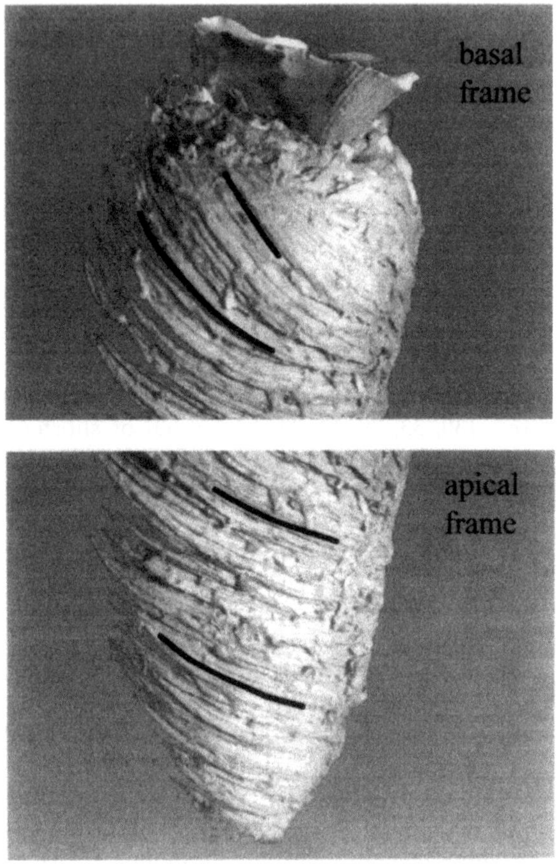

Fig. 3.1. Ventrolateral aspect of the left ventricular wall of a cow heart after removal of some superficial layers

down to the base. The ventricles were filled with a two-component resin (Technovit, Kulzer, Germany).

The hearts were boiled in tap water, to which 50 ml/5 l of 99.7% acetic acid was added to assist the dissolution of the connective tissue, for 2 h (±30 min). The subepicardial cushions of fat, the coronary vessels and the epicardial coating were removed. The hearts were analysed using the *fibre SPOT* and digitised by a manual method.

The preparation is begun by inserting one leg of a forceps 1–2 mm deep into the ventricular wall, then clamping the enclosed bundle and tearing it off from its surroundings (Fig. 3.1). The bundle is pulled along its more or less circular or spiraling pathway. When the strand is torn out of its grooved bed, countless connections with the neighbouring fibres are disrupted.

In deeper zones of the ventricular wall the strands grow in thickness over the distance along which they are pulled out of the myocardial mass. Fibre alignments on the two opposing surfaces of the slightly wedge-shaped strands are not arranged parallel to one another because the inclination angle increases with depth in the ventricular wall.

3.5 Digitising Technique

The grooves and crests on the displayed surfaces of the dilated (diastolic) pig heart were digitised using a three-dimensional magnetic-field digitising tablet (3 Draw Digitizer System, 3 SD 005, Polhemus, Cochester VTO 5446 USA). We digitised stepwise, starting from the subepicardium freed of its epicardial coating. Then the first CP coating was peeled off. The displayed striated surface was scanned by following with the stylus the grooved and salient surface structure. Both ventricles including the septum were prepared strand by strand, from the base to the apex and from the epicardium to the endocardium. In up to ten steps CP coatings were peeled off from the left ventricle and the resulting surfaces were digitised.

Manual digitising using the stylus and the magnetic tablet offers the advantage of instantly distinguishing between the individual contractile pathways. By following the well-delineated grooves and crests on the sequentially exposed surfaces with the stylus one mirrors the surface image of previously peeled-off contractile pathways.

The delineated CPs were processed by a software program which allowed the assessment of the continuously changing angle which each selected CP segment formed with the epicardial surface. For this purpose, the shortest distances to the epicardial surface of the given points on a CP segment were calculated, on the premise that the shortest possible junction between a CP point and a point on the epicardial surface is normal to the epicardial surface. The angle which the local CP tangent forms with the normal to the epicardium, minus 90°, was taken as the local inclination angle towards wall thickness.

3.6 Results

Starting from the subepicardium, after the epicardium and subepicardial fat had been removed, a clear surface graining appeared to the naked eye. This well-oriented structure became still more conspicuous when some subepicardial contractile pathways had been taken away using the fibre SPOT.

The main direction of the grain rotates from layer to layer upon an axis more or less normal to the epicardium (Fig. 3.2). Surface-specific rotation appears to vary quantitatively between areas. However, as a feature of our peel-off method, which allows us to follow also the transmural CP course, the surfaces displayed by successive peeling steps do not necessarily pertain to strictly surface-parallel continuous layers.

The first strands peeled off from the subepicardial myocardial mass appeared to be fairly homogeneous in thickness throughout their entire lengths, so the resulting surfaces were relatively parallel to the subepicardial myocardial surface. From the mid-wall on (third peeling), the peeled-off strands definitely increased in thickness with length and hence entered deeper wall zones. The resulting grooves and crests intruded along tortuous pathways into the inner ventricular wall until they reached the endocardium.

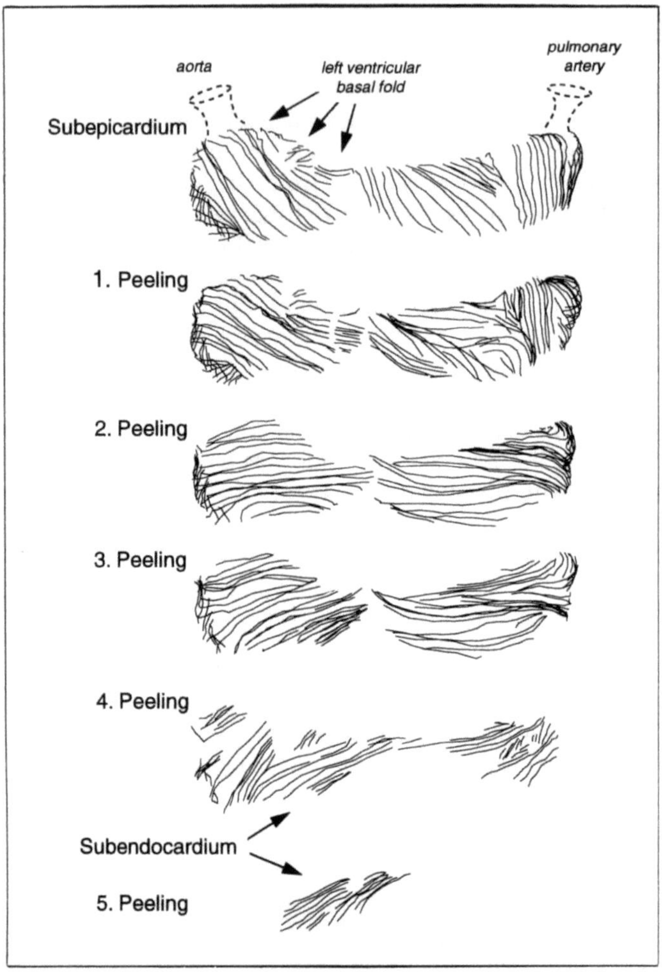

Fig. 3.2. Rotation of the main fibre orientation in a cow heart during preparation from the epicardium to the subendocardium

The displayed surfaces definitely inclined towards the endocardium, and with increasing depth they became more and more rugged. Preferential locations for pronounced CP strand inclination were confirmed to be the right and left ventricular basal fold, the apex, and the left ventricular inner layers. However, some transmural weave component was evident in any part and at any depth of the left ventricular wall.

The inclination angles of subepicardial CPS in the *dilated pig heart* are centred around the angle 0° only in the base (Fig. 3.3). With increasing wall depth the contractile pathways are inclined at rising angles and numbers only in the base and midportion, whereas in the apex the number of inclined CPs rather decreases with depth. Only a small number of fibres (<5%) reach an inclination angle amounting to +30°. Remarkable is the highest incidence

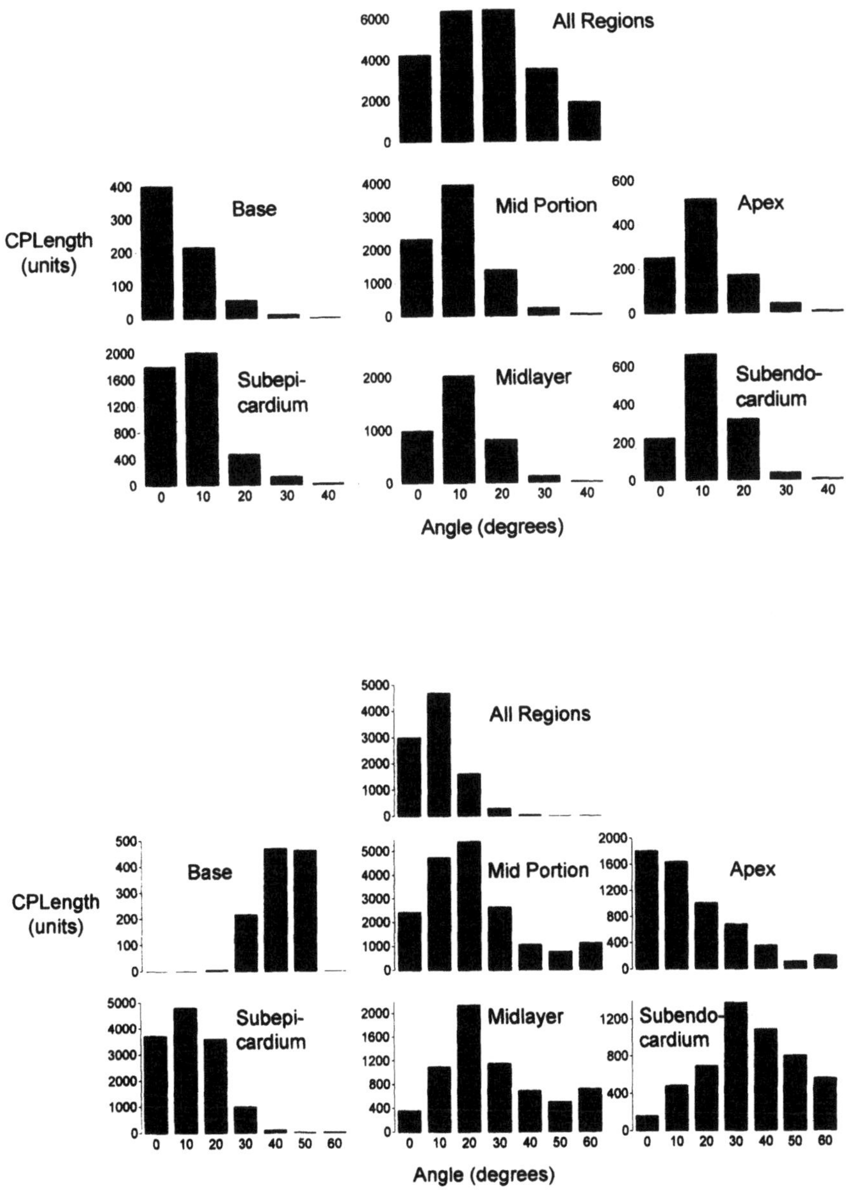

Fig. 3.3. Inclination angle in epiendocardial direction in a 'diastolic' pig heart (*above*) and a 'systolic' (rigor mortis) cow heart (*below*). The number of contractile pathways, listed on the *left*, is given in units of segment length

of the 10° inclination in all positions and wall depths except in the basal subepicardium and subendocardium.

The *constricted cow heart* has definitely more pronounced inclination angles than the dilated pig heart. Only in the apical subepicardium is the angulation centred around 0°. The highest angles of inclination are +60° and are concentrated (>10%) in the subendocardial midportion and apex. There is an inhomogeneous though remarkable shift to higher angles of inclination from the subepicardium to the subendocardium in all positions. Also remarkable is the highest incidence of 20° inclination in the midlayers and 30° in the subendocardium of the midportion and apex of the constricted cow heart.

3.7 Discussion

A wealth of anatomical work has been devoted to the study of fibre orientation with respect to the longitudinal, transverse and sagittal axes of the ventricles [23, 26, 28, 59]. However, fibre inclination towards wall thickness has received little attention.

SPOT confirms the rotation of mainly surface-parallel CPs about an axis normal to the epicardium, as known from preparations performed during the past centuries [6, 38, 48, 52]. Streeter [59] ultimately coined the expression "Japanese-fan-like" to describe this fibre alignment.

We expected and found confirmed (a) a higher degree of angulation in the constricted heart than in the dilated heart, (b) the thick-walled constricted cow heart to give a more detailed insight into the inhomogeneous distribution of the angles of inclination than the thin-walled dilated pig heart, and (c) higher angles of inclination in the subendocardium than in outer layers. This disparity of inclination angles (wide variation of angles) is evident in the midportion of the constricted cow heart but not in the dilated pig heart. The relatively high concentration of inclined CPs in the midportion is all the more interesting as the midportion, i.e. Krehl's *Triebwerk* [36] is understood to consist of an essentially circular, and hence mainly surface-parallel fibre weave.

The different results which were obtained from the constricted cow heart and dilated pig heart were, we believe, due mainly to the fact that the pig heart was thin-walled, whereas the cow heart was boiled in maximum rigor mortis and was therefore thick-walled. This suggests that the oblique transmural fibre weave becomes further erected in the epi-endocardial direction when ventricular wall thickness increases during the ejection period.

The digitised heart muscle [14, 15, 46] confirms Streeter's morphology insofar as it displays layered fibre rotation upon a transmural axis, erected in a normal direction to the epicardium. Yet, it also supplements Streeter's morphology, since the whole heart is analysed, including the septum and the right ventricle. Finally, it overcomes Streeter's morphology because it introduces an oblique, transmurally arranged netting component as being essential to the heart muscle structure.

Given the existence of an oblique, transmural netting component, we must answer the intriguing question of whether structural features displayed by any kind of contractile pathway bundle preparation are really operative. Are they functioning as force transmission pathways? For Streeter's morphology mathematicians have unconditionally assumed that the CP alignment corresponds to the stress transmission pathways [12, 59]. Likewise it is only logi-

Fig. 3.4. An auxotonic and a Laplacian (unloading) force signal in the left ventricular wall displaced together with the left ventricular intracavitary pressure and the ECG

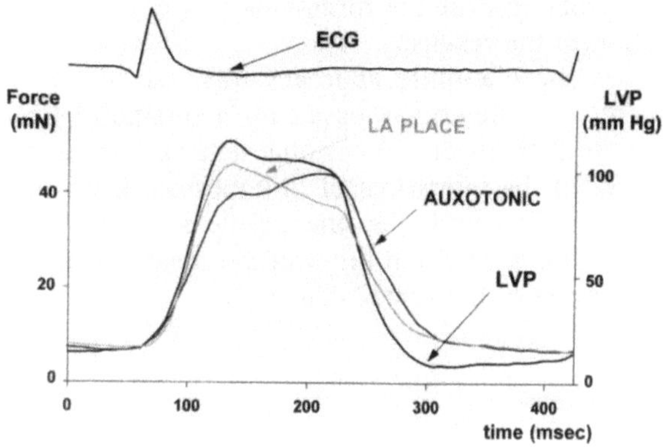

cal to assume that - until there is evidence to the contrary - the transmural netting component yields an endoepicardially oriented force vector which counteracts systolic wall thickening, and hence sustains ventricular dilation.

Of special interest is the pathophysiological aspect. If, for reasons to be further elucidated, the oblique, transmural mesh component is compelled to hypertrophy more than the tangential weave alignment, then the efficiency of ventricular mechanical performance should be decreased. Following this line of functional implication, we speculate that alterations in ventricular spatial mesh structure are related to defined clinical pathologies and may sensibly jeopardise the efficiency of ventricular mechanical performance.

The oblique transmural structure carries an *internal load*, which opposes systolic ventricular wall thickening and summons up energy stored in the elastic properties of the myocardium itself.

Measured mesh tension qualifies this opposing myocardial activity by a characteristic force recording displaying a continuous increase during the ejection period (auxotonic contraction = afterloaded type of local force signal) and a definitely delayed decay [44, 56] (Fig. 3.4). This load is primarily independent of haemodynamic pressure afterload. It is a function of *ventricular size* and *motion amplitude*. The forces thus stored during systole and persisting longer are, we believe, released at end-systole to give the first kick of ventricular unfolding. Late-systolic active wall thinning is thus regarded as one mechanism which initiates ventricular unfolding [41, 42].

The history of wall stress measurements documents the oversimplified understanding of ventricular wall structure and its function. Starting from the assumption that a multilayered, parallel contractile covering is wrapped around the intracavitary blood volume, strain gauges were sutured in a two-point fixation mode to [5, 13, 44], or implanted into, arbitrary wall segments [16–18, 20, 21, 30]. The inner (shortest distance between the two legs of the probe) and outer (embracing the whole ventricle in which wall stress was measured) muscle segments thus selected were understood to each act on the probe in a monodirectional but primarily opposing mode. Ultimately, the interaction of the 'inner' with the 'outer segment' was eliminated by destroying the inner myocardial segment by surgical resection. Spatial stress acting on the probe in different directions was not a matter of concern in the interpretation of the results.

We chose another approach to measuring local myocardial force development. Our method is based on a one-point fixation mode [33, 39, 44, 56]. Due to their three-dimensional netting, myocardial cells form a spatial meshwork. In the interstices of this meshwork we introduced a geometrically defined foreign body, i.e. the needle force probe, which is sensitive to *lateral compression forces*. In this way we measured the *mesh tension* at defined sites and layers of the ventricular wall.

3.8 Procedure

Lateral thoracotomy was performed through the 5th intercostal space. The heart was widely exposed by opening the pericardium from the base to the apex and by fixing it with sutures to the chest wall, thus forming a cradle.

A catheter-tip manometer (1.5 mm thick, Dr. M. Stroh, Magstadt, Germany) was implanted into the left ventricle by puncture via the apex. On the pretreated (banded aorta) hearts the pressure gradient between the aortic root and the post-stenotic segment of the ascending aorta was assessed by advancing the tip manometer into the aorta. Afterwards, the manometer was pulled back into the left ventricle and fixed in place.

A needle force probe (1.3 mm thick, 20 mm long) was inserted into seven measuring sites in the ventrolateral free wall of the left ventricle from base to apex. The probe was introduced into the wall in a direction strictly normal to the epicardial surface. It was progressively advanced in 1.5-mm steps from the epicardium to the endocardium. In the thus defined seven (eight) layers the probe was rotated upon its long axis until the maximum systolic signal was obtained. The signal was recorded and evaluated with respect to its shape and maximum during the ejection period.

In the control state (untreated dog hearts) the highest local force level was observed in the left ventricular base; the lowest level was measured in the apex (Fig. 3.5). The transmural force pattern in all functional states of the control hearts exhibited a force minimum in the middle layers. Subendocardial and subepicardial forces were similar during systole. During diastole the subepicardial wall stress was higher than the subendocardial stress. In the hypertrophied dog hearts the midlayer groove in the transmural diastolic and systolic force profile was somewhat flattened, and the longitudinal gradient was tempered, insofar as the basal forces did not increase as much as those in the midportion and the apex.

The signal measured by needle force probes in the various layers of the left ventricular wall is, in the outer layers, mainly an "unloading" type, which means that the peak force occurs in early systole (Fig. 3.4). With the onset of ventricular ejection the local force level begins to drop gradually until the end of ejection; then it drops sharply.

In an increasing number of measuring sites towards the inner third of the wall the local force signal keeps rising throughout the ventricular ejection period. This latter 'auxotonic' type of signal was found in histological con-

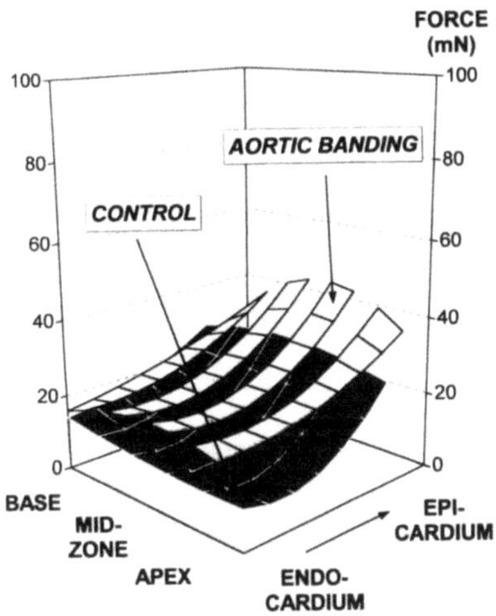

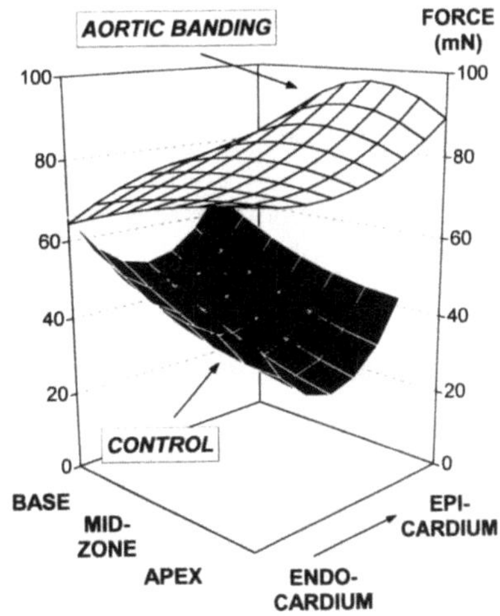

Fig. 3.5. The local force pattern determined by needle force probes in various areas and layers (mapping) of the left ventricular wall of the normal and hypertrophied dog heart during diastole (*left*) and systole (*right*)

trols to be associated with implantation sites aligned parallel to oblique transmural fibre populations. The 'auxotonic' type of signal characteristically keeps its active state longer than the 'unloading' type, which indicates that shortening in the 'auxotonic' myocardial weave compartment is delayed and/ or restricted [9, 34]. The persisting active state may contribute to a late contractile activity in the transmural direction, namely in the direction of late-systolic active wall thinning, resulting in a first dilator impetus [42].

3.9 Putative Functions of the Three-dimensional Weave

The promotion of dilating forces is one potential function of an oblique transmural netting component. The spatial netting feature of the heart muscle may also have the potential of measuring intraventricular pressure by sensing tangential stress in the prevailing surface-parallel netting component. Wall thickness, and hence ventricular diameter, could be measured by sensing stress in the oblique, transmurally aligned netting component. Likewise, stress in spatial directions could be measured by receptors coupled to the connective tissue. However, to our knowledge, the morphological substrate of stress receptors has not been identified in either coupling position.

Furthermore, the myocardial fibre arrangement in the interventricular septum is different from that in the free walls of the left ventricle, in that the turning in some layers of the fibre alignment upon a transmural axis is more abrupt between layers. Considering that superimposed layers in the septum are densely netted, we infer that shear stress must be high in the septum. This assumption is in keeping with our measurements. Microergometry has confirmed a particularly high level of mesh tension at some measuring sites of the septum, namely higher than at any measuring site in the free walls. High shear stress is in line with the relative lack of motion of the septum as compared with that in the free walls of the heart, as documented by various imaging methods [1, 4, 32]. Thus, the septum is likely to be a main site of action of internal, i.e. blind performance, resulting in septal (self-)stiffening [47]. The mechanism may be an important element of ventricular shaping, just as the sepia shell acts in the cuttle fish.

3.10 Clinical Implications

Any dualism in ventricular structure and function interferes with routine clinical diagnostics derived from ventricular pressure and volume data. This becomes still more conspicuous when the basic dualistic mechanisms are extended to the effect of connective tissue which parallels myocardial cells and intramural coronary vessels [10, 61]. Any pathological accumulation of connective tissue principally should mimic the effect of the heart muscle on ventricular mechanics. Thus a transmural, i.e. radial, perivascular fibrosis should impede systolic wall thickening, and hence systolic ventricular emptying. A surface-parallel accumulation of connective tissue, described by Hort [31] as "myocarditis constrictiva", should impede diastolic ventricular filling. Multiple microfocal fibrosis with interfocal connective tissue connexions should present a spatial impairment of wall motion, and hence should jeopardise systolic and diastolic ventricular function. This concept could lead to patient selection criteria for volume-reduction surgery [3, 49]. However, in 15 segments resected during Batista surgery we always found a mixture of all three archetypes of fibrosis. In any case, the cardiac surgeon has to select the appropriate segment of the left ventricular wall to be resected. He is well advised to determine beforehand what kind of pathology he is working on. This is why preoperative diagnostics should include the assessment of segmental ventricular motility. We recommend an acute loading and unloading manoeuvre such as i.v. vasodilator perfusion, followed by fast i.v. volume administration. Another mechanism which reduces local wall motion can be detected by stress echocardiography, namely myocardial contractile depression by hibernation, which may profit instantly from volume-reduction surgery because the resulting reduction in wall stress should be paralleled by at least a relative increase in coronary perfusion. However, fibrotic fettering of the ventricular wall is not instantly cured by volume-reduction surgery, but rather ends in low cardiac output failure. In this regard, based on recent results, the Texas group recommend 2–4 months of pretreatment [25] with a left ventricular assist device, which is assumed to induce connective tissue resolution [51].

References

1. Assad-Morell JL, Tajik AJ, Guiliani ER (1974) Echocardiographic analysis of the ventricular septum. Prog Cardiovasc Dis 17:219–237
2. Baird JR, Ameli FM (1971) The changes in intramyocardial pressure produced by acute ischemia. J Thorac Cadiovasc Surg 62:87–94

3. Batista RJV, Santos ILV, Takeshita N, Bocchino L, Lima L, Cunha MA (1996) Partial left ventriculectomy to improve left ventricular function in end-stage heart disease. J Cardiac Surg 11:96–97
4. Beolchi L, Kuhn M (1995) Mechanical imaging. In: Beolchi L, Kuhn M (eds) Studies in health technology and informatics, 19. ISO Press, Amsterdam
5. Boniface KJ, Brodie OJ, Walton RP (1953) Resistance strain gauge arches for direct measurement of heart contractile force in animals. Proc Soc Exp Biol Med 84:263–266
6. Borelli G (1681) De motu animalium. In: Bishop LF, Neilson J jr (eds) (1927) History of cardiology. Medical Life Press, New York
7. Brecher GA (1956) Experimental evidence of ventricular diastolic suction. Circ Res 4:513–518
8. Brücke E (1881) Physiologie des Kreislaufs, der Ernährung, der Absonderung, der Respiration und der Bewegungserscheinungen. Vorlesungen über Physiologie, vol 1. Wien, Wilhelm Braumüller, K.K. Hof- und Universitätsbuchhändler, pp 134–194
9. Brutsaert DL, Claes VA, Donders JH (1972) Effects of controlling the velocity of shortening on force-velocity-length and time relations in cat papillary muscle. Circ Res 30:310–315
10. Caulfield JB, Janicki JS (1997) Structure and function of myocardial fibrillar collagen. Technol Health Care 5:95–113
11. Chadwick RS (1981) The myocardium as a fluid-fiber continuum. Adv Biomed Eng 104:135–138
12 Chadwick RS (1982) Mechanics of the left ventricle. Biophys J 39:279–288
13. Cotton M (1953) Circulatory changes affecting measurement of heart force in situ with strain gauge arches. Am J Physiol 197:365–370
14. Cryer CW, Navidi-Kasmai H, Lunkenheimer PP, Redmann K (1996) Computation of the inclination angle of myocardial fibre strands. 12th Int Conf of the Cardiovascular System Dynamics Society, Nov. 7–10, Chapel Hill
15. Cryer CW, Navidi-Kasmai H, Lunkenheimer PP, Redmann K (1997) Computation of the inclination angle of manually and optically digitized myocardial fibre strands. Technol Health Care 5:79–93
16. Culler VH, Feldstein C, Lewis GW, Meerbaum S (1979) Trifunctional transducer for myocardial monitoring. Nasa Tech Briefs 4:517–518
17. Cushny AR (1910) Myocardiograph for the mammalian heart. Heart 2:1–4
18. Dieudonné JM (1967) Tissue-cavitary difference pressure of the dog left ventricle. Am J Physiol 213:101–106
19. Djavakhishvili N (1997) Significance of sinusoids for myocardial blood circulation. Technol Health Care 5:171–175
20. D'Silva JL, Mendel D, Winterton MC (1963) Effect of sympathomimetic amines on intramyocardial pressure in the rabbit. Am J Physiol 205:10–16
21. Dutertre J, Jean CF, Cartier R, Dieudonné JM (1972) Measurement of tissular strain with a tripod-like transducer. J Med Biol Eng 10:277–281
22. Ebstein E. (1904) Die Diastole des Herzens. Ergeb Physiol 3:123–194
23. Feneis H (1944/45) Das Gefüge des Herzmuskels bei Systole und Diastole. Gegenbaurs Morphol Jahrb 89:371–406
24. Frank O (1901) Isometrie und Isotonie des Herzmuskels. Z Biol 41:14–34
25. Frazier OH, Benedict CR, Radovancevic B, Bick RJ, Capek P, Springer WE, Macris MP, Delgado R, Buj LM (1996), Improved left ventricular function after chronic left ventricular uloading. Am Thorac Surg 62:675–682
26. Grant RP (1965) Notes on the muscular architecture of the left ventricle. Circulation 32:301–308
27. Gregg DE (1963) Effect of coronary perfusion pressure or coronary flow on oxygen usage of the myocardium. Circ Res 13:497–501
28. Greenbaum RA, Ho SY, Gibson DG, Becker AE, Anderson RH (1981) Left ventricular fibre architecture in man. Br Heart J 45:248–263
29. Harvey W (1628) Exercitatio Anatomica de Motu Cordis et Sanguinis in Animalibus. IV. Frankfurt
30. Hefner L, Sheffield T, Copbbs GC, Klip W (1962) Relation between mural force and pressure in the left ventricle of the dog, Circ Res 11:654–663
31. Hort W (1963) Morphologische Untersuchungen bei Myocarditis constrictiva. Verh Dtsch Ges Kreislaufforsch 29:262–267
32. Ingels NB (1997) Myocardial fiber architecture and left ventricular function. Technol Health Care 5:45–52

33. Ising H, Lunkenheimer PP, Dannenberg H (1974) Zur Messung der Myokardspannung. Biomed Tech 19:24–27
34. Jewell BR, Wilkie DR (1960) The mechanical properties of relaxing muscle. J Physiol Lond 152:30–47
35. Kirk ES, Honig CR (1964) An experimental and theoretical analysis of myocardial tissue pressure. Am J Physiol 207:361–367
36. Krehl L (1891) Beiträge zur Kenntnis der Füllung und Entleerung des Herzens. In: Abhandlungen der Mathematisch-Physischen Classe der Königlich Sächsischen Gesellschaft der Wissenschaften, Siebzehnter Band, Leipzig
37. Lochner W, Arnold G, Müller-Ruchholz E (1968) Metabolism of the artificially arrested heart and of the gas-perfused heart. Am J Cardiol 22:299–311
38. Lower R (1669) The anatomy of the heart. London
39. Lunkenheimer PP, Graham G, Stroh N, Welham K, Scharsich M (1976) Assessment of local force in myocardium disproving the distinctness of contractility parameters derived from left ventricular pressure. Eur Surg Res 8:[Suppl] 104–105
40. Lunkenheimer PP, Stroh N, Scharsich M, Koubenec J, Schmuziger M, Achatzy R, Dittrich H, Welham K, Graham G (1977) Continuous assessment of myocardial force during heart surgery. Curr Top Crit Care Med 3:28–38
41. Lunkenheimer PP, Lunkenheimer A, Stroh N, Köhler F, Welham K, Graham G, Kirk E, Sonnenblick EH, Kröller J (1982) Vergleich klassischer und neuer methodischer Zugänge zum intramyokardialen Kraftverteilungsmuster. Rev Zentralbl Vet Med [A] 29:557–601
42. Lunkenheimer PP, Lunkenheimer A, Torrent-Guasp F (1985) Kardiodynamik: Wege zur strukturgerechten Analyse der Myokardfunktion. In: Beitr Kardiol 33
43. Lunkenheimer PP, Merker HJ (1973) Morphologische Studien zur funktionellen Anatomie der "Sinusoide" im Myokard. Z Anat Entw Gesch 142:65–90
44. Lunkenheimer PP, Lunkenheimer A, Whimster WF, Edel G, Stroh N, van Aken H (1986) Local myocardial and global ventricular function compared during positive inotropic medication. Basic Res Cardiol 81:[Suppl 1] 59–71
45. Lunkenheimer PP, Redmann K, Stroh N, Richter K-H, Niederer P, Cryer C (1997) The assessment of intramural stress alignment on the beating heart in situ using micro-ergometry. Technol Health Care 5:115–122
46. Lunkenheimer PP, Redmann K, Dietl K-H, Cryer C, Richter K-D, Whimster WF, Niederer P (1997) The heart's fibre alignment assessed by comparing two digitizing systems. Methodological investigation into the inclination angle towards wall thickness. Technol Health Care 5:65–77
47. Maughan WL, Sunagawa K, Sagawa K (1987) Ventricular systolic interdependence: volume elastance model in isolated canine hearts. Am J Physiol 253:H1381-H1390
48. McCallum JB (1900) On the muscular architecture and growth of the ventricles of the heart.Welch Festschrift, John Hopkins Hosp Rep 9
49. McCarthy PM (1997) The Cleveland Clinic experience. Cardiac Volume Reduction Forum 1997, Tokyo, October 4
50. Meesmann W (1958) Nachweis der diastolischen Sogwirkung der Herzkammern und deren Einfluß auf die intrakardialen Druckabläufe. Z Kreislforsch 47:534–551
51. Müller J, Wallukat G, Weng Y-G, Dandel M, Spiegelsberger S, Semrau S, Brandes K, Theodoridis V, Loebe M, Meyer R, Hetzer R (1997) Weaning from mechanical cardiac support in patients with idiopathic dilated cardiomyopathy. Circulation 96:542–549
52. Pettigrew JB (1860) On the arrangement of the muscular fibres in the ventricular portion of the heart of the mammal (Coonian lecture). Proc R Soc 10:433–444
53. Puff A, Langer H (1965) Das Problem der diastolischen Entfaltung der Herzkammern. Morphol Jahrb 107:184–212
54. Rabbany SY, Kresh JY, Noordergraaf A, (1989) Intramyocardial pressure: interaction of myocardial fluid pressure and fiber stress. Am J Physiol 257:H357-H364
55. Rabbany SY, Kresh JY, Noordergraar A (1997) Differentiation of intramyocardial fluid pressure from fiber stress. Technol Health Care 5:145–157
56. Redmann K, Lunkenheimer PP, Scheld HH, Fischer S, Cryer C, Whimster WF, Stroh N (1997) Inhomogeneities in wall stress measured by microergometry in the heart muscle in situ. Technol Health Care 5:123–134
57. Schaper J, Mollnau H, Hein S, Scholz D, Münkel B, Devaux B, (1995) Wechselwirkungen zwischen Kardiomyozyten und der extrazellulären Matrix im insuffizienten menschlichen Herzen. Z Kardiol 84:33–38
58. Sonnenblick EH, Parmley WW, Urschel CW (1969) The contractile state of the heart as expressed by force-velocity relations. Am J Cardiol 23:488–503

59. Streeter DD jr, Spotnitz HM, Patel DP, Ross J jr, Sonnenblick EH (1969) Fiber orientation in the canine left ventricle during diastole and systole. Circ Res 2:4 339–347
60. Walton P, Brodie OJ (1947) The effect of drugs on the contractile force of a section of the right ventricle under conditions of an intact circulation. J Pharmacol Exp Ther 90:26–41
61. Weber KT (1989) Cardiac interstitium in health and disease: the fibrillar collagen network. J Am Coll Cardiol 13:1637–1652

CHAPTER 4

Methods of Nuclear Medicine to Verify Vitality and Efficacy of TMLR

H. EICHSTÄDT

4.1 Summary

Nuclear medicine diagnosis of myocardial vitality is of particular importance to decision-making on indication in preparation for TMLR therapy and for prognostic appraisal of patients concerned. Among four pathophysiologically distinguishable forms of contractile dysfunction, no differentiation is possible between hibernating myocardium and scar with pure perfusion indicators. However, on account of determinants for activity distribution in advanced-phase images, above all in the wake of ^{201}TI injection, this radiopharmaceutical has proved helpful in many cases to differentiate myocardial ischaemia at rest from scar, which is of major importance to indication for transmyocardial laser revascularisation. Owing to the perfusion indicators nowadays available, myocardial "stunning" can be differentiated without any problem from ischaemia at rest or scar. While the results of vital diagnosis obtainable from ^{201}TI scintigraphy with optimised test protocol come close to those obtainable from positron emission tomography with ^{18}F-FDG, the latter has remained to be the reference method, primarily in cases of high-severity left-ventricular dysfunction and known coronary occlusion.

4.2 Introduction

The severity of ventricular dysfunction is of major prognostic relevance in the course of coronary heart disease, especially when it comes to decision-making on indications for recanalisation interventions. Interest has been increasingly focused at differentiated function diagnosis of the myocardium, ever since many cases had become known in which improved contractility was exhibited by akinetic post-stenotic myocardial segments in response to reoxygenation. Particular attention has been given to the question for potentially functional myocardium in akinetic wall segments. Vitality of a sufficient number of myocytes in the affected wall area is a prerequisite for restoration of the contractile function, with an intact structure-maintaining metabolism being essential to myocyte vitality. However, the point must be made that "vitality" is a necessary but not always sufficient prerequisite for reversibility of functional impairment.

The discussion of possibilities and limits of perfusion scintigraphy as pre-interventional and post-interventional parameters, consequently, gives rise to the question if and under what conditions differentiation between intact or non-existent structure-maintaining metabolism would be possible in akinetic

Table 4.1. Segmental contractile dysfunctions in CHD

Type of dysfunction	Clincial consequence	Outcome
Regional flow inadequate for energy demand	Early ischaemic contractile dysfunction	Reversible after removal of triggering cause
Energy demand adapted to low flow	Hibernating myocardium	Reversible after revascularisation, e.g. TMLR
Inadequate use of energy after reperfusion	"Stunned" myocardium	Reversible after variable periods of time
No energy metabolism	Fibrosis/ necrosis/scar	Irreversible

wall segments of the ventricle by means of the radiopharmaceuticals available today. What are the pathophysiological conditions of ventricular dysfunction which must be distinguished from each other in this context?

4.3 Forms of Segmental Contractile Dysfunction in Coronary Heart Disease (CHD)

Ischaemia-induced metabolic alterations of the myocardium may be characterised by different courses which are summarised in Table 4.1. They are pathophysiological conditions which are not necessarily separable from each other with regard to localisation. The tissue volume in one scintigraphic image element is made up of several strata and, consequently, may correspond to several forms, as are distinguished from each other in Table 4.1.

4.4 Early Ischaemic Contractile Dysfunction

Myocardial ischaemia is characterised by disproportion between supply of and demand for energy. Short-time imbalance of demand for and supply of energy due to reduced coronary circulation causes loss of contractile function which will be proportional to the amount by which circulation is reduced [38, 39, 96]. This process may be attributable either to ischaemia-induced reduction of ATP concentration [43] or defect in energy transfer [50] or upcoming action of other mediators [49, 51, 53, 55].

While the causative role played by various biochemical alterations has not been elucidated as yet [46], evidence has been provided to the effect that early ischaemic contractile dysfunction is accompanied by loss of the creatine phosphate level in the myocardium [23, 42, 43, 50]. Creatine phosphate is an energy reservoir in the cell and may be utilised by transfer of phosphate linkage to ADP via creatine kinase of myofibrils.

4.5 Hibernating Myocardium

In cases of myocardial ischaemia in which residual circulation is reduced but still is above a critical value, contractile dysfunction may persist over a long period of time without causing irreversible damage [66, 78]. A condition of this kind, different from early ischaemic contractile dysfunction, is characterised by metabolic adaptation [2, 35, 72]. Such adaptation obviously leads to normalisation of the myocardial creatine phosphate level. Other metabolic parameters, too, seem to undergo normalisation in the course of persistent ischaemia and contractile dysfunction. Inotropic stimulation (by administration of dobutamine), as a matter of principle, is possible under such circumstances [85], which may offer an explanation for the clinically promising results of dobutamine or arbutamine stress echocardiography in vitality diagnosis of hibernating myocardium [3, 64, 73]. However, it is uncertain for how long the ischaemic myocardium is capable of maintaining its reactivity to inotropic stimulation. Long-time ischaemia, after all, notwithstanding general reversibility of contractile dysfunction, leads to considerable morphological alterations, including loss of myofibrils, disorganisation of sarcomeres and disappearance of the sarcoplasmic reticulum [36].

4.6 "Stunned" Myocardium

"Stunning" occurs in the wake of myocardial ischaemia, no matter whether it is short-time high-severity ischaemia or a condition following hibernation. "Stunned" myocardium is characterised by absence of a relationship between contractile function and current regional circulation of the myocardium. In a "stunned" myocardium, circulation has been fully or almost fully restored. The contractile dysfunction, however, will continue to exist, although it is, basically, reversible [17]. The length of time needed for recovery of the contractile function after reperfusion depends on severity and duration of the preceding ischaemia [13, 44]. The following underlying mechanisms of myocardial "stunning" currently are under discussion:

- Increased cytosolic calcium concentration, leading to reduced myofibrillar calcium sensitivity [33, 56, 63];
- Membrane damage by free radicals [12, 15];
- Dysfunction of sarcoplasmic reticulum [54].

With regard to energy metabolism of "stunned" myocardium, persistent myocardial dysfunction is accompanied by delayed refilling of the ATP reservoir [27, 42, 92], but there are certain clues to suggest that there is no direct causative interconnection between these phenomena [47].

The post-ischaemic myocardium, notwithstanding contractile dysfunction, obviously is capable of responding to inotropic substances [3, 6, 13, 34, 45, 48, 57, 68, 80], which, in turn, enables vitality diagnosis by means of dobutamine stress echocardiography [74, 88]. Therefore, contractile dysfunction may possibly result from a defect in energy utilisation rather than from inadequate energy availability [46].

The possibilities of vitality diagnosis by means of radiopharmaceuticals are determined by mechanisms which have an impact on the kinetics of the latter, and they also depend on changes of those mechanisms in response to the different forms of contractile dysfunction.

4.7
Kinetics of Radiopharmaceuticals for Perfusion Scintigraphy prior to and after TMLR

4.7.1
Conventional Thallium Scintigraphy

Absorption of ^{201}TI by the myocardium is proportional to the three parameters of local myocardial blood flow, myocardial mass and extraction fraction [41, 76, 90, 91, 99]. Extraction is based on ^{201}TI crossing the capillary wall, interstitium and cell membrane, with both passive and active transport processes being involved. Active transport is initiated by means of the ATP-dependent sodium-potassium pump. Hence, cellular ATP loss might lead to reduced extraction of ^{201}TI and, consequently, to underestimation of viable myocardial volume. However, experimental studies have shown that the normal extraction fraction of approximately 85% is not or not substantially reduced by cellular acidosis or hypoxia as long as there is no development of myocardial necrosis [41, 60, 61, 71, 99].

Initial distribution of ^{201}TI is proportional, above all, to flow on account of the high extraction fraction. This is followed by continuous interchange between myocardial and intravasal ^{201}TI. Hence, the activity concentration of a given myocardial area several hours after injection is governed by the following factors:

- Initial regional blood flow (at the time of injection);
- Local blood flow in time interval up to advanced-phase imaging;
- ^{201}TI efflux from myocardium;
- Recirculating amount of activity which, in turn, strongly depends on intravasal activity.

Injection of ^{201}TI at rest is a special case in which regional blood flow may be considered as being constant over the entire period of time. It is due to the ^{201}TI kinetics that perfusion of vital myocardium is reflected only by early images (immediately after injection), whereas advanced-phase images, as time goes by, are getting increasingly independent of perfusion effects and tend to reflect the distribution of the vital myocardial volume [7, 9, 75]. The lower the deviation of initial activity from vitality distribution and the longer the period for interchange processes and the higher the recirculating activity concentration, the higher will be the accuracy with which the vital myocardial mass is represented [20, 21]. The conditions for vitality diagnosis are less favourable if ^{201}TI is injected during exercise ischaemia, above all for two reasons: an initial local activity deficit and relatively low amount of recirculating activity due to the firm bond of ^{201}TI to the peripheral musculature. Pharmacological intervention, on the other hand, which we perform with arbutamine and adenosine is followed by considerable availability of recirculating activity, among others, from the enteral and pulmonary activity pools which are higher by magnitudes immediately after injection than following injection under ergometric loading [59].

These considerations are likely to show that a four-hour interval after exercise injection – especially physical ergometry – may be insufficient for vitality-related distribution. In other words, vitality would be more clearly reflected in activity distribution measured after an extended period of time, say, 24 hours after injection. On the other hand, the practicability of 24-hour imaging should be seriously questioned unless a repeat injection was applied, as residual activity is as low as about 25%.

Vital myocardium will not be underrepresented by injection of ^{201}TI at rest unless the blood flow at rest is reduced. Myocardial ischaemia at rest was found to develop in cases of instable angina pectoris and in marginal infarction zones. The kinetic considerations appear to suggest that imaging long time after injection at rest is superior to early imaging in representing vitality distribution and that vitality diagnosis should always go together with an examination under anti-anginal medication.

In both *early-ischaemic contractile dysfunction* and *hibernating myocardium* early imaging of ^{201}TI will merely reflect reduced blood flow and will fail to provide conclusive information on the dimensions of vital myocardium. True, advanced-phase or long-interval images are affected by local perfusion but widely reflect the distribution of vital myocardium. In cases of "*stunning*", the distribution of vital myocardium is reflected in both short-interval and long-interval images. Activity is reflected neither in early nor advanced phases in cases of *necrosis* and *fibrosis* which, therefore, are not eligible for TMLR at all.

Our own experiments with thallium solutions through different membranes showed thallium might not be suitable for discrimination of vital against scared tissue.

4.7.2 ^{99m}Tc-MIBI

The extraction fraction of isonitriles is relatively low (approx. 65%). These are compounds that reach the myocardial cell primarily through passive diffusion and are subject merely to low efflux from the myocardium. Myocardial absorption, above all, is determined by blood flow and integrity of the sarcolemma membrane. A minor role is played by hypoxia or integrity of the Na^+/K^+ pump [8, 30], notwithstanding differentiated concentration in necrotic or fibrotic tissue. Quite independent of different mechanisms of concentration, relations experimentally found to exist between ^{201}TI and ^{99m}Tc levels in the myocardium were in a similar way correlated with blood flow, i.e. across the full range between normal flow and occlusion [24, 65].

Hence, when it comes to clinical requirements, the information obtainable from ^{99m}Tc-MIBI scintigraphy following injection under the impact of exercise or at rest is comparable to early imaging after ^{201}TI injection under corresponding conditions. The magnitude of vitality in hibernating myocardium usually is underestimated in the same way (dependence of concentration on flow), whereas in **"stunned" myocardium** the amount of vital tissue volume is reflected in activity distribution. The informative potential of ^{201}TI and

Table 4.2. Informative potential of ^{201}TI and ^{99m}Tc-MIBI scintigraphy with regard to vitality (+)

	Early ischaemic contractile dysfunction	Hibernating myocardium	"Stunned" myocardium	Fibrosis/ necrosis
^{201}TI (rest) early	+	–	+	–
^{201}TI (rest) late	+	(+)	(+)	(+)
^{99m}Tc-MIBI (rest)	+	–	+	–
Vitality information	+ secured (+) widely reliable			

^{99m}Tc-MIBI scintigraphy for vitality assessment under various pathophysiological conditions is summarised in Table 4.2.

4.8 Clinical Results

4.8.1 Indications

The protocol of ^{201}TI scintigraphy after injection with exercise and with short-interval and long-interval imaging, as has been used over the past 20 years, may give rise to considerable underestimation of vital myocardium, as has been explained. Evidence has been provided to such method-related limitation both by follow-up checks after bypass surgery [11, 40, 62, 79] as well as by comparative ^{18}F-FDG positron emission tomography [18, 82]. It has proved hard to estimate how often myocardial vitality has been and still is underestimated by using the standard exercise protocol, because it depends strongly on the given selection of patients and definition of "persistent defect". More than 50% of all patients referred for coronary bypass operations or selected for TMLR were believed to exhibit myocardial segments with FDG absorption after four hours of persistent ^{201}TI defects [18, 82]. Here, defects characterised merely by incomplete reversibility were obviously rated as "persistent".

There are some cases in which vitality can be proven by means of 24-hour interval images, notwithstanding severe reduction of photon flux after 24 hours and associated deteriotation of image quality [25, 52, 69, 101].

The diagnostic benefit obtainable from ^{201}TI re-injection at rest has been subject of comprehensive studies in recent years. Even without specific subdivision and classification of different re-injection protocols, data so far published suggest that in about 35% of all persistent ^{201}TI defects, according to the standard exercise protocol, persuasive evidence was provided to reversibility following re-injection, which was accompanied by parallel PET evidence to vitality [16, 31, 32, 77, 93, 94]. Reversibility quite often is an expression of pronounced collateralisation due to chronic high-severity stenosis [4, 84].

The question for exercise-induced ischaemia may quite often be of minor relevance to cases of high-severity left-ventricular dysfunction. It rather is the question for the extent of vitality which is very much in the focus of diagnostic interest. In such cases, scintigraphy with ^{201}TI or ^{99m}Tc-MIBI should be performed only at rest, and impulse density across affected wall segments should be related to maximum impulse density of the image concerned. With such approach, 85 to 90% of defects with relative impulse density above 50% will be associated with myocardial areas which were classified as being vital [16]. Agreement between ^{18}F-FDG-PET and ^{201}TI scintigraphy amounted to 89%.

It is on account of the above flow dependence of activity distribution that despite fair agreement with PET data limitations may be imposed on vitality assessment by means of ^{201}TI early imaging (about ten minutes after injection). That flow dependence, in cases of ischaemia at rest, tends to result in underrepresentation of vital myocardium. Ischaemia at rest is rarely recordable from those patients who generally are selected prior to or after TMLR. That is why reversibility of initial defects may be realised only in 11% of the myocardial segments affected by comparison of early with late images after injection at rest [26, 28, 67].

Reference should as well be made, in this context, to the phenomenon of inverse redistribution. Deterioration of a defect in an advanced phase, according to current knowledge and on the basis of the above kinetic effects, is attributable to decrease in local vital myocardial mass along with normalised local perfusion [58, 86, 100]. The obtainability of comparable physiological information from ^{201}TI early images and ^{99m}Tc-MIBI scintigrams seems to explain why ^{99m}Tc-MIBI scintigrams at rest have proved to be suitable for assessment of myocardial vitality [5, 37, 87]. The only limitation on vitality diagnosis by ^{99m}Tc-MIBI as well as by ^{99m}Tc-tetrophosmin lies in underestimation of vitality in cases of ischaemia at rest (**hibernating myocardium**), as has been shown by comparison not only with ^{201}TI late images at rest but also with ^{18}F-FDG-PET [1, 22, 29, 70, 83]. No problem, on the other hand, is faced in vitality diagnosis in cases of **"stunned" myocardium**. That is why advantage may be taken of a stable myocardial concentration, following injection of ^{99m}Tc-MIBI, for efficiency control, for example, of thrombolysis. The protocol provides for injection of the radiopharmaceutical prior to thrombolysis, while scintigraphy will have to be performed only after haemodynamic stabilisation. The extent to which perfusion has dropped prior to thrombolysis may thus be realised. Subsequent re-injection, followed by scintigraphy, will provide an image of the change to perfusion by thrombolysis. Comparison of scintigrams recorded in the two phases shows the amount of thrombolysis-rehabilitated myocardium in an early phase in which the contractile function still may be short of normalisation [10, 89, 97, 98].

4.9 Follow-up Study of Myocardial Perfusion in Patients before and after Transmyocardial Laser Revascularization (TMLR)

4.9.1 Patients and methods

Our investigations of 42 out of total 134 patients [6f., 36 m.; age 53–76 ys) who underwent a TMLR since Nov. 1994 were analysed before and three months after TMLR. After intravenous application of 90–110 MBq ^{201}Tl-images were obtained 10 min. after dynamic exercise on a supine bicycle ergometer and three hours later.

Images were performed with a single head gamma camera. Corresponding examinations before and after TMLR were made under equal conditions.

Visual analysis and semiquantitative computerized analysis in bullseye technique (five segments: apical, anterior, lateral, inferior, septal) was made.

The CO_2-Heart-Laser (800 W) was used for TMLR, an average number of 30 channels [15–50] was applied in each patients.

The septal segment has never been lasered and the relativ uptake was used as a perfusion reference for the lasered segments (Fig. 4.1).

4.9.2 Results

Visual analysis of ^{201}TI-scintigraphies showed comparable results in 30/42 pat., improvement in 6/42 and an aggravation in 6/42 pat. (Table 4.3, Table 4.4).

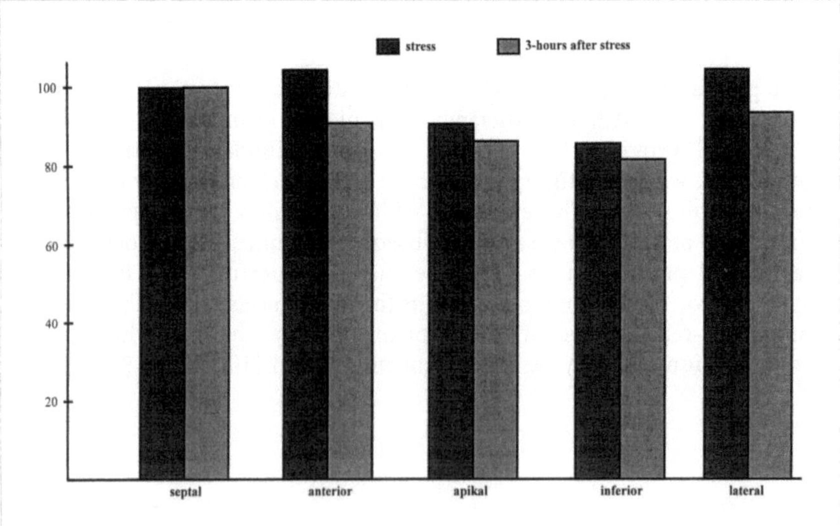

Fig. 4.1. Semiquantitative analysis of myocardial ^{201}TI-uptake in the lasered and unlasered septal segment

Table 4.3. Visual analysis of myocardial ^{201}Tl-scintigraphies

	pre TMLR	3 months after
Ischemia	28	25
Intramural scar	35	33
Transmural scar	21	21

Table 4.4. Comparision of patients' complaints and myocardial ^{201}Tl-scintigraphies

	+	=	-
Patients' complaints	19	19	4
Visual-analysis	6	30	6
Semiquantitative	8	30	4

Patients' complaints improved in 45%, remained unchanged in 45% and were aggravated in 10% (Table 4.4).

The pulmonary uptake under stress conditions as an indirect parameter of left ventricular function increased from 43.6% before to 44.8% after TMLR ($p>0.05$).

Correlation of laser channel quantity and ^{201}TI-uptake showed sometimes a significant (t-Test, $p<0.05$) decrease of ^{201}TI-uptake and sometimes not (Fig. 4.2). In total all lasered segments without correlation of channel quantity showed a significant decrease of ^{201}TI-uptake after bicycle ergometer stress after TMLR if compared with the unlasered septal segment (Fig. 4.3).

4.9.3 Conclusion

Although a clinical improvement three months after TMLR was observed in 45% of all our patients, there was no increase of myocardial perfusion shown by ^{201}TI-myocardial scintigraphy by means of visual or semiquantitative computerized analysis.

Further investigations 6 and 12 months after TMLR must show if an improvement of myocardial perfusion can be visualized by ^{201}TI-scintigraphy.

4.10 Comparison with ^{18}F-FDG-PET

Fair agreement between PET results, on the one hand, and findings recorded from early images following ^{201}TI re-injection, on the other, i.e. approximately 85% [93], should not be allowed to deceive examiners about the fact that in few cases a ^{201}TI defect had been classified as vital by PET. If in such cases the postulation was made of ischaemia at rest, which could not be differentiated from cicatrisation by means of ^{201}TI early imaging after injection at rest, it would make sense to compare the PET findings to the results of the ^{201}TI injection protocol at rest with early and late images in concomi-

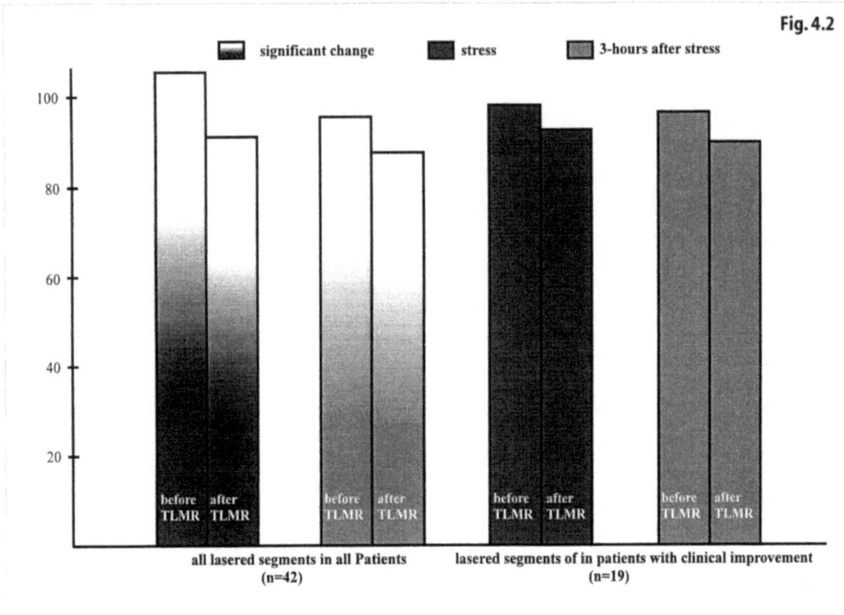

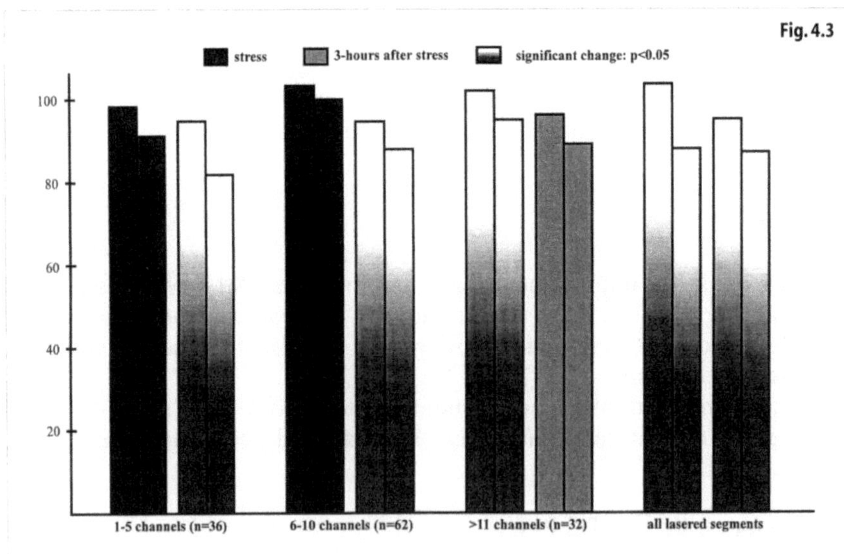

Fig. 4.2. ^{201}TI-uptake in all lasered segments in comparision to the lasered segments in patients with clinical improvement

Fig. 4.3. Relative uptake of ^{201}TI in comparison to the number of laser channels before (*left column*) and three months after TMLR (*right column*)

tance with anti-anginal combination therapy. However, such comparative studies so far have rarely been conducted, though in small numbers of patients retention of metabolic activity was postulated in segments with irreversible ^{201}TI deficit after injection at rest, and superiority of ^{18}F-FDG PET was concluded from those findings [19]. However, it should be borne in mind that the SPECT images - different from those obtained from PET - were not quantified. On the other hand, reference has been made to more recent data based on quantitative SPECT evaluation for vitality classification of myocardial segments to demonstrate the equivalence of the method to ^{18}F-FDG-PET [28].

4.11 Which Protocol under which Conditions?

Pathophysiological considerations, kinetics of radiopharmaceuticals and empirical data provide a background against which certain methods are preferred in scintigraphic protocols, depending on the specific clinical situation which calls for vitality diagnosis. Here is a brief summary of those clinical situations together with the protocols adequate to them on account of current insights:

1. Previous infarction; patient sustains exercise; question for vital residual myocardium and occurrence of ischaemic responses, e.g. prior to TMLR: Either ^{201}TI standard exercise protocol or standard MIBI protocol. No need for re-injection at rest if decline in relative impulse density is recordable from late images of ^{201}TI infarction area. Need for re-injection at rest in the case of minor but not unambiguous increase in impulse density. No need, in general, for re-injection at rest in the case of clearly visible increase in impulse density (redistribution), but in cases of high-severity incomplete redistribution a differentiated approach should be taken, depending on the therapeutic consequence for the case at hand.
2. Following fresh infarction and recanalisation (no indication in the context of routine diagnostics): ^{201}TI or ^{99m}Tc-MIBI, following injection at rest.
3. Following acute infarction without recanalisation (no indication in the context of routine diagnostics): ^{201}TI injection at rest followed by early and late imaging.
4. Instable angina pectoris (no indication in the case of routine diagnostics): ^{201}TI injection at rest followed by early and late imaging.
5. TMLR worthwhile even after high-severity left-ventricular dysfunction with known coronary occlusions? ^{201}TI injection at rest followed by early and late imaging, perhaps PET.

An exercise-associated protocol should generally be preferred as long as there is no contra-indication to ergometric or pharmacological exposure, since additional diagnostic and prognostic information is obtainable from exercise-associated myocardial scintigraphy and should not be ignored. Also, re-injection at rest will not be necessary in most cases after thorough evaluation of scintigrams of the standard protocol, provided clear-cut definition of the clinical problem (see Item 1).

Examinations for vitality should be accompanied by optimum therapeutic medication unless there is a contra-indication. Medication may be initiated, perhaps, after exercise-associated injection.

4.12 Conclusions

The possibility of scintigraphic evidence to vital myocardium with perfusion indicators prior to TMLR results from the fact that myocardial metabolism or integrity of the cell membrane are prerequisites for accumulation of radiopharmaceuticals. Flow-limited myocardial absorption is the reason why methods applied to cases of ischaemia may lead to underestimation of vital myocardial mass. However, local ischaemia is relatively rare under conditions of rest and anti-anginal medication. In such cases, the distribution of myocardial mass tends to be reflected in late images of ^{201}TI distribution following injection at rest. No definite answer can yet be given to the question for possible superiority of PET with ^{18}F-FDG over ^{201}TI injection at rest with late imaging for diagnosis of vital myocardium, although PET is part of some TMLR protocols. There is no generally accepted position either on the question whether procedures of nuclear medicine for vitality diagnosis might be replaced by echocardiography prior to and along with dobutamine or dobutamine/atropine stimulation because of basically existing inotropic reactivity of reperfused or hibernating myocardium. In any discussion about the reliability of diagnostic procedures for vitality diagnosis, especially in evaluating potential success of TMLR, one should not forget that there are general limits on its clinical relevance. TMLR or revascularisation may remain unsuccessful even with availability of vital residual myocardium in an occlusion-affected wall area, if regional circulation cannot be improved because of the vascular morphology distal from the point of bypass insertion. On the other hand, a patient with severe symptoms should receive a bypass or PTCA of an affected coronary vessel even in a situation in which no vitality is detectable in the typical circulation area of that vessel. Late control of wall motility and the overall clinical pattern after intervention, therefore, are the ultimate criteria by which to evaluate the clinical conclusions drawn from the results obtained from the examination methods that are available to the examiner. Surprising achievements, in this context, have been noticed in the wake of TMLR.

References

1. Altehöfer C, vom Dahl J, Biedermann M (1994) Significance of defect severily in technetium 99m-MIBI SPECT at rest to assess myocardial viability: comparison with fluorine-18-FDG PET. J Nucl Med 35:569–574
2. Arai AE, Pantely GA, Anselone CG, Bristow J, Bristow JD (1991) Aclive downregulation of myocardial energy requirements during prolonged moderate ischemia in swine. Circ Res 69:1458–1469
3. Baer FM, Voth E, Deutsch HJ et al. (1994) Assessment of viable myocardium by dobutamine transesophageal echocardiography and comparison with fluorine-18-fluorodeoxyglucose positron emission tomography. J Am Coll Cardiol 24:343-353
4. Bartenstein P, Schober O, Hasfeld M et al. (1992) Thallium-201 single photon emission tomography of myocardium:Additional information in reinjection studies is dependent on collateral circulation. Eur J Nucl Med 19:790–795
5. Beanlands RS, Dawood F, Wen WH el al. (1990) Are kinetics of technetium-99m methoxyisobutyl isonitrile affected by cell metabolism and viability? Circulation 82:1802–1843

6. Becker LC, Levine JH, DiPaula AF, Guarnieri T, Aversano T (1986) Reversal of dysfunction in postischemic stunned myocardium by epinephrine and postextrasystolic potentiation. J Am Coll Cardiol 7:580–589
7. Beller GA, Holzgrefe HH, Watson DD (1983) Effects of dipyridamole-induced vasodilation on myocardial uptake and clearance kinetics of thallium-201. Circulation 68:1328–1338
8. Beller GA, Sinusas AJ (1990) Experimental studies of the physiologic properties of technetium-99m isonitriles. Am J Cardiol 16:66:5E–8E
9. Beller GA, Watson DD, Ackell P et al. (1980) Time course of thallium-201 redistribution after transient myocardial ischemia. Circulation 61:791–797
10. Beller GA (1993) Myocardial reperfusion imaging: Basic principles and clinical applications. Am J Card Imaging, pp 11–23
11. Berger BC, Watson D, Burbell LR et al. (1979) Redistribution of thallium at rest and in patients with stable and unstable angina and the effect of coronary artery bypass surgery. Circulation 60:1125–1131
12. Bolli R, Jeraudi MO, Patel BS et al. (1989) Direct evidence that oxygen-derived free radicals contribute to postischemic myocardial dysfunction in the intact dog. Proc Natl Acad Sci USA 86:4695–4699
13. Bolli R, Zhu W-X Myers ML, Hartley CJ, Roberts R (1985) Beta-adrenergic stimulation reverses postischemic myocardial dysfunction without producing subsequent deterioration. Am J Cardiol 56:964–968
14. Bolli R, Zhu W-X, Thornby Jl, O'Neill PG, Roberts R (1988) Time course and determinations of recovery of function after reversible ischemia in conscious dogs. Am J Physiol 254:H 102–H114
15. Bolli R (1988) Oxygen-derived free radicals and postischemic myocardial dysfunction ("stunned myocardium"). J Am Coll Cardiol 12:239–249
16. Bonow RO, Dilsizian V, Cuocolo A et al. (1991) Identification of viable myocardium in patients with chronic ischemic coronary artery disease and left ventricular dysfunction: Comparison of thallium scintigraphy with reinjection and PET imaging with 18-F-fluorodeoxyglucose. Circulation 83:26–37
17. Braunwald E, Kloner PA (1982) The stunned myocardium: prolonged, postischemic ventricular dysfunction. Circulation 66:1146–1149
18. Brunken R, Schwaiger M, Grover-McKay M et al. (!987) Positron emission tomography detects tissue metabolic activity in myocardial segments with persistent thallium defects. J Am Coll Cardiol 10:557–567
19. Brunken RC, Kottou S, Nienaber CA et al. (1989) PET detection of viable tissue in myocardial segments with persistent defects at Tl-201 SPECT. Radiology 65:65–73
20. Budinger TF, Knittel BL (1987) Cardiac thallium redistribution and model. J Nucl Med 25:588
21. Budinger TF, Pohost GM (1986) Thallium "redistribution" – An explanation. J Nucl Med 27:996
22. Bell U, Altehoefer C (1974–1992) (1993) Die Tl-201 Myokardszintigraphie: Vom Perfusionsdefekt zum Vitalitätsnachweis. Nucl-Med; 32:1–5
23. Camacho SA, Lanzer P, Toy BJ et al. (1988) In vivo alterations of high-energy phosphates and intracellular pH during reversible ischemia in pigs: a 31P magnetic resonance spectroscopy study. Am Heart J 116:701–708
24. Canby RC, Silber S, Pohost GM (1990) Relations of the myocardial imaging agents Tc-99m-MIBI and Tl-201 to myocardial blood flow in a canine model of myocardial ischemic insult. Circulation 81:289–296
25. Cloninger KG, DePeuy EG, Garcia EV et al. (1988) Incomplete redistribution in delayed thallium-201 single photon emission computed tomographic images: An over estimation of myocardial scarring. J Am Coll Cardiol 12:955–963
26. Dae MW, Botvinick EH, Starksen NF et al. (1991) Do 4-hour reinjection thallium images and 24-hour thallium images provide equivalent information? J Am Coll Cardiol 17:29
27. DeBoer LWV, Ingwall JS, Kloner RA, Braunwald E (1980) Prolonged derangements of canine myocardial purine metabolism after a brief coronary artery occlusion not associated with anatomic evidence of necrosis. Proc Natl Acad Sci USA 77:5471–5475
28. Dilsizian V, Bacharach SL, Perrone-Filardi P et al. (1991) Concordance and discordance between rest-redistribution thallium imaging and thallium reinjection after stress redistribution imaging for assessing viable myocardium: Comparison with metabolic activity by PET. Circulation 84:89
29. Dilsizian V, Arrighi JA, Diodati JG et al. (1994) Myocardial viability in patients with chronic coronary artery disease. Comparison of Tc-99m-Sestamibi with thallium reinjection and (18F) fluoro-deoxyglucose. Circulation 89:578–587

30. Dilsizian V, Rocco T, Strauss W et al. (1989) Technetium-99m isonitrile myocardial uptake at rest. l. Relation to severity of coronary artery stenosis. J Am Coll Cardiol 14:1673–1677
31. Dilsizian V, Rocco TP, Freedman NM et al. (1990) Enhanced detection of ischemic but viable myocardium by the reinjection of thallium after stress-redistribution imaging. N Engl J Med 323:141–146
32. Dilsizian V, Smeltzer W, Freedman NM et al. (1991) Thallium reinjection after stress redistribution imaging. Does 24-hour delayed imaging after reinjection enhance detection of viable myocardium? Circulation 83:1247–1255
33. Ehring T, Heusch G (1991) Postextrasystolic potentiation does not distinguish ischaemic from stunned myocardium. Pfluegers Arch 418:453–461
34. Ellis SG, Wynne J, Braunwald E et al. (1984) Response of reperfusion-salvaged, stunned myocardium to inotropic stimulation. Am Heart J 107:13–19
35. Fedele FA, Gewirtz H, Capone RJ, Sharaf B, Most AS (1988) Metabolic response to prolonged reduction of myocardial blood flow distal to a severe coronary artery stenosis. Circulation 78:729–735
36. Flameng W, Suy R, Schwarz F et al. (1981) Ultrastructural correlates of left ventricular contraction abnormalities in patients with chronic ischemic heart disease: Determinants of reversible segmental asynergy post vascularization surgery. Am Heart J 102:846–857
36a. Frazier OH, Cooley DA, Kadipasaoglu KA (1995) Myocardial Revascularization With Laser. Circulation 92:58–65
37. Freeman I, Grunwald A, Hoory S et al. (1991) Effect of coronary occlusion and myocardial viability on myocardial activity of technetium-99m Sestamibi. J Nucl Med 32:292–298
38. Gallagher KP, Kumada T, Koziol JA et al. (1980) Significance of regional wall thickening abnormalities relative to transmural myocardial perfusion in anesthetized dogs. Circulation 62:1266–1274
39. Gallagher KP, Matsuzaki M, Osakada G et al. (1983) Effect of exercise on the relationship between myocardial blood flow and systolic wall thickening in dogs with acute coronary stenosis. Circ Res 52:716–729
40. Gibson RS, Watson DD, Taylor GJ et al. (1983) Prospective assessment of regional myocardial perfusion before and after coronary revascularization surgery by quantitative thallium-201 scintigraphy. J Am Coll Cardiol 1:804–815
41. Grunwald AM, Watson DD, Holzgrefe HH Jr et al. (1981) Myocardial thallium-201 kinetics in normal and ischemic myocardium. Circulation 64:610–618
42. Guth BD, Martin JE, Heusch G (1987) Regional myocardial blood flow, function and metabolism using phosphorus-31 nuclear magnetic resonance spectroscopy during ischemia and reperfusion. J Am Coll Cardiol 10:673–681
43. Hearse DJ (1979) Oxygen deprivation and early myocardial contractile failure: a reassessment of the possible role of adenosine triphosphate. Am J Cardiol 44:1115–1121
44. Heusch G, Guth BD, Gilpin E et al. (1987) Determinants of recovery of regional contractile function after exercise-induced ischemia in conscious dogs. Fed Proc 46:834
45. Heusch G, Schäfer S, Kröger K (1988) Recruitment of inotropic reserve in "stunned" myocardium by the cardiotonic agent AR-L57. Basic Res Cardiol 83:602–10
46. Heusch G (1992) Hibernation, stunning, ischemic preconditioning – neue Paradigmen der koronaren Herzkrankheit. Z Kardiol 81:596–609
47. Hoffmeister HM, Mauser M, Schaper W (1985) Effect of adenosine and AICAR on ATP content and regional contractile function in reperfused canine myocardium. Basic Res Cardiol 80:445–458
48. Ito BR, Tate H, Kobayashi M et al. (1987) Reversibly injured, postischemic canine myocardium retains normal contractile reserve. Circ Res 61:834–846
49. Jacobus WE, Pores IH, Lucas SK et al. (1982) Intracellular acidosis and contractility in normal and ischemic hearts examined by 31P NMR. J Mol Cell Cardiol 14:13–20
50. Kammermeier H (1963) Verhalten von Adenin-Nukleotiden und Kreatinphosphat im Herzmuskel bei funktioneller Erholung nach länger dauernder Asphyxie. Verh Dtsch Ges Kreislaufforsch 30:206–211
51. Kentish JC (1986) The effects of inorganic phosphate and creatine phosphate on the force production in skinned muscle from rat vesicle. J Physiol 370:585–604
52. Kiat H, Berman DS, Maddahi J et al. (1988) Late reversibility of tomographic myocardial thallium-201 defects: An accurate marker of myocardial viability. J Am Coll Cardiol 12:1456–1463
52a. Krabatsch T, Dörschel K, Tülsner J, Hempel B, Hofmeister J, Lieback E, Hetzer R (1995) Transmyokardiale Laserrevaskularisation – Erste Erfahrungen in der Therapie der diffusen koronaren Herzerkrankung. Lasermedizin 11:192–198

53. Krause S, Hess ML (1984) Characterization of cardiac sarcoplasmic reticulum dysfunction during short-term, normothermic, global ischemia. Circ Res 55:176–184
54. Krause SM, Jacobus WE, Becker LC (1989) Alterations in cardiac sarcoplasmic reticulum calcium transport in the postischemic "stunned" myocardium. Circ Res 65:526–530
55. Kübler W, Katz AM (1977) Mechanism of early "pump" failure of the ischemic heart: possible role of adenosine triphosphate depletion and inorganic phosphate accumulation. Am J Cardiol 40:467–471
56. Kusuoka H, Koretsune Y, Chacko VP et al. (1990) Excitation-contraction coupling in postischemic myocardium. Does failure of activator Ca^{++} transients underly stunning? Circ Res 66:1268–1276
57. Kusuoka H, Porterfield JK, Weisman HF et al. (1987) Pathophysiology and pathogenesis of stunned myocardium: Depressed Ca 2+ activation of contraction as a consequence of reperfusion-induced cellular calcium overload in ferret hearts. J Clin Invest 79:950–961
58. Langer A, Burns RJ, Freeman MR et al. (1992) Reverse redistribution on exercise thallium scintigraphy: relationship to coronary patency and ventricular function after myocardial infarction. Can J Cardiol 26:707–710
59. Lee J. Shung CC, Lee K et al. (1994) Biokinetics of thallium-201 in normal subjects: comparison between adenosine, dipyramidole, dobutamine and exercise. J Nucl Med 35:535–541
60. Leppo JA, Macneil PB, Moring AF et al. (1986) Separate effects of ischemia, hypoxia, and contractility on thallium-201 kinetics in rabbit myocardium.J Nucl Med 27:66–74
61. Leppo JA (1987) Myocardial uptake of thallium and rubidium during alterations in perfusion and oxygenation in isolated rabbit hearts. J Nucl Med 28:878–885
62. Liu P, Kiess MC, Okada RD et al. (1985) The persistent defect on exercise thallium imaging and its fate after myocardial revascularization: Does it represent scar or ischemia? Am Heart J 110:996–1001
62a. Maisch B, Funck R, Schönian U, Moosdorf R (1996) Indikationen zur transmyokardialen Lasertherapie. Z Kardiol 85:269–279
63. Marban E (1991) Myocardial stunning and hibernation. The physiology behind the colloquialisms. Circulation 83:681–688
64. Mazullo P, Parodi O, Reisenhofer B et al. (1993) Value of rest thallium-201/technetium-99m sestamibi scans and dobutamine echocardiography for detecting myocardial viability. Am J Cardiol 71:166–172
65. Marshall R, Leidholdt E, Zhang DY et al. (1991) The effect of flow on technetium-99m Teboroxime (SQ30217) and thallium-201 extraction and retention in rabbit heart. J Nucl Med 32:1979-1988
66. Matsuzaki M, Gallagher KP, Kemper WS et al. (1983) Sustained regional dysfunction produced by prolonged coronary stenosis: gradual recovery after perfusion. Circulation 68:170–182
67. McCallister BD, Clemments IP, Hauser ME et al. (1991) The limited value of 24-hour images following 4-hour reinjection thallium imaging. Circulation 84 (suppl II):II-533
68. Mercier JC, Lando U, Kanmatsuse K et al. (1982) Divergent effects of inotropic stimulation on the ischemic and severely depressed reperfused myocardium. Circulation 66:397–400
68a. Moosdorf R, Maisch B, Höffken H (1996) Transmyokardiale Laserrevaskularisation – Grenzen und Möglichkeiten. Z Kardiol 85:281–285
68b. Moosdorf R, Schoebel FC, Hort W (1997) Transmyokardiale Laserrevaskularisation – morphologische, pathophysiologische und historische Grundlagen der indirekten Revaskularisation des Herzmuskels. Z. Kardiol. 1997, 86:149–164
69. Mori T, Minamiyi K, Kurogane H et al. (1991) Rest injected thallium-201 imaging for assessing viability of severe asynergic regions. J Nucl Med 32:1718–1724
69a. Nägele H, Kalmar P, Nienaber CA, Rödiger W, Stubbe HM (1997) Stellenwert der transmyokardialen Laser-Revaskularisation bei therapiefraktärer koronarer Herzkrankheit. Dtsch med Wschr 122:1117–1120
69b. Nägele H, Kalmar P, Lübeck M, Marcsek P, Nienaber CA, Rödiger W, Stiel GM, Stubbe HM (1997) Transmyokardiale Laserrevaskularisation – Behandlungsoption der koronaren Herzerkrankung? Z Kardiol 86:171–178
70. Nakajima K, Taki J, Shuke N et al. (1993) Myocardial perfusion imaging and dynamic analysis with technetium-99m-tetrofosmin. J Nucl Med 34:1478–1484
71. Nielsen A, Morris K, Murdock R et al. (1980) Linear relationship between the distribution of thallium-201 and blood flow in ischemic and nonischemic myocardium during exercice. Circulation 4797–4801

72. Pantely GA, Malone SA, Rhen WS et al. (1990) Regeneration of myocardial phosphocreatine in pigs despite continued moderate ischemia. Circ Res 67:1481–1493
73. Picano E, Marzullo P, Gigli G et al. (1992) Identification of viable myocardium by dipyridamol-induced improvement in regional left ventricular function by echocardiography in myocardial infarction and comparison with thallium scintigraphy at rest. Am J Cardiol 70:252–258
74. Pierard L, Landsheere C, Berthe C, Rigo P, Kulbertus H (1990) Identification of viable myocardium by echocardiography during dobutamine infusion in patients with myocardial infarction after thrombolytic therapy: Comparison with positron emission tomography. J Am Coll Cardiol 15:1921–1931
75. Pohost GM, Okade RD, O'Keefe DD et al. (1981) Thallium redistribution in dogs with severe coronary artery stenosis of fixed caliber. Circ Res 48:439–446
76. Pohost GM, Zir LM, Moore RH et al. (1977) Differentiation of transiently ischemic from infarcted myocardium by serial imaging after a single dose of thallium-201. Circulation 55:294–302
77. Rocco TP, Dilsizian V, McKusick KA et al. (1990) Comparison of thallium redistribution with rest "reinjection" imaging for the detection of viable myocardium. Am J Cardiol 66:158–163
78. Ross Jr J (1991) Myocardial perfusion-contraction matching. Implications for coronary heart disease and hibernation. Circulation 83:1076–1083
79. Rozanski A, Berman DS, Gray R et al. (1981) Use of thallium-201 redistribution scintigraphy in the preoperative differentiation of reversible and nonreversible myocardial asynergy. Circulation 1981; 64:936–944
80. Schäfer S, Heusch G (1990) Recruitment of a time dependent inotropic reserve by postextrasystolic potentiation in normal and reperfused myocardium.
Basic Res Cardiol 85:257–269
81. Schäfer S, Lindner C, Heusch G (1990) Xamoterol recruits an inotropic reserve in the acutely failing, reperfused canine myocardium without detrimental effects on its subsequent recovery. Naunyn-Schmiedebergs Arch Pharmacol 342:206–213
82. Schelbert X, Buxton D (1988) Insights into coronary artery disease gained from metabolic imaging. Circulation 78:496–505
83. Schneider CA, Voth E, Theissen P et al. (1994) Vitalitätsbeurteilung chronischer Myokardinfarkte durch F-18-FluoroD-Glukose-Positronenemissionstomographie und Tc-99m-MIBI-SPECT. Z Kardiol 83:124–131
84. Schober O, Hasfeld M, Matheja P, Schäfers M, Breithardt G (1991) Thallium reinjection vs redistribution in severe stenosis of coronary arteries dependent on the collateralization. Eur J Nucl Med 18:538
85. Schulz R, Guth BD, Pieper K et al. (1992) Recruitment of an inotropic reserve in moderately ischemic myocardium at the expense of metabolic recovery: a model of shortterm hibernation. Circ Res 70:1282–1295
86. Silberstein EB, DeVries DE (1985) Reverse redistribution phenomenon in thallium-201 stress tests: angiographic correlation and clinical significance. J Nucl Med 26:707–710
87. Sinusas A, Wason D, Cannon J et al. (1989) Effect of ischemia and post ischemic dysfunction on myocardial uptake of technetium-99m labeled methoxybutyl isonitrile and thallium-201. J Am Coll Cardiol 14:1785–1793
88. Smart S, Sawada S, Ryan T et al. (1993) Low-dose dobutamine echocardiography detects reversible dysfunction after thrombolytic therapy of acute myocardial infarction. Circulation 88:405–415
88a. Smith JA, Dunning JJ, Parry AJ, Large SR, Wallwork, J (1995) Transmyocardial Laser Revascularization. Journal of Cardiac Surgery 10:569–672
89. Sinusas AJ, Trautmann KA, Bergin JD ct al. (1990) Quantification of area at risk during coronary occlusion and degree of myocardial salvage after reperfusion with technetium-99m methoxyisobutyl isonitrile. Circulation 82:1424–1437
90. Strauer BE, Bürger S, Büll U (1978) Multifactorial determination of Thallium-201 uptake of the head: an experimental study concerning the influence of ventricular mass, perfusion and oxygen consumption. Basic Res Cardiol 73:298–306
91. Strauss HW, Harrison K, Langan JK et al. (1975) Thallium-201 for myocardial imaging. Relation of thallium-201 to regional myocardial perfusion. Circulation 51:641–645
92. Swain JL, Sabina RL, McHale PA et al. (1982) Prolonged myocardial nucleotide depletion after brief ischemia in the open-chest dog. Am J Physiol 242:H818–H826
93. Tamaki N, Othani H, Yamashita K et al. (1991) Metabolic activity in the areas of new fill-in after thallium-201 reinjection: Comparison with positron emission tomography using fluorine-18-deoxyglucose. J Nucl Med 32:673–678

94. Tamaki N, Othani H, Yonekura Y et al. (1990) Significance of fill-in after thallium-201 reinjection following delayed imaging: Comparison with regional wall motion and angiographic findings. J Nucl Med 31:1617–1623
95. Tamaki N, Yonekura Y, Yamashita K et al. (1988) Relation of left ventricular perfusion and wall motion with metabolic activity in persistent defects on thallium-201 tomography in healed myocardial infarction. Am J Cardiol 52:202–208
96. Vatner SF (1980) Correlation between acute reductions in myocardial blood flow and function in conscious dogs. Circ Res 47:201–207
97. Verani MS, Jeroudi MO, Mahmarian JJ et al. (1988) Quantification of myocardial infarction during coronary occlusion and myocardial salvage after reperfusion using cardiac imaging with technetium-99m hexakis 2-methoxyisobutyl isonitrile. J Am Coll Cardiol 12:1573–1581
98. Wackers FJTh, Gibbons RJ, Verani MS et al. (1989) Serial quantitative planar technetium-99m isonitrile imaging in acute myocardial infarction: Efficacy for noninvasive assessment of thrombolytic therapy. J Am Coll Cardiol 14:861–873
99. Weich HF, Strauss HW, Pitt B (1977) The extraction of thallium-201 by the myocardium. Circulation 56:188–191
100. Weiss AT, Maddahi J, Lew AS et al. (1986) Reverse redistribution of thallium-201: a sign of nontransmural myocardial infarction with patency of the infarct-related coronary artery. J Am Coll Cardiol 7:61–67
101. Yang L, Berman DS, Kial H et al. (1990) The frequency of late reversibility in SPET thallium-201 stress-redistribution studies. J Am Coll Cardiol 15:334–340

PART II

Treatment Strategies for Coronary Heart Disease

CHAPTER 5

Medical Treatment in the Case of Severe Coronary Artery Disease

O. Oldenburg · R. Erbel

5.1 Introduction

In Europe, every year up to 63,500 patients undergo coronary bypass surgery and more than 147,700 patients percutaneous transluminal coronary angioplasty (PTCA) [1]. Additionally, the thrombolytic therapy of acute myocardial infarction results in an increasing number of patients surviving coronary artery disease (CAD) with and without heart failure. Repeated coronary interventions and coronary bypass surgerys are common. The treatment of these patients imposes special demands on the physician. In the following we describe the medical therapy of patients with advanced CAD with and without heart failure.

5.2 Patients with Severe Coronary Artery Disease and without Cardiac Failure

The combined therapy with nitrates, β-blockers and calcium channel blockers is the first choice in the medical treatment of patients with severe CAD and without heart failure.

During the therapy with nitrates it has to be ensured that the dosage is adapted to the individual condition. The effectiveness of the medical treatment has to be tested again and again because of the possible onset of nitrate tolerance. Acute administration of nitroglycerin and elevation of the dosage may overcome this effect. The emphasis should rely more on practical than on theoretical considerations. The main point is that drugs that will cause less tolerance side effects are available, like e.g. molsidomine [2, 3].

There are several methods to evaluate the success of the therapy: recording of the number of angina pectoris attacks per day or week, the result of stress tests or the recording of the frequency and duration of ST-segment-depressions in the 24h-Holter-ECG.

If a patient under therapy develops angina pectoris again, two reasons have to be considered: on one hand an unstable angina pectoris may be present, on the other hand a nitrate tolerance has to be taken into account. In this context Bassenge and coworkers showed that acetylsalicylacid [4] and angiotensin converting enzyme-inhibitors [5], as well as N-acetylcystein [6] can block the development of a nitrate tolerance.

The therapy with β-blockers is a secondary preventive treatment and should be given to all patients without contraindications. Because of other preexisting CAD risk factors, possible side effects of the β-blocker therapy

Table 5.1. Medical treatment in the case of severe CAD: Therapy aims.

Therapy	Therapy control
β- blockers	Resting heart rate <60/min
Diuretics	Daily weight assessment
Nitrates	Number of angina pectoris episodes ST-segment analysis Stress testing
ACE-inhibitors	Blood pressure: 110–130 mmHg Serum creatinine
CSE-inhibitors	Cholesterol <160 mg/dl LDL <100 mg/dl
Niacin	Triglycerides <160 mg/dl

have to be considered. Usually there is no danger of an impairment of glucose tolerance [7], except for patients who have developed a nephropathy or neuropathy. Dietary and/or medical treatment of a hyperlipoproteinemia can be difficult while patients are receiving β-blockers. Therefore β_1-selective blockers should be used, e.g. metoprolol, bisoprolol or nisoprolol [8].

The heart rate is an outstanding predictor for control of therapy. The resting heart rate should not exceed 60 bpm, the heart rate under stress should be less than 120 bpm, considered as signs of a good treatment regimen (Table 5.1).

Medical treatment with calcium channel blockers is important in patients in whom β-blockers can not be given. Second generation calcium channel blockers like nisoldipine or amlodipine and calcium antagonists with negative chronotropic effects like verapamil or diltiazem are drugs of the first choice in these cases [9]. The aim of this treatment is to lessen the oxygen consumption of the heart, therefore the absence of angina pectoris attacks and an opimal blood pressure level are good parameters for control of optimal treatment.

5.3 Cardiovascular risk factors

The reduction of cardiovascular risk factors is one of the first aims of the treatment. Here not only such well known risk factors as hypertension, diabetes mellitus, hyperlipidemia, uric acidaemia and nicotine abuse are important: recently identified factors like hyperfibrinogenemia, hyperhomocysteinemia, hyperinsulinemia and a high level of lipoprotein (a) are of special interest.

5.3.1 Hyperlipidemia

The first step in therapy is to optimize the diet. In this context it is important to reduce especially cholesterol rich food [10, 11]. Most of the time this diet has to be not only low in fat, in addition it is important to have a balance in the calories uptake. Software for such dietary planning is now available. A regime called "Mediterranean diet" is a good example. This diet is mostly vegeterian and involves the consumption of small servings of alcohol (<15g alcohol per day). The advantage of this Mediterranean diet can be seen in the different parts of Europe. There is a remarkably higher cardiovascular mortality in the northern parts of Europe than in the southern or the mediterranean countries. These differences can even be seen by comparison of the cholesterol blood levels of the northern and southern parts of Germany.

5.3.1.1
Cholesterol is the "killer number one"

Recent studies like the 4S- [12], the WOS- [13] and the CARE-Study [14] clearly documented, that lowering the cholesterol blood level reduces the overall mortality and the amount of coronary events. A one percent reduction in the cholesterol level seems to reduce coronary events by two percent. In this context it is remarkable, that this benefit is independent of age. Under the assumption of a reduction in the cholesterol level of 23.2mg/dl, the reduction in coronary events are 54% in the age group of 35 to 45 year old men and 20% at the age of 70 years. In summary there is a benefit in lowering the cholesterol blood level, which does not depend on age, gender or the left ventricular ejection fraction [15].

A nutritional change on its own rarely reduces a high cholesterol blood level. The reduction of the cholesterol level might be 5% to 10% or less in most cases. Since the introduction of HMG-coenzyme A reductase-inhibitors (CSE-inhibitors), there is the opportunity of a greater reduction. With first generation CSE-inhibitors like lovastatin, simvastatin, pravastatin and fluvastatin, a reduction of the cholesterol level between 30% and 35% is possible. New generation drugs like atorvastatin are able to reduce this level by up to 60% [16].

If a significant reduction in the cholesterol level cannot be achieved with CSE-inhibitors, resins like cholestyramin or cholestipol should be given. Alternatives to these substances are sitoserine and pectine. In the United States oat meals have been preferred since it received publicity in the media.

The reduction of the cholesterol blood level encompasses an improvement in endothelial function together with a better perfusion [17, 18]. Whereas the effects on atherosclerosis is a long lasting effect, the effect on the endothelial function is a short-term one. First effects on the intima can be seen after weeks, in contrast to an impaired endothelial function and perfusion which can occur in minutes [19].

Lowering cholesterol levels leads to a reduction in PTCAs and coronary artery bypass surgery between 20% and 35% in the studies mentioned above. For the first time in internal medicine a drug treatment was able to reduce the number of revascularisation procedures. This has important economic consequences, so that the cholesterol reduction must be achieved by all means. In addition to this, the CARE-Study [14] shows that this reduction in the cholesterol blood level is not only necessary at high levels (>240mg/dl), but also at moderatly elevated levels between 190 mg/dl to 240 mg/dl.

Special benefits of a cholesterol reduction can also be seen in heart transplant patients. As Kobashigawa and coworkers reported, the one year survival rate during a pravastatin medication was more than 94% comparely to 78% in the control group [20]. The number of acute rejections went down. This effect can be related to a lower cytotoxic effect of killer cells. As the study mentioned above showed, this cytotoxic effect of the killer cells is less in the group treated with pravastatin than in the placebo group.

So far it remains unresolved whether the reduction is to be made aggressively or moderately to reach the recommended cholesterol levels. To answer this question a follow up study after CABG-surgery was developed. In this study lovastatin was given in a low and in a high dosage (2,5mg to 5mg per day or 40mg to 80mg per day). The results of this study were a more pronounced lowering of the total cholesterol and the LDL-cholesterol and an increase of HDL-cholesterol with the more aggressive treatment. Additionally, a progression in artheriosclerosis was seen in only 27% compared to 39% and revascularisation proceedings were necessary in 6.5% compared to 9.2% of patients. The differences of these results were between 18% and 39% [21]. Similar results were provided by the Munich Bypass Study: the more the cholesterol level was depressed the better was the myocardial infarction- and survival-rate, Seidel reported at the hotline session during the spring convention of the German Cardiology Association in 1997.

The efficacy of the treatment can be monitored by determining total cholesterol-, LDL- and HDL-blood levels (Table 5.1).

To optimize this therapy, we recommend a self-monitored therapy by the patient similar to hypertension or diabetes mellitus therapy. In special lessons, patients are taught to use the cholesterol testing equipment. A test every 10 to 14 days is recommended, later on every 3 to 4 weeks.

5.3.1.2
Hypertriglyceridemia

An elevation in the triglycerid blood level is often combined with a high cholesterol level and can be treated by dietary changes in most patients. If the hypertriglyceridemia persists, a drug treatment with nicotinic acids is necessary (xantinol, e.g. complamin®). The blood level of triglycerids should be below 160mg/dl (Table 5.1). New generation CSE-inhibitors are a therapeutic alternative in the case of an combined hypercholesterolemia and hypertriglyceridemia, because these drugs are able to lower the triglycerid-level as well.

5.3.2
Hyperinsulinemia

Hyperinsulinism is an independent risk factor that was identified a few years ago. Despres and coworkers [22] have shown, that there is an increasing number of ischemic heart disease cases with an increasing level of fasting insulin. With a blood level of less than 67pmol/l only one percent of patients suffered from ischemic heart disease, compared to seven percent with a level above 96pmol/l. These findings were independent of the gender. The authors came to the conclusion that the determination of the fasting insulin level has to be a part of the risk factor analysis.

5.3.3 Hyperfibrinogenemia

Recent studies have confirmed that an elevated fibrinogen level is a risk factor for CAD [23]. Lowering the fibrinogen level causes an activation of the fibrinolysis, which can be a part of the desintegration of microthrombosis and a reduction of blood viscosity, which can lead to an improvement in the microvascular circulation.

5.3.3.1 *Fibrates*

Fibrates are effective drugs to lower the fibrinogen level. To verify the treatment with fibrates, in the BECAIT-Study bezafibrate was given for a period of five years in a dosage of 200mg three times a day [24]. Besides a reduction of the cholesterol of 14% and of triglycerids of 26%, there was a reduction in the fibrinogen blood level of 13% compared to placebo. Looking at the long term results, the effects of a therapy with benzofibrates can be settled between the effects of simvastatin and pravastatin [25]. Thus fibrinogen can be lowered with an orally available drug that can also be combined with CSE-inhibitors and resins if necessary.

5.3.3.2 *Urokinase*

Urokinase is more efficient than benzofibrates. This therapy is well known as an effective treatment of acute myocardial infarction. Leschke and coworkers in Düsseldorf first started with this therapy in the event of an unstable angina pectoris [26]. They found that 500,000 I.E. urokinase which is given three times a week for 12 weeks is more effective than 50,000 I.E. three times a week. The group which received the higher dosage clearly demonstrated a more favorable effect. This regimen was able to reduce the clinical symptoms (angina events per week) by approxymately 75%, the fibrinogen blood level fell by about 35%, the red blood cell aggregation by 18%. The myocardial perfusion improved as shown by MIBI-SPECT analysis [27, 28]. Within a period of approxymately 14 months the occurrence of angina pectoris was reduced or an absence of these attacks in 66% of the patients was achieved. Gastrointestinal bleeding was observed in only 0.8%. No effect was found in 3.3% of all patients and 0.8% of patients developed an intolerance. A recurrence of unstable angina was observed in 35%. Cardiac mortality was 12% [29]. Further studies are necessary to investigate if this therapy is superior to the conventional drug treatment.

5.3.4
Lipoprotein (a)

Lipoprotein (a) has been described as an independent risk factor as well [30]. Lipoprotein (a) was found in atherosclerotic plaques. It reduces the activity of plasminogen. 90% of all cases with an elevated lipoprotein (a) level are genetically determined. There are also elevated levels in case of kidney failure and diabetes mellitus [31]. Haemodialysis, estrogen substitution and treatment with tamoxyfen reduces the lipoprotein (a) blood level. Therapeutic options are physical activity, fishoil- and moderate alcohol-consumption. Nicotinic acid is another therapeutic option. LDL-apheresis is particulary effective. Thiery and coworkers succeeded in reducing LDL by 51%, Apolipoprotein B by 46% and Lipoprotein (a) by 45% using a heparin-induced extracorporeal LDL precipitation (HELP) once a week. Under this regimen the fibrinogen decreased by minus 46%. An influence of a combined therapy with CSE-inhibitors on fibrinogen and lipoprotein (a) was not found, whereas the LDL-cholesterol levels decreased by 70–80% [32]. The treatment of patients with severe, life-threatening hypercholesterinemia with the HELP-systems, rather than with liver transplantation, is recommended by Lees and coworkers [33].

There are other systems than the HELP-system to carry out LDL-apheresis. In the LAARS-study one group was treated with, the other group without a LDL-apheresis but both groups were given 40mg of simvastatin every day. The LDL-apheresis led to a higher cholesterol reduction than treatment with simvastatin only. The lipoprotein (a) level decreased remarkably in the group treated with the combined therapy. The number of coronary artery stenoses, evaluated by quantitative coronary angiography (QCA), decreased significantly in the LDL-apheresis group than in the group that was treated with drugs only. Very important in daily life is the fact that there was a continuous increase in maximal exercise capacity in the LDL-apheresis group. For a period of two years the authors investigated the length of time before an exercise induced ST-segment depression in the ECG occurred. The time before the onset of a ST-segment depression lengthened and the total number of ST-segment depression was reduced, even though there was no change in the drug treated group [34].

5.3.5
Homocysteine

High levels of homocysteine have been identified as another independent risk factor for vascular, especially cardiovascular diseases [35]. Major factors influencing homocysteine levels are age, gender, genetics, nutrition, vascular disease state and medication. Homocysteine increases with age and is higher in men than in age-matched women, increases with serum creatinine and is lowered by haemodialysis. There is also a wide rage in the blood levels between citizens of different countries with a high level in Scandinavia and low levels in Japan [36]. An imbalanced nutrition with Vitamin B_6 or B_{12} deficiency or folate deficiency are negatively correlated to homocysteine levels even in healthy persons. Methotrexate, azaribine, phenytoin, carbamazepine and nitrous oxide, which inactivates vitamin B_{12}, and estrogen containing oral contraceptives were recognized to have a increasing effect on homocysteine plasma levels [37].

Therefore various factors are important for the treatment of hyperhomocysteinemia. Homocysteine levels in folate-deficient patients can be lowered by oral folic acid replacement [38], whereas only the combined replacement of vitamin B_6 and B_{12} is able to reduce the homocysteine level in general [37]. Further studies are not only necessary to establish the exact dosage for treatment, but also to evaluate the effect of the drug therapy on patients' prognosis.

5.4 Medical Treatment in Case of Severe Coronary Artery Disease and Cardiac Failure

Diuretics, angiotensin converting enzyme (ACE)-inhibitors and cardiac glycosides are elements of the first choice in drug treatment. Furosemide alone or in combination with thiazide diuretics or spironolactone is the cornerstone of diuretic therapy. An easy way to control the efficacy of this therapy is the daily control of body weight and renal function (Table 5.1).

5.4.1 ACE-Inhibitors

ACE-inhibitors are of special interest, because large multicenter studies have confirmed a better outcome with these drugs in case of a heart failure due to left ventricular systolic dysfunction [39, 40, 41]. The guideline of the American Heart Association [42] suggest the use of ACE-inhibitors in all cases if no special contraindications exist. In this context it has to be noticed, that (1) these positive effects were observed with a dosage of 50mg captopril given three times a day or other ACE-inhibitors in equally high dosages, e.g. enalapril, and (2) the total effect was seen not earlier than 6–8 weeks after starting this treatment.

To start a therapy with ACE-inhibitors, it is recommended to start with short acting ACE-inhibitors like captopril in a small initial dosage, and switch to long acting drugs, e.g. enalapril, ramipril or cilazapril later on. Frequent evaluation of the blood pressure during the start of the therapy is essential. After the initial phase of treatment, the systolic blood pressure should be between 110–130 mmHg. The weight should be constant and the dosage of diuretics should be adapted. In case of simultaneous renal failure the dosage must be adapted to the renal function and during the initial administrations, blood pressure should be taken in short time intervals and serum creatinine levels must be monitored.

5.4.2 Cardiac glycosides

Cardiac glycosides can be given as digitoxin and digoxin. Serum levels should be taken to recognize an overdosage, in addition the heart rate and e.g. the reduction of a preexisting pulse deficit are good markers for an effective therapy. Recent studies have confirmed, that higher dosages of cardiac glycosides are not more effective than a treatment resulting in low- or medium- blood levels, in contrary, a higher dosage causes more side effects like additional arrhythmias [43].

Medical treatment in case of heart failure today follows the guidelines of the American Heart Association. There is no doubt that angiotensin-converting enzyme inhibitors are drugs of the first choice, an alternative are nitrates and angiotensin-II-receptor antagonists, e.g. losartan. In addition, diuretics are recommended. Cardiac glycosids should be used, if ACE-inhibitors and diuretics are insufficient or in case of atrial fibrillation in order to lower heart rate. An anticoagulation in patients with atrial fibrillation and a medical treatment with β-blockers after acute myocardial infarction are important additional considerations [44, 45]. An interesting alternative in case of a severe CAD and heart failure is outpatient treatment with dobutamine or enoximone, but general advices can not be given today.

5.5 Prognosis

In patients with severe CAD and heart failure optimized drug therapy has to be balanced with heart transplantion and CABG. Yancy and coworkers determined the maximal oxygen uptake during cardiopulmonary exercise testing, left ventricular ejection fraction and filling pressure [46]. In case of vital myocardium and a suitable coronary anatomy, they described good results for CABG in the case of an oxygen uptake above 15 ml/kg/min assessed by spiroergometry. A heart transplantion was performed in case of an unsuitable coronary anatomy, a left-ventricular filling pressure above 20 mmHg and an oxygen consumption below 15 ml/kg/min. A medical treatment was chosen in case of a left-ventricular filling pressure below 20 mmHg and an oxygen uptake above 15 ml/kg/min. Figure 5.1 shows a modified concept. In table 5.2 the results of an observation period of one year are shown. There are similar results in the medical treatment group compared to CABG or heart transplantion, the mortality was 7.7% compared to 8.3% and 6.1% [46].

Table 5.2. Results of patients management according to the strategy given in figure 5.1.

	n	1-year mortality [%]	LVEF [%]	VO_{2max} [ml/kg/min]	PCW [mmHg]
Drug treatment	26	7.7	0.24	20	21
CABG	12	8.3	0.28	21	19
Heart transplantation	31	6.1	0.17	13	29
Waiting for heart transplantation	10	70.0	0.19	13	32

n: number of patients; *LVEF*: left ventricular ejection fraction;
VO_{2max}: peak oxygen uptake during cardiopulmonary exercise testing; *PCW*: pulmonary capillary wedge pressure (modified to [46]).

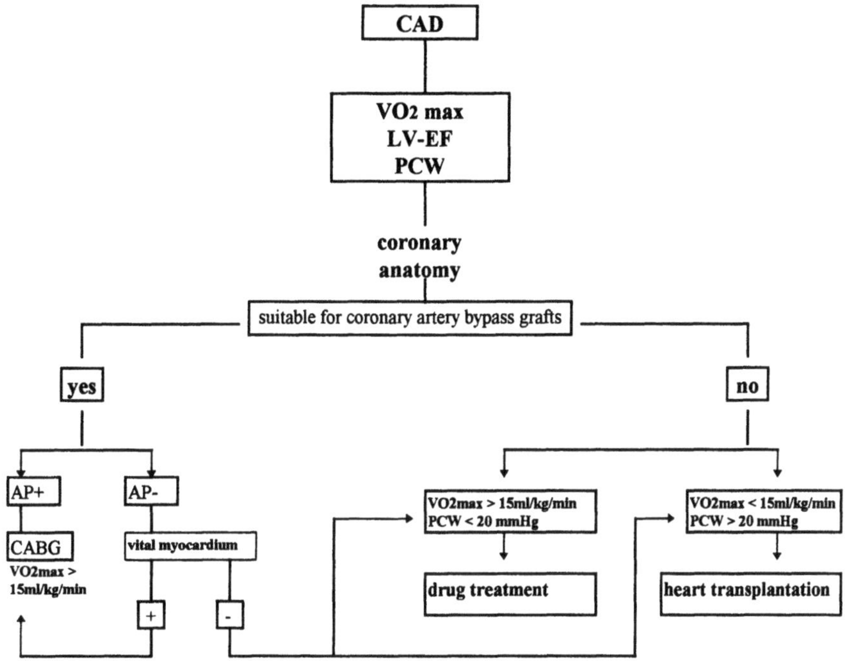

VO2 max: peak oxygen uptake during cardiopulmonary stress testing; LV-EF: left ventricular-ejection fraction; PCW: pulmonary capillary wedge pressure; AP: angina pectoris; modified to [46]

Fig. 5.1. Management strategy in severe CAD with heart failure

5.6 Summary

In case of severe coronary artery disease, a reduction of risk factors in combination with an optimized drug treatment is essential. New aspects are the reduction of recent identified risk factors like fibrinogen, homocysteine and lipoprotein (a). The recommendations of the American Heart Association are guidelines of an effective treatment. This article represents a strategy concept and clinical practice guideline.

References

1. Röthlisberger C, Meier B (1995) Coronary interventions in Europe 1992. Eur Heart J 16:922–929
2. Rudolph W, Dirschinger J (1991) Clinical comparison of nitrates and sydnonimines. Eur Heart J 12 (Suppl E):33–41
3. Große-Heitmeyer W (1994) Modsidomin intravenös bei Herz-Kreislauf-Erkrankungen – Zusammenfassende Übersicht. Med Klinik 89:62–63
4. Bassenge E, Personal communication
5. Münzel T, Bassenge E (1993) Chronic angiotensin converting enzyme-inhibition retards nitrate tolerance and prevents coronary rebound constriction (Abstract). Circulation 88:I–90

6. Boesgaard S, Iversen HK, Wroblewski H et al. (1994) Altered peripheral vasodilator profile of nitroglycerin during long-term infusion of N-acetylcystein. J Am Coll Cardiol 23:163–169
7. Sawicki PT, Berger M (1992) Metabolische Wirkungen von β-Rezeptorenblockern. Dtsch med Wschr 117:875–879
8. Leschke M, Strauer BE (1995) Wie selektiv sind kardioselektive β-Rezeptorenblocker. Dtsch med Wschr 120:45–46
9. Dargie HJ (1996) Angina and left ventricular dysfunction. Eur Heart J 17 (Suppl G):2–7
10. Ritter MM, Richter WO (1995) Gesundheitliche Auswirkungen einer vegetarischen Lebensweise. Fortschr Med 113:239–242
11. Watts GF, Lewis B, Jackson P et al (1995) Relationships between nutrient intake and progression/regression of coronary atherosclerosis as assessed by serial quantitative angiography. Can J Cardiol 11 (Suppl G):110G–114G
12. The Scandinavian Simvastatin Survival Study Group (1994) Randomised trial of cholesterol lowering in 4444 patients with coronary heart disease: The Scandinavian Simvastatin Survival Study (4S); Lancet 344:1383–1389
13. Shepherd J, Cobbe SM, Ford I et al. (1995) Prevention of coronary heart disease with pravastatin in men with hypercholesterinemia. N Engl J Med 333:1301–1307
14. Sacks FM, Pfeffer MA, Moye LA et al. (1996) The effect of pravastatin on coronary events after myocardial infarction in patients with average cholesterol levels. N Engl J Med 335:1001–1009
15. Law MR, Wald NJ, Thompson SG (1994) By how much and how quickly does reduction in serum cholesterol concentration lower risk of ischaemic heart disease? BMJ 308:367–372
16. Nawrocki JW, Weiss SR, Davidson MH et al (1995) Reduction of LDL cholesterol by 25% to 60% in patients with primary hypercholesterinemia by atorvastatin, a new HMG-CoA reductase inhibitor. Arterioscler Thromb Vasc Biol 15:678–682
17. Zeiher AM, Drexler H, Wollschläger H, Just H (1991) Modulation of coronary vasomotor tone in humans, progressive endothelial dysfunction with different early stages of coronary atherosclerosis. Circulation 83:391–401
18. Vogel RA, Corretti MC, Plotnick GD (1996) Changes in flow-mediated brachial artery vasoactivity with lowering of desirable cholesterol levels in healthy middle-aged men. Am J Cardiol 77:37–40
19. Stroes ESG, Rabelink TJ (1997) Hyperlipidemia and endothelial function; in: Born GVR, Schwartz CJ. Vascular endothelium, Schattauer, Stuttgart, pp 311–328
20. Kobashigawa JA, Katznelson S, Laks H et al (1995) Effects of pravastatin on outcomes after cardiac transplantation. New Engl J Med 333:621–627
21. The post coronary artery bypass graft trial investigators (1997). The effect of aggressive lowering of low-density lipoprotein cholesterol levels and low-dose anticoagulation on obstructive changes in saphenous-vein coronary artery bypass grafts. N Engl J Med 336:153–163
22. Despres JP, Lamarche B, Mauriege P et al (1996) Risk factors for ischaemic heart disease: is it time to measure insulin? Eur Heart J 17:1453–1454
23. Wilson PWF (1994) Established risk factors and coronary artery disease: The framingham study. Am J Hypertens 7:7S–12S
24. de Faire U, Ericsson CG, Grip L et al. (1996) Secondary preventive potential of lipid-lowering drugs. The bezafibrate coronary atherosclerosis intervention trial (BECAIT). Eur Heart J 17 (Suppl F):37–42
25. de Faire U, Ericsson CG, Grip L et al. (1997) Retardation of coronary atherosclerosis: the bezafibrate coronary atherosclerosis intervention trial (BECAIT) and other angiographic trials. Cardiovasc Drugs Ther 11 (Suppl 1):257–263
26. Leschke M, Höffken H, Vogt M et al. (1989) Intermittent urokinase therapy as a new strategy concept in untracable angina pectoris (Abstract). J Am Coll Cardiol 13:16A
27. Leschke M, Schoebel FC, Mecklenbeck W, Strauer BE (1993) Intermittent urokinase therapy in symptomatic end-stage coronary artery disease (Abstract). J Am Coll Cardiol 21:452A
28. Schoebel FC, Leschke M, Stein D et al. (1995) Chronic-intermittent urokinase therapy in refractory angina pectoris. Fibrinolysis 9 (Suppl 1):121–125
29. Schoebel FC, Leschke M, Strauer BE (1995) Therapierefraktäre Angina pectoris. Pathophysiologische Grundlagen und alternative Therapieansätze. Dtsch med Wschr 120:301–307
30. Schreiner PJ, Morrisett JD, Sharret AR et al (1993) Lipoprotein (a) as a risk factor for preclinical atherosclerosis. Arterioscler Thromb 13:826–833

31. Haffner SM, Gruber KK, Aldrete G et al (1992) Increased lipoprotein (a) concentrations in chronic renal failure. J Am Soc Nephrol 3:1156–1162
32. Thiery J, Seidel D (1992) Neue Strategien in der Behandlung der schweren Hypercholesterinämie koronarkranker Patienten: HMG-CoA-Reduktase Inhibitoren und H.E.L.P.-LDL-Apherese. Versicherungsmedizin 44:186–192
33. Lees RS, Holmes NN, Stadler RW et al. (1996) Treatment of hypercholesterolemia with heparin-induced extracorporeal low-density lipoprotein precipitation (HELP). J Clin Aphereses 11:132–137
34. Kroon AA, Aengevaeren WRM, van der Werf T et al. (1996) LDL-Apheresis atherosclerosis regression study (LAARS). Effect of aggressive versus conventional lipid lowering treatment on coronary atherosclerosis. Circulation 93:1826–1835
35. Clarke R, Daly L, Robinson K et al. (1991) Hyperhomocysteinemia: an independent risk factor for vascular disease. N Engl J Med 324:1149–1155
36. Alfthan G, Aro A, Gey F (1997) Plasma homocysteine and carcdiovascular disease mortality. Lancet 349:397
37. Mayer EL, Jacobsen DW, Robinson K (1996) Homocysteine and coronary atherosclerosis. J Am Coll Cardiol 27:517–527
38. Stabler SP, Marcell PD, Podell ER et al. (1988) Evaluation of total homocysteine in the serum of patients with cobalamin or folate deficiency detected by capillary gas chromatography - mass spectometry. J Clin Invest 81:466–474
39. SOLVD Investigators (1991) Effect of enalapril on survival in patients with reduced left ventricular ejection fractions and congestive heart failure. N Engl J Med 325:293-302
40. SOLVD Investigators (1992) Effect of enalapril on mortality and the development of heart failure in asymptomatic patients with reduced left ventricular ejection fraction. N Engl J Med 327:685–691
41. CONSENSUS Trial Study Group (1987). Effects of enalapril on mortality in severe congestive heart failure: Results of the Cooperative North Scandinavian Enalapril Survival Study (CONSENSUS). N Engl J Med 316:1429–1435
42. ACC/AHA Task Force Report: Guidelines for the evaluation and management of heart failure. Circulation 92:2764–2784
43. Slatton ML, Irani WN, Hall SA et al. (1997) Does digoxin provide additional hemodynamic and autonomic benefit at higher doses in patients with mild to moderate heart failure and normal sinus rhythm? J Am Coll Cardiol 29:1206–1213
44. Koefoed BG, Gullov AL, Petersen P (1997) Prevention of thromboembolic events in atrial fibrillation. Throm Haemost 78:377–381
45. First International Study of Infarct Survival (ISIS-I) Collaborative Group (1986) Randomised trial of intravenous atenolol among 16,027 cases of suspected acute myocardial infarction: ISIS-I. Lancet 57–65
46. Yancy C, Escobar J, Solomon M et al. (1997) Management of ischemic heart disease in patients reffered for cardiac transplantation. J Am Coll Cardiol 29:28 A

CHAPTER 6

Potential and Limitations of PTCA in Severe Coronary Artery Disease

N. Reifart · S. Göhring

6.1 Introduction

In the late seventies coronary angioplasty was limited to the treatment of simple lesions only (i.e. type A or type B 1 according to the classification of the American Heart Association). The method was also restricted to patients with single-vessel-disease. The success-rate in these short, non calcified, non thrombotic lesions of rather straight segments was about 70%. Severe complications (Q-infarction, emergency CABG, death) happened in 5 to 10% of the patients, and restenosis occured in 20 to 40%. Today, more complex lesions (type B 2 and C following the AHA-classification) are treated and patients with multi-vessel-disease are the majority. Operator experience and an incredibly rapid development of technology resulted in a success rate of 99% in type A and B 1 lesions and 90% with more complex stenoses. Chronic old occlusions can now be recanalized in about 70% of the patients. Severe complications (Q-wave myocardial infarction, emergency coronary bypass operation, or death) happen in no more than 1% of the patients treated today.

A reccurrence however might occur in 20% to 60% of the cases despite stenting, very much depending on the lesion morphology.

Severe coronary artery disease means to face a significantly higher risk during and following PTCA. Among those are patients with unstable angina pectoris (at rest, despite anti-anginal medication) as well as patients with acute myocardial infarction, severe left-ventricular dysfunction („last remaining vessel"), diffuse coronary disease, complex multi-vessel-disease and severe left main stenosis. Today, these patients can be treated with balloons and newer devices with acceptable results and complication rates.

Figures 6.1 a and b show a patient unstable angina pectoris and a proximal stenosis of the left anterior descending (LAD) as well as a large thrombust at the distal end of the lesion. The patient is treated following an acute anginal attack by immediate PTCA. Following balloon inflation a major dissection had to be covered with a stent.

This combination of balloon and stent enabled us to discharge the patient two days later. Stent implantation and the additional anti-platelet therapy (especially Ticlopidine) made the treatment of patients with acute ischemic syndromes much easier.

Some patients further receive Glycoprotein II b III a inhibitors.

The availability of stents and other second generation devices (figure 6.2) did not only increase the success rate, but also enabled us to do more complex lesions than in the past. Thus the amount of patients with multivessel disease is now exceeding 75%.

Fig. 6.1 a, b. Proximal subtotal stenosis of the left arterial descending coronary artery with a poststenotic thrombus. The patient was unstable despite a combination of beta-blockers, nitrates, and calcium antagonists. After PTCA and stenting the stenosis was reduced from 86% to 6% and the patient could be discharged without complications and symptoms

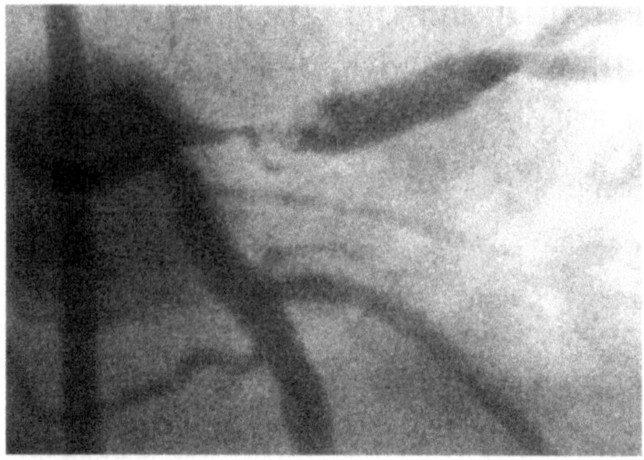

a

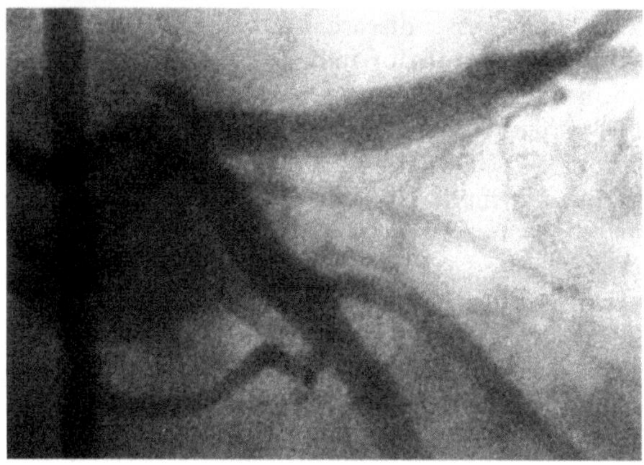

b

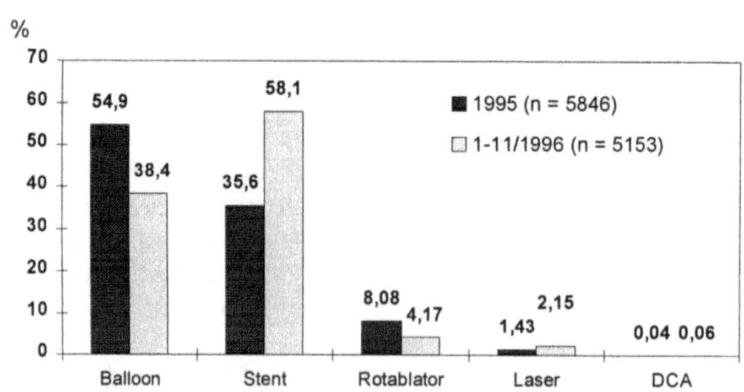

Fig. 6.2. Use of plain balloon angioplasty and second generation devices in our institution in 1995 and the first 11 months of 1996

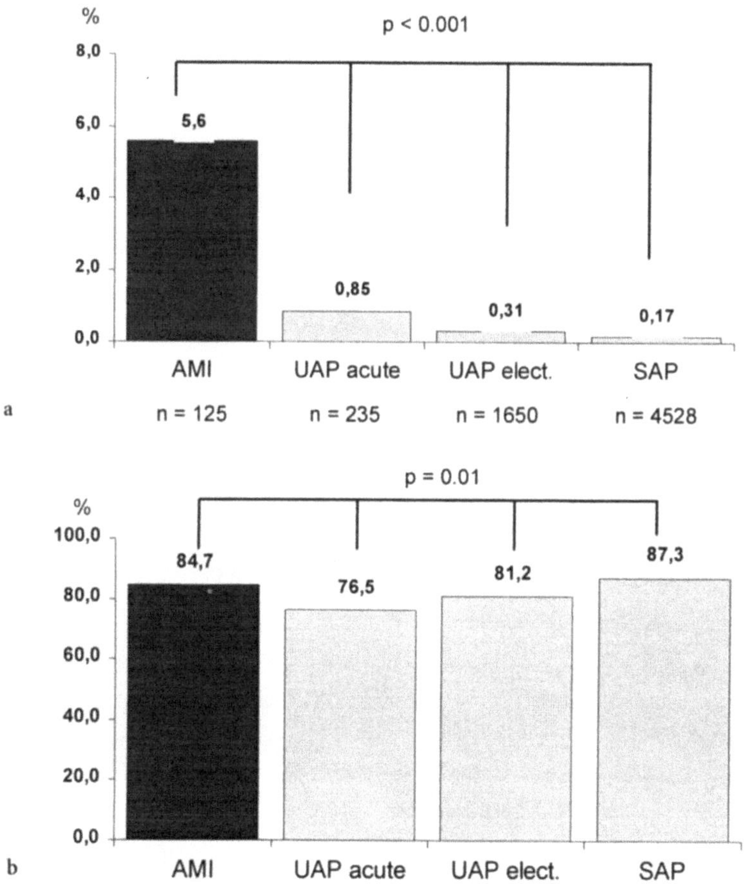

Fig. 6.3 a, b. Mortality and long term success of PTCA without stenting 1988–90 in the Red-Cross-Hospital Frankfurt

6.2 Unstable Angina Pectoris and Acute Myocardial Infarction

A few years ago PTCA was applied only in stable patients "cooling off" was recommended for unstable angina prior to dilatation. Figure 6.3 a shows our results of PTCA in the pre-stent era (1988–90) in patients with acute myocardial infarction, unstable angina pectoris (immediate PTCA), unstable angina pectoris (stabilizing medication first), and patients with stable angina pectoris. Mortality was not significantly different between the groups without myocardial infarction. Figure 6.3 b shows the long term results after 12 months. As expected, patients with stable angina pectoris (SAP) have the best outcome. We could speculate that, with stenting, these results might further improve.

The superiority of PTCA in acute myocardial infarction compared with thrombolysis has been demonstrated in several studies [1–8]. This is especially true for patients with prior coronary-bypass-surgery, reinfarction, large infarction, anterior infarction, and patients in cardiogenic shock, or elderly.

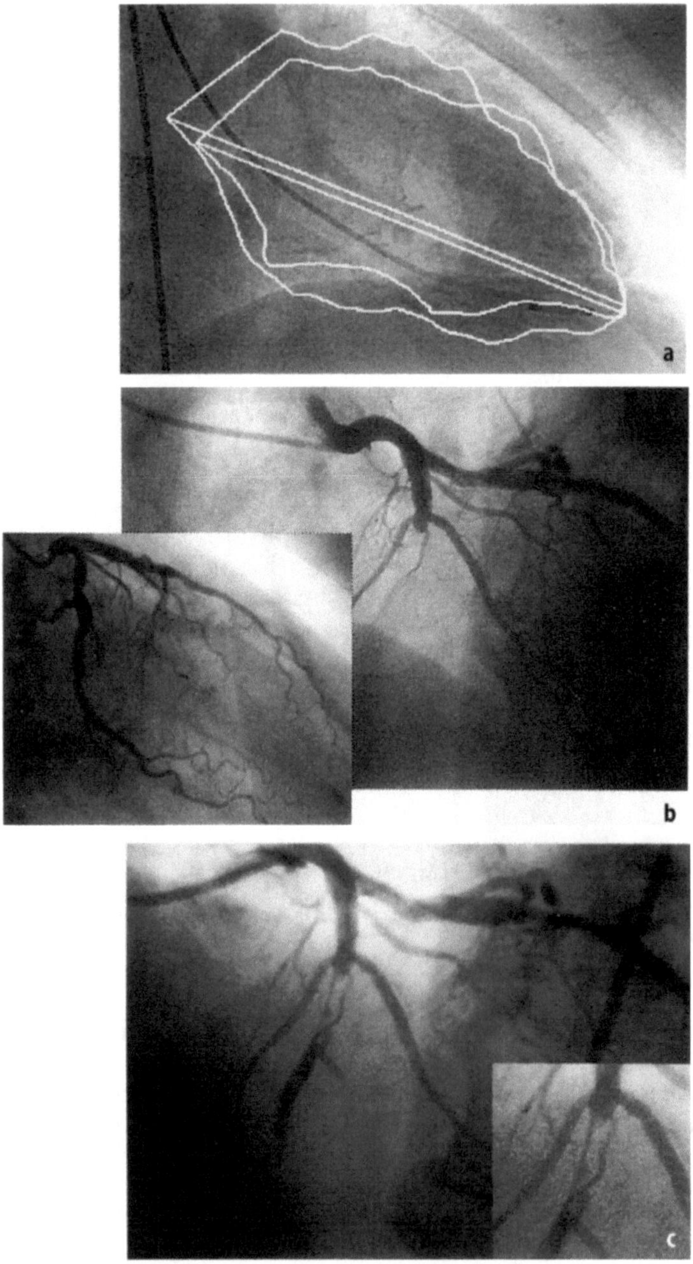

Fig. 6.4 a–e. Large anterior infarction with ejection fraction of 38%. The LAD is occluded right behind the take off of the first diagonal. **c** shows a large thrombus and **d** Markedly reduced flow after balloon angioplasty. **e** Final result after stent implantation. Residual stenosis less than 10%

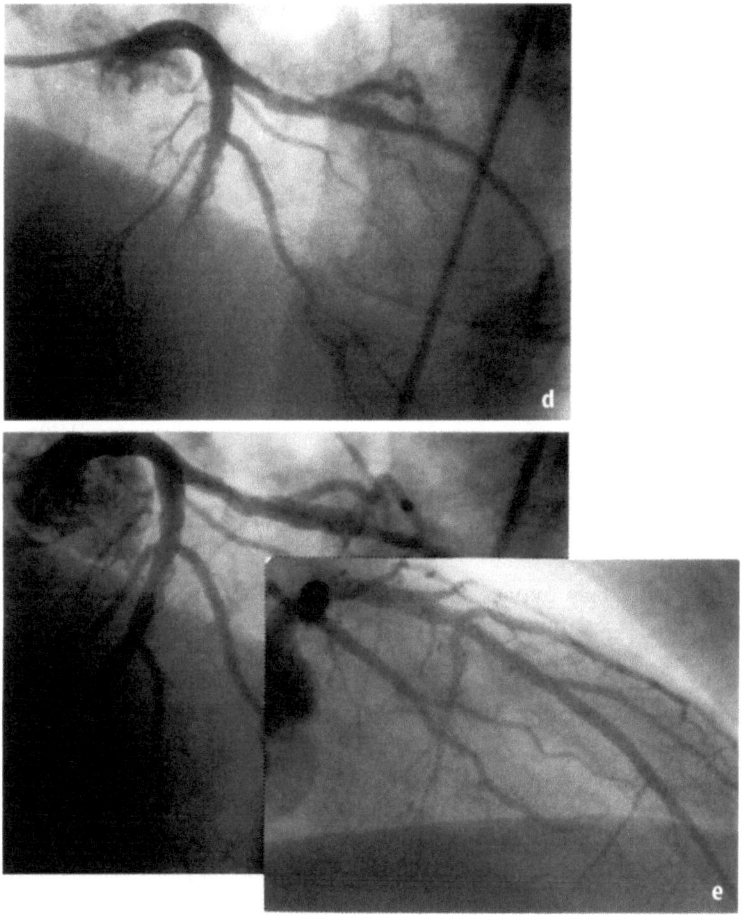

Fig. 6.4 d–e

Patients with shock have a chance to survive of 10% when treated conservatively, 30% after thrombolysis, and between 40 and 86% after PTCA [9–11].

More recently, stents appear to further improve results in acute myocardial infarction. Figures 6.4 a to e show a patient with anterior infarction and cardiogenic shock (ejection fraction 38%) who still suffers from slow flow because of large thrombus after opening the vessel with a wire and a balloon. After injection of Reopro 10 mg the thrombus is markedly reduced. Then, the thrombus was completely pressed against the vessel wall with a stent. The residual stenosis was 8%, and blood flow was reestablished. The patient rapidly recovered from shock. The clue to success was a combination of fast mechanical reopening, medical treatment of thrombus, and the restoration of the lumen with a stent. Today, it is obvious that PTCA in unstable angina pectoris and acute myocardial infarction is successful in 90% of cases, with severe complications in 3–5%. Especially in patients with high risk (old age,

Table 6.1. Results of PTCA in cases with an ejection fraction of less than 40%

Author	Year	N	Success	Death	MI	CABG	Survival
Eltchaninoff	1994	343	95%	2.6	2.6	3.2	82% (3 Y)
Holmes	1993	1802	–	0.8	4.9	4.5	87% (1 Y)
Stevens	1991	845	93%	4	–	2	87% (1 Y)
O'Keefe	1991	100	–	3	–	–	84% (1 Y)
Seifart	1992	645	93%	1.3	1.1	0.2	85% (1 Y)

Table 6.2. PTCA of high risk patients (e.g. last remaining vessel, unprotected left main) and severe comorbidity. The surgical risk of these patients was considered to exceed 10% according to judgment of cardiac surgeon and cardiologist

Angiographic Success	37/40 = 92.5%
Death	3/40 = 7.5%
Emergency-CABG	1/40 = 2.5%
Q-MI	1/40 = 2.5%
Non-Q-MI	1/40 = 2.5%
Clinical Success	35/40 = 87.5%

reinfarction, coronary bypass surgery, limited hemodynamics) PTCA is superior to all other treatment modalities.

6.3 Reduced Left-Ventricular Dysfunction. Last Remaining Vessel. Severe Comorbidity

According to literature [12–13] the success rate of patients with an ejection fraction of less than 40% is about 90%, mortality about 3%, and infarction rate about 2%. Emergency coronary bypass surgery appears necessary in 2% of these patients (Table 6.1).

In patients with severe comorbidity and complex lesion morphology and a significant stenosis in one of the major vessel, supplying more than 50% of the viable myocardium, or in patients with last remaining vessel and an ejection fraction of less than 30%, or in patients with an unprotected left main, we perform PTCA with support or standby of heart-lung-machine. In these patients the mortality of an elective cardiac surgical procedure was estimated above 10% according to the cardiac surgical conference. Table 6.2 shows our acute results of 40 high risk patients treated with PTCA and support or standby of a heart-lung-machine. Most of them could be discharged within 4 days. This close cooperation of cardiac surgeons, anesthesiologists, and interventional cardiologists offers an option to patients with an otherwise desperate prognosis.

6.4 Diffuse Coronary Artery Disease (Stenoses longer than 20 mm and Diffuse Calcification and Tortuosity)

In these patients results of balloon angioplasty are unfavourable. Sometimes, balloons or wires don't cross the stenosis, or the balloon doesn't open com-

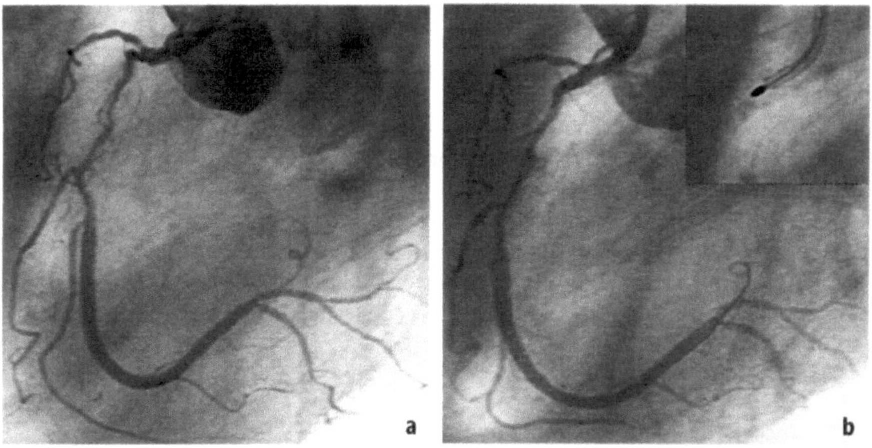

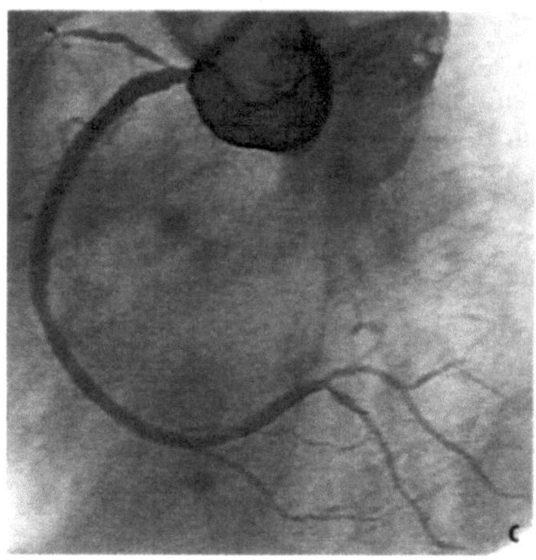

Fig. 6.5 a–c. Long lesion of the right coronary artery (36 mm) pretreated with 1.75 mm Rotablator (**b**) followed by balloon angioplasty with a 3.5 mm long balloon and a stent resulting in residual stenosis of less than 10% (**c**). Rotablation was necessary because of calcification and proximal tortuosity

Table 6.3. Randomized trial comparing balloon angioplasty, laser angioplasty, and rotablator in complex coronary lesions (ERBAC). Stents were used in less than 2%. Subgroup analysis on long lesions (>10 mm). Rotablator is significantly more successfull than laser and balloon angioplasty. Restenosis rate, however, exceeds that of balloon angioplasty alone

	PTCA	ELCA	PTRA	p
n	92	109	101	
Angiographic Success (%)	70	70	87	<0.01
Major Complications (Q-MI, Emergency CABG, Death, %)	3	5	3	n.s.
Restenosis (%)	46	49	58	n.s.

pletely. Long dissections are frequent, and stent implantation is difficult because of remaining long diffuse plaque material and tortuosity.

Without stent implantation, however, abrupt closure with infarction or emergency coronary bypass surgery may follow. In addition, long lesions are accompanied by restenosis exceeding 50%.

Especially when stent implantation appears difficult, percutaneous transluminal rotational angioplasty (PTRA) is used to ablate fibrotic calcified mass, prior to balloon dilatation. Under, these circumstances stent implantation is easier than without debulking. Table 6.3 shows the results of a randomized study (ERBAC, 14), in which balloon angioplasty, laser assisted angioplasty, and rotablator assisted angioplasty were compared in complex coronary lesions (subgroup long stenoses). Rotablation is superior as a treatment, but, is followed by a higher recurrence rate at one year follow-up.

Figures 6.5 a to c show an example of a successful rotational angioplasty of a long lesion of the right coronary artery followed by a stent. This combination of PTRA and stent might finally reduce the restenosis rate from 60% to 40%.

6.5 Multi-Vessel Disease

Since many years multi-vessel disease is no longer a taboo for PTCA. Many randomized studies have shown that early results are at least as good as those of coronary bypass operation. But, PTCA is complicated by a restenosis rate of about 30% that leads to repeated angioplasty in the following months [15]. Most of these randomized studies, however, excluded stents and debulking devices and may therefore not reflect the current practice and results. The decision whether to perform PTCA or to prefer CABG is very much dependent on lesion morphology and operator experience (both cardiologist and cardiac surgeon).

6.6 Left Main Stenosis

Without doubts unprotected left main stenosis is an indication for coronary bypass operation. But, PTCA may be an alternative in patients with significant comorbidity. Figure 6.6 shows an example of a left main stenosis and diffuse disease of the right coronary artery before and one year after atherectomy and PTCA (O. Katoh, M.D.). The success rate of PTCA for left main stenoses may exceed 90% with a rate of major complications less than 2%. But, long term prognosis is clearly worse compared to coronary bypass surgery. Acute cardiac death appears the main problem (about 5 to 10% in the first year), even with stents. Therefore PTCA of unprotected left main disease is contraindicated in patients suitable for CABG.

6.7 Limitations of PTCA in 1998

There are still a few limitations of PTCA. Chronic occlusions older than 12 months are successfully treated in up to 50% of the cases only. However, new wires and sophisticated techniques are required to achieve even these results. Figures 6.7 a–e show the reopening of an eight months old occlusion by a new hydrophilic wire. Figure 6.8 shows the recanalization of a 24 years old

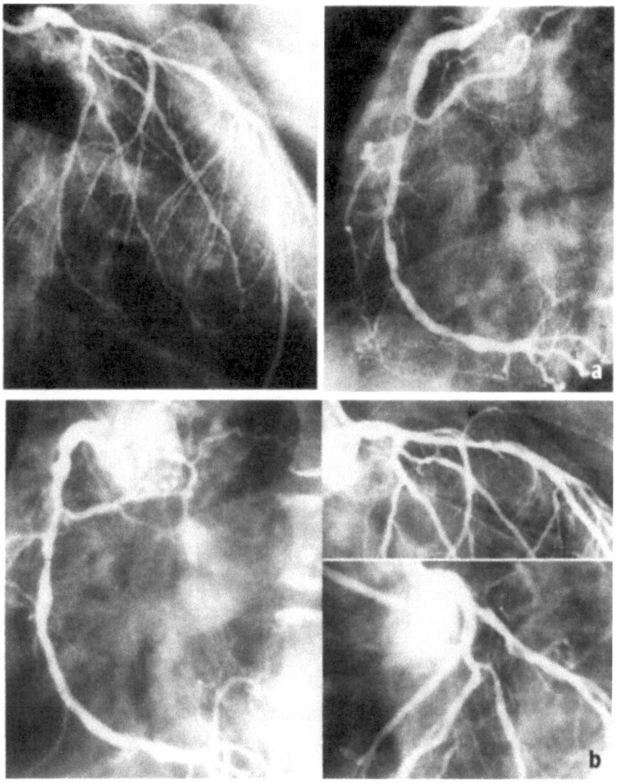

Fig. 6.6 a, b. Left main stenosis and diffuse disease of all three major vessels treated by DCA and balloon angioplasty with good result at one year follow up (O. Katoh, M.D.)

occlusion by a laser wire. This new technique allows in some cases the re-opening of very old occlusions that could not be crossed with conventional wires.

Another limitation are old venous grafts, because of embolization in 3% of cases and the restenosis rate of more than 50%.

An increasing problem is restenosis within a stent. Although stents have proven to decrease restenosis following balloon angioplasty by 10% (from 42% to 32%, [16]), significant proliferation may occur and has then to be treated by redilatation or a debulking technique. However, if restenosis within a stent is diffuse (approximately 70% of the cases), the likelihood of a second restenosis is between 50 and 80% [17–18].

6.8
Future directions

Alternative treatment modalities are tested to reduce proliferation: locally delivered antiproliferative drugs, local radiation (β, γ, infra-red laser), and PTFE-covered stents. Figure 6.9 a and b show that a stent covered with a layer may successfully be implanted into coronary arteries.

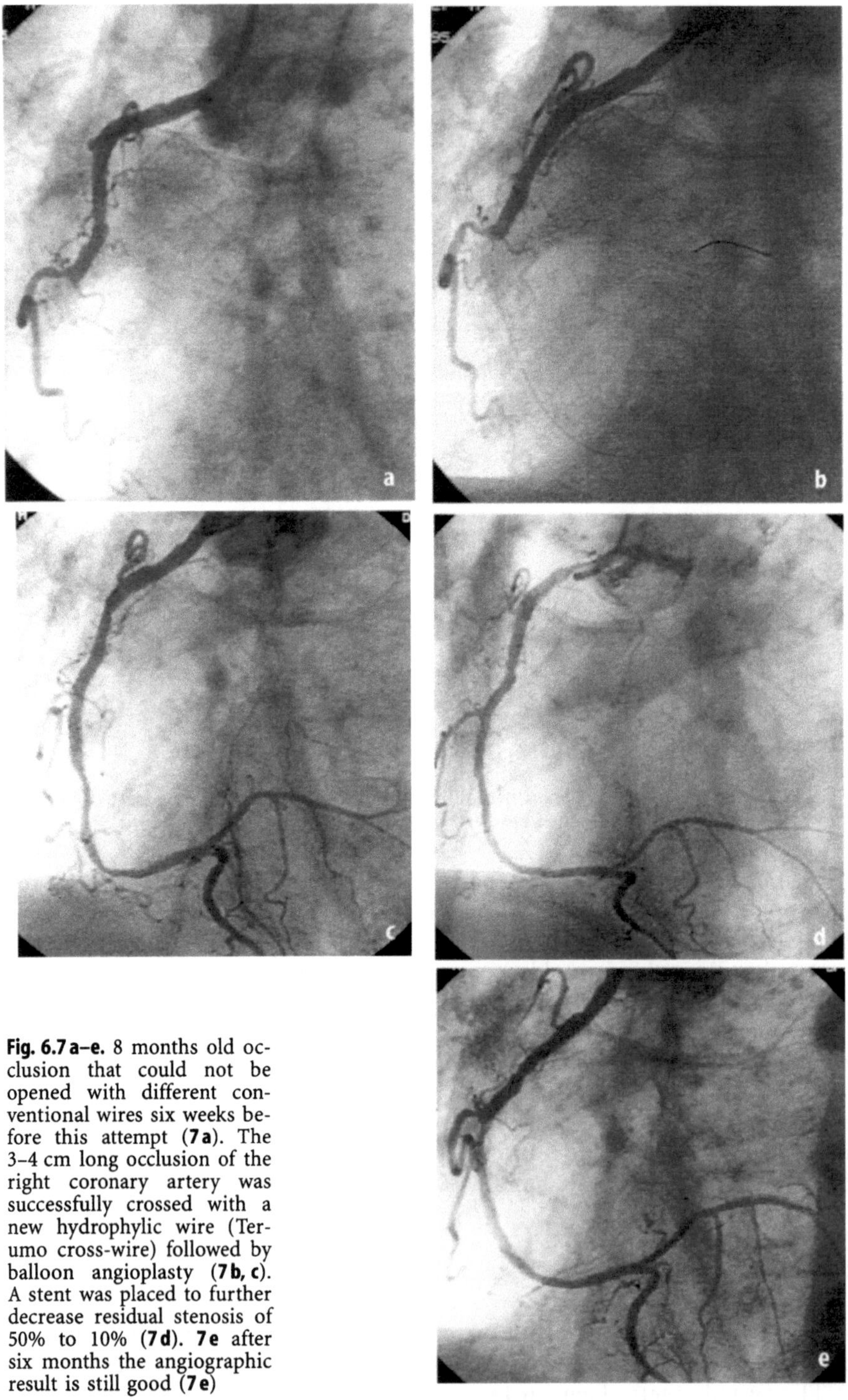

Fig. 6.7 a–e. 8 months old occlusion that could not be opened with different conventional wires six weeks before this attempt (**7 a**). The 3–4 cm long occlusion of the right coronary artery was successfully crossed with a new hydrophylic wire (Terumo cross-wire) followed by balloon angioplasty (**7 b, c**). A stent was placed to further decrease residual stenosis of 50% to 10% (**7 d**). **7 e** after six months the angiographic result is still good (**7 e**)

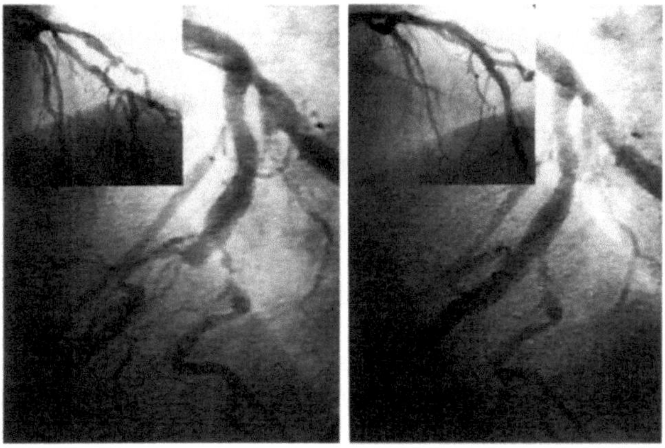

Fig. 6.8. A 24-years old 1.5 cm long occlusion of the LAD that could not be opened with conventional wires was successfully recenalized with a laser wire followed by a laser catheter, balloon, and a stent. The residual stenosis is less than 10%

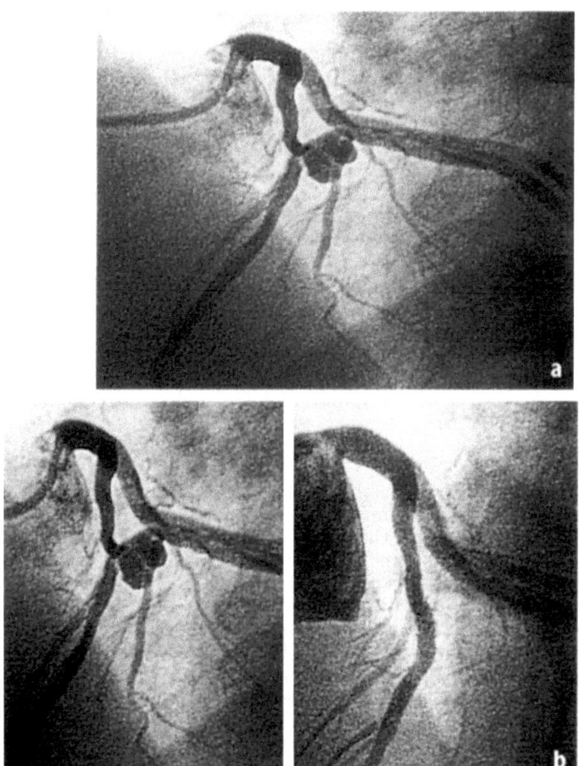

Fig. 6.9 a, b. High grade stenosis of the LAD with a coronary aneurysm is successfully treated by a vein-covered stent. A good long term result could be documented 4 months later

Transmyocardial laser revascularization is applied by cardiac surgeons to improve perfusion of areas that can not be bypassed. In November 1996, we performed the first percutaneous laser myocard revascularization in a patient. So far six of seven patients have been treated successfully without major complications. Five patients experienced significant improvement of symptoms and work capacity after four months.

Since 1977 PTCA as an alternative treatment to coronary artery bypass surgery and medication has overcome many problems, namely acute complications in the cath lab and failure to revascularize complex coronary lesions and treat patients with multi-vessel-disease. While cardiac surgeons proceed with huge steps to minimally invasive techniques, the interventional cardiologists become more and more "aggressive". This means continuous competition, but also a chance for a closer cooperation. To my view, eventually many patients will be treated by combined procedures and by a physician called "interventional cardiac surgeon" or "interventional surgical cardiologist".

References

1. RITA (1993) Trial Participants. Coronary angioplasty versus coronary artery bypass surgery: the Randomized Intervention Treatment of Angina (RITA) trial. Lancet 341:573–580
2. Goy JJ, Eckhout E, Burnand B et al. (1994) Coronary angioplasty versus left internal mammary artery grafting for isolated proximal left anterior descending artery stenosis. Lancet 343:1449–1453
3. Hamm CW, Reimers J, Ischinger T, Rupprecht H-J, Berger J, Bleifeld W (1994) A randomuized study of coronary angioplasty compared with bypass surgery in patients with symptomatic multivessel coronara disease. N Engl J Med 331:1037–1041
4. King SB III, Lembo NJ, Weintraub WS et al. (1994) A randomized trial comparing coronary angioplasty with coronary bypass surgery. N Engl J Med 331:1044–1050
5. CABRI Trial Participants. First-year results of CABRI (coronary Angioplasty versus Bypass Revascularisation Investigation). Lancet 346:1179–1184
6. The Bypass Angioplasty Revascularization Investigation (BARI) Investigators (1996) Comparison of coronary bypass surgery with angioplasty in patients with multivessel disease. N Engl J Med 335:217–225
7. Pocock SJ, Henderson RA, Rickards AF et al. (1995) Meta-analysis of randomized trials comparing coronary angioplasty with bypass surgery. Lancet 346:1184–1189
8. Sim I, Gupta M, McDonald K, Bpourassa MG, Hlatky MA (1995) A meta-analysis of randomized trials comparing coronary artery bypass grafting with percutaneous transluminal coronary angioplasty in multivessel coronary artery disease. Am J Cardiol 76:1025–1029
9. Holmes DR Jr, Bates ER, Kleiman NS, Sadowski Z, Horgan JH, Morris DC, Califf RM, Berger PB, Topol EJ (1995) Contemporary reperfusion therapy for cardiogenic shock: the GUSTO-I trial experience. The GUSTO-I Investigators. Global Utilization of Streptokinase and Tissue Plasminogen Activator for Occluded Coronary Arteries. J Am Coll Cardiol 26:668–674
10. O'Keefe JH Jr, Bailey WL, Rutherford BD, Hartzler GO (1993) Primary angioplasty for acute myocardial infarction in 1,000 consecutive patients. Results in an unselected population and high-risk subgroups. Am J Cardiol 72:107G–115G
11. Lee L, Erbel R, Brown TM, Laufer N, Meyer J, O'Neill WW (1991) Multicenter registry of angioplasty therapy of cardiogenic shock: initial and long-term survival. J Am Coll Cardiol 17:599–603
12. Stevens T, Kahn JK, McCallister BD, Ligon RW, Spaude S, Rutherford BD, McConahay DR, Johnson WL, Giorgi LV, Shimshak TM et al. (1991) Safety and efficacy of percutaneous transluminal coronary angioplasty in patients with left ventricular dysfunction. Am J Cardiol 68:313–319
13. Eltchaninoff H, Franco I, Whitlow PL (1994) Late results of coronary angioplasty in patients with left ventricular ejection fraction<or=40%. Am J Cardiol 73:1047–1052

14. Reifart N, Vandormael M, Krajcar M, Göhring S, Preusler W, Schwarz F, Störger H, Hofmann M, Klöpper J, Müller S, Haase J (1997) Randomized comparison of angioplasty of complex coronary lesions at a single center. Excimer laser, Rotational atherectomy, and Ballon Angioplasty Comparison (ERBAC) study. Circulation 96:91–98
15. Bittl JA (1996) Advances in coronary angioplasty. N Engl J Med 335:1282–1289
16. Fischman DL, Leon MB, Baim DS, Schatz RA, Savage MP, Penn I, Detre K, Veltri L, Ricci D, Nobuyoshi M, Cleman M, Heuser R, Almond D, Teirstein PS, Fish RD, Colombo A, Brinker J, Moses J, Shaknovich A, Hirshfeld J, Bailey S, Ellis S, Rake R, Goldberg S (1994) A randomized comparison of coronary-stent placement and balloon angioplasty in the treatment of coronary artery disease: Stent Restenosis Study Investigators. N Engl J Med 331:496–501
17. Topaz O, Vetrovec GW (1996) The stenotic stent: mechanisms and revascularization options. Cathet Cardiovasc Diagn 37:293–299
18. Hoffmann R, Mintz GS, Dussaillant GR, Popma JJ, Pichard AD, Satler LF, Kent KM, Griffin J, Leon MB (1996) Patterns and mechanisms of in-stent-restenosis. A serial intravascular ultrasound study. Circulation 94:1247–1254

CHAPTER 7

Possibilities and Limits of Cardiac Surgery in Patients with Severe Coronary Artery Disease

C. Schmid · B. Asfour · M. Kondruweit · T.D.T. Tjan · H.H. Scheld

7.1 Introduction

Within the past 10 years, the treatment of patients with coronary artery disease (CAD) has changed dramatically. Various cardiological and surgical procedures have been introduced into clinical practice. Meanwhile, mild CAD is a domain of the cardiologist, whereas patients with severe CAD are referred predominantly to the cardiac surgeon [1, 15]. However, there is no clear borderline: many cases may be treated by either surgeon or cardiologist.

7.2 Indications

In most patients with isolated proximal coronary artery stenosis, percutaneous transluminal coronary angioplasty (PTCA) is simple and effective. Still a contraindication for PTCA, and thus an indication for surgery, is left main stem stenosis and proximal stenosis of the left anterior descending artery. Furthermore, in patients with 3-vessel disease with or without impaired left ventricular function surgical revascularisation is preferred, since long-term results are superior to those obtained with medical therapy [5, 9, 24]. All other patients undergo surgical procedures only if medical or interventional treatments fail or are not applicable. Complications of myocardial infarction may also promote surgery. A large aneurysm of the left ventricular wall with consecutive thromboembolism and ventricular tachycardia can be resected, and tachycardias ablated (Fig. 7.1). Significant mitral incompetence due to ruptured papillary muscles can be treated by various reconstructive techniques or valve replacement. Ventricular septal defect following acute myocardial infarction usually necessitates emergency surgery, with the patients frequently being in poor overall condition. Rhythm disturbances additional to CAD may be treated with antitachycardiac surgery guided by intraoperative mapping, or by implantation of a cardioverter/defibrillator [11, 12]. However, bypass surgery is neither indicated nor possible in all cases. A diameter of the involved vessel of more than 2 mm and a sufficient peripheral run-off are prerequisites for successful coronary revascularisation. Moreover, extreme calcification may necessitate a large endarterectomy or even render an anastomosis impossible; the latter can also be true for an intramural course of a coronary vessel [19, 21]. Nevertheless, even with optimal conditions for surgery, there is still a certain risk. In the best case, it is less than 1%, but it may increase to more than 50%, depending on the patient's condition [16]. Many institutions use a score system to estimate the risk prior to surgery

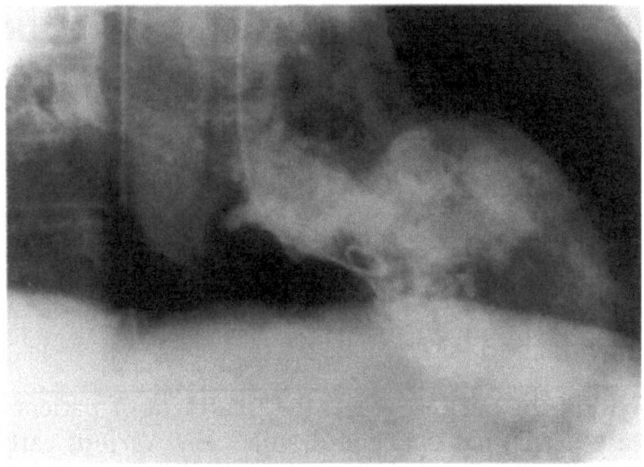

Fig. 7.1. Angiography of a huge left ventricular aneurysm

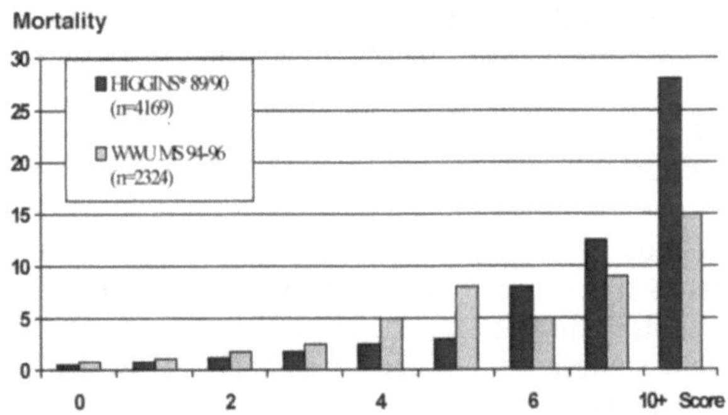

Fig. 7.2. Münster Score in comparison to the Cleveland Score. *Higgins*, Reference 14; *WWUMS*,

[14]. In Münster, we use a modification of the Cleveland Score as depicted in Fig. 7.2, which compares well with that of the Cleveland Clinic and also allows identification of high-risk procedures [17].

7.3 Complications

The limits of bypass surgery are also evident when one looks at complications. Most hazardous is graft occlusion with consecutive myocardial infarction and haemodynamic compromise. Rhythm disturbances, especially atrial fibrillation, are much more frequent but easy to handle. To keep the incidence of postoperative complications as low as possible, optimal patient management has to be initiated prior to surgery. The patients are requested to eliminate their risk factors. We aspire not to operate on patients who are significantly obese or have not terminated their nicotine abuse, except in emergency situations. Lipid levels and antiangina medication should be optimised and carotid arteries investigated by ultrasound or angiography. In case of significant stenosis of an internal carotid artery, we endarterectomise the vessel prior to cardiac surgery. Scintigraphy and positron emission tomography (PET) are used to assess the vitality of the myocardium involved. Only

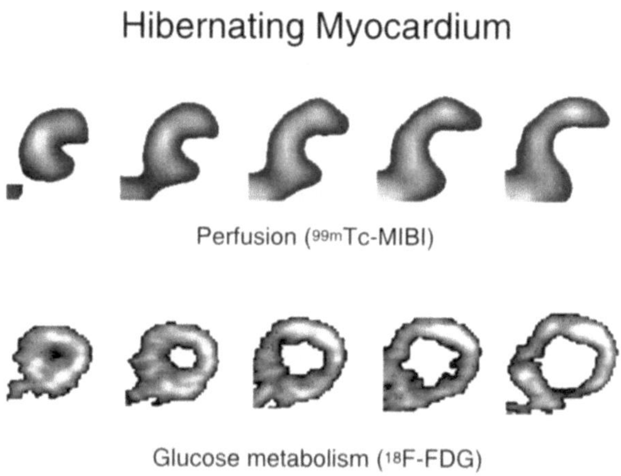

Fig. 7.3. PET demonstrating 'hibernating myocardium': lack of perfusion with still existing metabolism

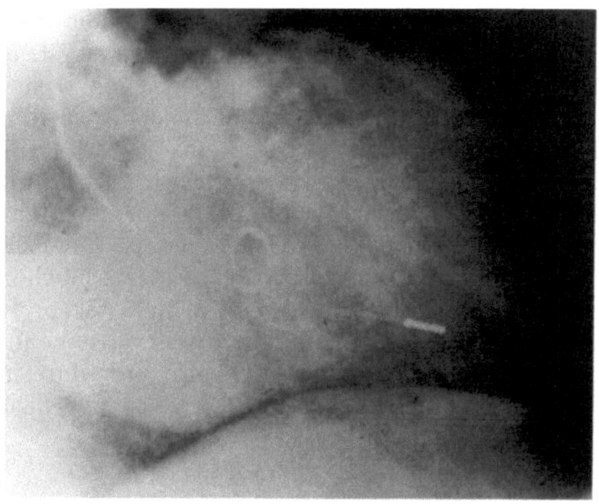

Fig. 7.4. Angiography of severly impaired left ventricular function

PET allows for differentiation of scar and 'hibernating myocardium' (Fig. 7.3), which is of overall importance in borderline indication and high-risk surgery [2, 20].

A further tool for lowering the risk in patients with severely impaired left ventricular pump function is preoperative insertion of an intra-aortic balloon pump (IABP) (Fig. 7.4). The value of prophylactic IABP use has been well demonstrated not only at our institution, but also in many other places [6]. Meanwhile, 10% of all patients have placement of an IABP in our institution, where the preoperative use is as frequent as a postoperative implantation. Thus, not only the perioperative risk, but also the stay on the intensive care ward and the postoperative need for catecholamines can be lowered. Of course, the IABP may also be inserted during surgery.

Further intraoperative means in patients with severe CAD are of a technical nature. We routinely use blood cardioplegia in these patients, which improves myocardial preservation during aortic cross-clamping. Moreover, in these cases we prefer to perform an additional bypass graft rather than omitting one. Nevertheless, we think that more than five bypass grafts are normally not indicated [3, 18]. In selected cases, we perform high-risk surgery with left ventricular assist stand-by. However, this is true only for transplant candidates and will not be further discussed here.

7.4 Postoperative Management

Postoperatively, patients should be mobilised as quickly as possible. During intensive care, patients must be stabilised with catecholamines and vasodilative treatment and should be extubated as early as possible to prevent development of pneumonia. Apart from physical therapy, adequate analgesia is important for mobilisation, as thoracic drains are rather unpleasant [10]. Our anaesthetists use peridural anaesthesia combined with an external pump system, which enables patients to apply an additional bolus of analgetics if pain persists or increases. These drug-delivery systems guarantee more or less freedom from pain for most patients and seem to facilitate rehabilitation considerably in difficult cases. Such sophisticated analgesia is very important in combination with short-term anaesthesia during minimally invasive surgery and 'fast-track recovery', which has found broad use all over the world within a short period of time [8]. Major intentions have been and remain to lower costs and improve cosmetic results. However, there are also advantages for a special subgroup of patients. Patients in whom the use of extracorporeal circulation is associated with a high risk or is even impossible may be provided with a mammary artery graft, in some institutions even with multiple grafts [4]. In a so-called hybrid procedure, minimally invasive bypass surgery is combined with consecutive balloon dilatation at a different site in the coronary system.

7.5 Current Situation

There is no definitive cure for patients with CAD, as the latter progresses steadily. Bypass grafts occlude with time, and long-term results and the superiority of arterial over venous bypass grafts are well known [13]. Recurrent angina may ensue and reoperation is indicated. Redo surgery and third-stage procedures are becoming more and more frequent, and less graft material is available with each operation. If the first bypass procedure was performed many years ago one may use the current standard, the mammary artery; during the past 5–10 years venous bypass grafts have been performed almost exclusively. Use of bilateral mammary arteries should be limited to patients without diabetes mellitus, of the gastroepiploic artery to those without previous abdominal surgery. The radial and epigastric artery can be used only as a free graft, which enhances the surgical task. For venous grafts, not only the major but also the minor saphenous veins may be harvested, even if it is somewhat troublesome with the patient in a supine position. In rare cases we use veins from the forearm; however, these grafts have a weak vessel wall and a large calibre, i.e. are unsuitable in most cases [22]. An increasing number of patients are being referred for surgical revascularisation in whom both mammary arteries have been used during previous operations and there are no further vein grafts to harvest. As artificial grafts have lead to disappointing results over many years, we use a PTFE graft with a Venturi mechanism in these patients. This artificial graft is anastomosed to the aorta at its proximal end; the coronary anastomoses are performed side-to-side, and the end of the graft with the Venturi mechanism is attached to the right atrial appendage or superior vena cava [7, 23].

7.6 Conclusion

In conclusion, the use for surgical revascularisation of patients with CAD has shifted towards more interventional procedures. However, severe CAD remains a domain of the cardiac surgeon. Multiple technical improvements have increased the possibilities and lowered the risk for surgery. Nevertheless, there is a certain threshold beyond which no bypass surgery is possible. To date it is not known whether transmyocardial laser revascularisation or only heart transplantation may be helpful under these end-stage conditions.

References

1. Guidelines and indications for coronary artery bypass graft surgery. A report of the American College of Cardiology/American Heart Association task force on assessment of diagnostic and therapeutic cardiovascular procedures (subcommittee on coronary artery bypass graft surgery). J Am Coll Cardiol 17:543–589
2. Braunwald E, Rutherford JD (1986) Reversible ischemic left ventricular dysfunction: evidence for the "hibernating myocardium". J Am Coll Cardiol 8:1467–1470
3. Buckberg GD (1990) Oxygenated cardioplegia: blood is a many splendored thing. Ann Thorac Surg 50:175–177
4. Califiore AM, Di Giammarco G, Luciani N, Maddestra N, Di Nardo E, Angelini R (1994) Composite arterial conduits for a wider arterial myocardial revascularization. Ann Thorac Surg 58:185–190
5. CASS principal investigators and their associates (1983) Coronary Artery Surgery Study (CASS), a randomized trial of coronary artery bypass surgery survival data. Circulation 68:939–950
6. Dietl C, Berkheimer MD, Woods EL, Gilbert CL, Pharr WF, Benoit CH (1996) Efficacy and cost-effectiveness or preoperative IABP in patients with ejection fraction of 0.25 or less. Ann Thorac Surg 62:401–409
7. Emery RW, Joyce LD, Arom KV, King RM, Nicoloff DM (1994) Operative considerations in implantation of the Perma-Flow graft. Ann Thorac Surg 58:1770–1773
8. Engelman RM (1996) Mechanisms to reduce hospital stays. Ann Thorac Surg 61 [Suppl 2]:S26-S29
9. European Coronary Surgery Study Group (1982) Long-term results of prospective randomized study of coronary artery bypass surgery in stable angina. Lancet 2:1173–1180
10. Glass PS (1995) Pharmacokinetic and pharmacodynamic principles in providing "fast-track" recovery. J Cardiothorac Vasc Anesth 9 [Suppl 1]:16–20
11. Hammel D, Block M, Konertz W, Borggrefe M, Isbruch F, Asfour B, Geiger A, Breithardt G, Scheld HH (1993) Surgical experience with defibrillators using nonthoracotomy leads. Ann Thorac Surg 55:685–693
12. Hammel D, Borggrefe M, Scheld HH, Möllhoff T, Schmid C (1996) Hat die VT-CHirurgie im Zeitalter transvenöser Defibrillatoren noch einen Stellenwert? Thorac Cardiovasc Surg 44 [Suppl I]:92

13. Hannan RL, Gersh BJ (1995) Recent reports on long-term results of coronary artery bypass grafting. Curr Opinion Cardiol 10:549–555
14. Higgins TL, Estafanous FG, Loop FD, Beck GJ, Blum JM, Paranandi L (1992) Stratification of morbidity and mortality outcome by preoperative risk factors in coronary artery bypass patients. JAMA 26:2344–2348
15. Muhlbaier LH, Pryor DB, Rankin JS, Smith LR, Mark DB, Jones RH, Glower DD, Harrell FE, Lee KL, Califf RM, Sabiston DC (1992) Observational comparison of event-free survival with medical and surgical therapy in patients with coronary artery disease: 20 years of follow-up. Circulation 86 [Suppl II]:198–204
16. Nashef SAM, Carey F, Silcock MM, Oommen PK, Levy RD, Jones MT (1992) Risk stratification for open heart surgery: trial of the Parsonnet system in a British hospital. Br Med J 305:1066–1067
17. Roeder N, Kondruweit M, Köpcke W, Scheld HH (1996) Scoresysteme zur Charakterisierung von Patientenprofilen. In: Baur M, Fimmers R (eds) GMDS 96. MMV Medizin Verlag: Munich
18. Scheld HH, Deng MC, Schmid C, Hammel D (1995) Koronarchirurgie - Münsteraner Konzept. Z Herz-, Thorax-, Gefäßchirur 9:1–8
19. Scheld HH, Görlach G, Mulch J, Loskot F, Stein A (1986) Kann die PTFE-Prothese zur Revaskularisation der rechten Koronararterie verwendet werden? Thorac Cardiovasc Surg 34:25
20. Scheld HH, Soeparwata R, Deng MC, Deiwick M, Roeder N (1996) Operationen bei eingeschränkter linksventrikulärer Pumpfunktion. Z Kardiol 85 [Suppl 6]:287–301
21. Schmid C, Hammel D, Kerber S, Schober O, Scheld HH (1996) Indikation zur operativen koronaren Revaskularisation. Chir Praxis 51:477–483
22. Schmid C, Scheld HH (1996) Trends and strategies for myocardial revascularization. Thorac Cardiovasc Surg 44:113–117
23. Schmid C, Weyand M, Kerber S, Breithardt G, Scheld HH (1996) The use of a Perma-Flow graft for coronary artery bypass surgery. Eur J Cardiothorac Surg 10:284–286
24. The Veterans Administrations Coronary Study Group (1984) Eleven-year survival in the Veterans Administration randomized trial of coronary bypass surgery for stable angina. N Engl J Med 311:333–339

CHAPTER 8

Borderline Indications for Heart Transplantation and Alternative Measures

M. M. KOERNER · G. TENDERICH · R. KOERFER

8.1 Introduction

At the present time, approx. 1–2% of the population of the Western world contract cardiac insufficiency, usually therapy-resistant and terminal. Orthotopic heart transplantation (HT) represents the only currently available curative form of therapy with a justifiable 5-year survival prognosis (Ref. 12). The growing mismatch between donor pool and recipient group has provoked constant discussion about the criteria for inclusion and exclusion in these groups (Refs. 18, 28). Whereas in the initial stages of HT recipient age and concomitant diseases were crucial criteria for recipient selection, improved chances of survival caused these criteria to be relaxed (Ref. 12). Biological age is becoming more and more predominant in the selection of recipients. Concomitant diseases, such as diabetes mellitus, hepatitis B/C, secondary amyloidosis, condition following neoplasia beyond the 5-year recurrence rate no longer represent contraindications (Refs. 23, 26, 16, 17). Current contraindications for orthotopic HT include fixed pulmonary hypertension (>5 Wood units), active acute infections and HIV infections.

According to a saying, thought to be from the Chinese philosopher Confucius (551-479 B.C.), "*there are three ways of acting intelligently: through thinking, which is the most noble; through imitating, which is the most simple; through experience, which is the most bitter*". Bitter experience could also apply to the field of endstage heart failure treatment.

Nowadays, alternative measures and bridging procedures in cases of borderline indications for HT are differentiated and in a constant state of expansion and improvement, in line with the status of terminal cardiac insufficiency. In special cardiac insufficiency/cardiac failure programs, the following procedures are applied before a possible HT or in combination as alternative measures. Some of these methods, such as the Batista operation with or without cardiomyoplasty, are to be viewed as experimental procedures, the uncritical and euphoric application of which has been warned against by the American Society of Thoracic Surgeons (Ref. 32). Which therapeutic methods are actually applied and which benefits the individual patient actually receives frequently depend upon the experience and estimation of the individual centers involved:

1) Bridging with drugs: beta-blockers, e.g. carvedilol, alpha-blockers, e.g. prazocine, angiotensin-receptor T1- or -receptor T2-antagonists, growth hormone antagonists, brainnatiuretic peptide analogs, intermittent or long-term, also out-patient, iv medication with phosphodiesterase inhibitors, catecholamines, prostaglandins, urokinase (Ref. 20), NO respiration.

2) 'High-risk' interventions and/or cardiac preservation measures: Norwood procedure, mitral valve valvuloplasty or replacement in cases of dilatative cardiomyopathy (DCM) (Ref. 21), partial left-ventricular resection surgery – Batista operation – in cases of DCM (Refs. 3, 8), dynamic cardiomyoplasty (Ref. 29), cardiomyopexy, cardioomentopexy, cardiopericardiopexy, Vineberg operation, bypass grafting and/or transmyocardial laser revascularization (TMLR) attempts, spinal cord stimulation in cases of refractory angina pectoris (Refs. 11, 24, 25, 36, 37).
3) Bridging with devices: four chamber pacing (Refs. 5, 10), automatic implantable cardioverter defibrillator (AICD) (Ref. 34), continuous veno-venous high-volume hemofiltration (CVVH) (Ref. 13), heparin-mediated extracorporeal low-density lipoprotein cholesterol precipitation (HELP apheresis) (Ref. 4).
4) Mechanical circulatory support: intraaortic balloon counterpulsation, femoro-femoral mechanical circulatory support (MCS) with oxygenator, non-pulsatile MCS (centrifugal pump) as left-ventricular assist device (LVAD), right-ventricular assist device (RVAD) or biventricular assist device (BVAD), intrathoracic and/or extrathoracic MCS with/without oxygenator as bridging (temporary) or permanent LVAD/RVAD/BVAD. IVOX/Hemopump are currently being tested.

The total artificial heart is currently undergoing approval in its mechanical version for its effectiveness and benefit as a long-term MCS for the candidate (Refs. 22, 30). Xenografts are not yet justified for clinical use (Refs. 33, 9, 2, 27).

8.2 The indications for HT

An indication fundamentally exists whenever the risk of the intervention, as well as the long-term risks following HT, are lower than the individually estimated risk of the terminal therapy-resistant severe cardiac insufficiency, especially true when the maximum O_2 consumption is 10–12 ml/kg/min/m^2, the cardiac index is <2.0 l/min/m^2, the left-ventricular ejection fraction (EF) is <20% and the pulmonary pressure increases to pathological ranges under stress (Refs. 23, 35, 26, 14, 15, 16, 17).

The Thoracic Organ Transplantation Committee of the United Network of Organ Sharing proposed the following guidelines for placing adult patients on the waiting list (Ref. 35) which are continually under discussion:

I) Heart failure
a. Cardiogenic shock or low output state with reversible end-organ dysfunction requiring MCS.
b. Low output state or refractory heart failure requiring continuous inotropic support.
c. Advanced heart failure signs and symptoms (NYHA Classes III and IV) with objective documentation of marked functional limitation and poor 12 month prognosis despite maximized medical therapy.
d. Recurrent or rapidly progressive heart failure symptoms unresponsive to maximized vasodilatators and a flexible diuretic program.

e. Severe hypertrophic or restrictive cardiomyopathy with NYHA Class IV heart failure or anginal symptoms.

II) Refractory angina pectoris
a. Severe ischemic symptoms consistently limiting day-to-day activity and not amenable to conventional revascularization, with objective evidence for angina pectoris and extensive myocardial ischemia after optimization of medical therapy.
b. Recurrent unstable myocardial ischemic syndromes requiring multiple hospitalizations in patients unable to undergo conventional revascularization.
c. Life threatening coronary anatomy (such as a critical left main stenosis), not amenable to conventional coronary revascularisation.

III) Life-threatening refractory ventricular arrhythmia
a. Recurrent symptomatic life-threatening ventricular arrhythmias that cannot be controlled by all appropriate conventional medical and surgical modalities.
b. Prolonged periods of documented-electromechanical disassociation following AICD conversion of ventricular tachycardia or ventricular fibrillation to normal sinus rhythm.

IV) Cardiac tumor
a. Tumor confined to the myocardium.
b. No evidence for distant disease revealed by an extensive metastatic work-up. Tumors with a very high likelihood of metastasis despite an initial negative work-up should preclude transplant listing.

To list infants and children for heart transplantation, the patient must have one of the following:

I) Hypoplastic left heart syndrome
II) Complex congenital heart disease not amenable to conventional surgical repair or palliation with progressive ventricular failure or progressive cyanosis.
III) Cardiomyopathy with supportive findings outlined in the guidelines.

8.3 Alternative measures in Cases of Borderline Indications for Orthotopic HT: Some Comments

Cardiac insufficiency may occur in three different forms: systolic, diastolic and combined.

In the case of *ischemic heart disease* (IHD) with an EF ≥30% and/or angina pectoris and/or arrhythmia, the following alternative therapies may be attempted:

- Re-CABG with VAD readiness
- PTCA/rotablation
- Laser/with simultaneous revascularization as required
- Cardiomyoplasty

- Cardiomyopexy, Vineberg operation
- AICD
- Four chamber pacing
- (Spinal cord blockade)

In the case of a *primary mitral insufficiency*:
- Mitral valve replacement
- Reconstruction or valvuloplasty

In cases of extinguished vitia with EF ≤30%, thin left-ventricular walls or pulmonary hypertension, HT is the only viable option.

In the case of a *secondary mitral regurgitation* with IHD or DCM:
- Mitral valve replacement or reconstruction/valvuloplasty, except when:
  1. global systolic dysfunction (EF ≤30%) exists
  2. LV walls are thinner than 8 mm without profiting from volume reduction
  3. in the echo the transmitral flow is more than 1 m/sec and the isovolumetric relaxation phase is <70 ms
  4. in the stress echo (dobutamine iv or exercise) the EF does not increase or the walls thicken: in this case we believe HT to be the only viable option.

In the case of an *aortic vitia with normal blood pressure*:
- combined aortic vitia: the operation should be carried out earlier than with isolated aortic stenosis or insufficiency due to the volume and pressure burden
- aortic regurgitation: to be evaluated similarly to mitral valve insufficiency. If a structural dilatation exists, a remodeling is improbable so that HT is the only viable option.
- hypertrophic obstructive cardiomyopathy: myectomy/ catheter ablation with controlled infarction: only when indicated

TMLR is only applied in our hospital in selected individual cases. 16 interventions are currently carried out in 6 operating rooms using extracorporeal circulation with the help of the heart-lung machine, amounting to an annual rate of 4000 interventions. In cases of a vascular finding which can no longer be revascularized and an EF ≤30%, evidence of ischemia is required in the surface electrocardiogram, the positron emission tomogram and myocardial scintigraphy.

At least one well perfused myocardial area must be objectifiable. This was possible 6 times within a follow-up of 1–11 months. The following findings resulted:

- no improvement in EF, segmental wall contractility or ergometric performance
- evidence of restricted perfusion under stress in one patient (TMLR in combination with CABG).

8.4 Bad Oeynhausen's Heart Transplant Program

8.4.1 Experience with Borderline Indications and Results

From 3/89 to 5/97, 834 HT were carried out in our center in 699 male and 135 female recipients aged between 2 days and 77 years (mean 49.6 years). Donor age ranged from 1 day to 66 years (mean 33 years). The causes for terminal therapy-resistant cardiac insufficiency were DCM in 414 (49.6%), IHD in 317 (38%), valvular heart disease in 47 (5.6%), congenital heart disease in 27 (3.2%), acute or chronic graft failure in 13 (1.6%) and miscellaneous in 16 (1.9%). The current survival curve according to Kaplan Meyer reveals a 1-year survival rate for women and men of 80% and a 5-year survival rate of 75% (see Fig. 1). The recipient group aged under 16 years even demonstrated a 5-year survival rate of 85%, observed in isolation in the presence of DCM. In contrast, the comparable age group with congenital heart defects demonstrated a 1-year survival of just 70%, caused by the necessity of an already complicated procedure with HT due to potentially co-existent vascular deformities or status following one or more pallations (see Fig. 2). The HT of 60-year olds is the exception at practically all the centers worldwide: firstly because of the age itself, then the potential concomitant diseases and also the higher de novo malignancy rate under immunosuppression. And yet the short and long-term results of our center, approaching a 5-year survival rate of 70% for the age group >60 years (n=240), justify the diagnosis and performance of HT, especially considering the fact that hearts from donors aged 55 to 66 years have also been successfully implanted (see Fig. 3; Ref. 14). Through intensive individual care and training, the 5-year survival rate for insulin-dependent diabetics in our center following HT is 70% (n=35; 10 deaths). The re-transplantation results are not encouraging - in accordance with the international results (1-year survival just 40%), the indication exists only in cases of early graft failure within the first 7 days, or in special recipients several years, after primary HT.

HT is not a contraindication in patients with a 5-year prognosis of ≥70% for a pre-existing malignancy after chemotherapy, radiation and/or surgery, especially if there has been a recurrence-free interval of about a year and if extended donor criteria are applied (Ref. 17).

For a later HT, the implantation of a VAD as bridging or in cases of post-cardiotomy syndrome has significant advantages within the first 3 years after HT, insofar as with the MCS no complications such as infections, thromboembolisms or apoplexy occur, explained best by the possibility of organ recovery from multi-organ failure caused by cardiac insufficiency and/or cardiogenic shock: from 117 patients with previous MCS, nearly 90% are still alive one year later, albeit 75% after 5 years, as for the conventional, direct heart recipients (see Fig. 4; Ref. 19).

Permanent VAD support in cases of borderline indications or contraindications for HT is reserved for special patients, since only a few case reports about individual successful LVAD therapies over a period of up to 2 years,

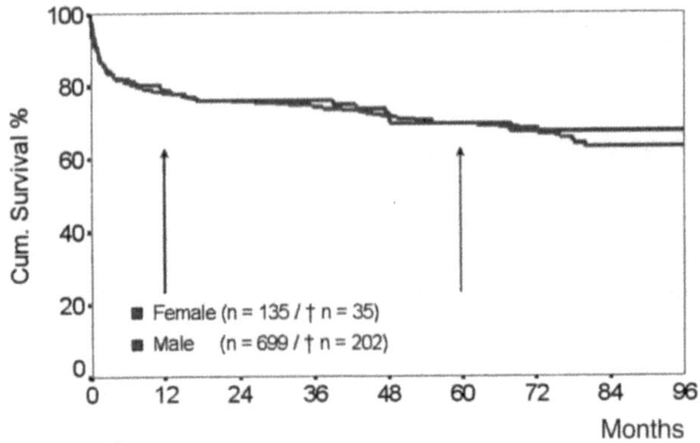

Fig. 8.1

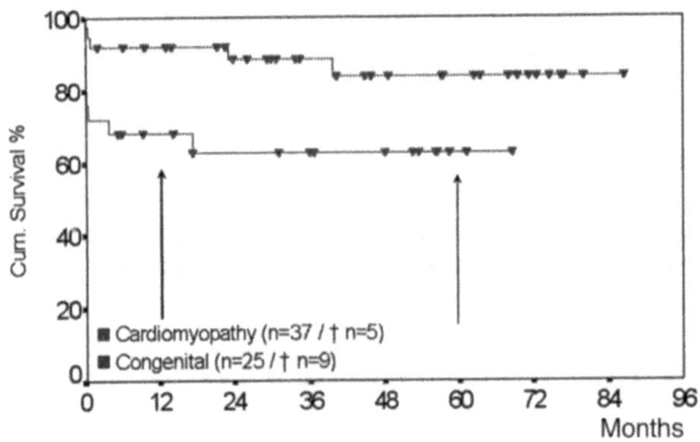

Fig. 8.2

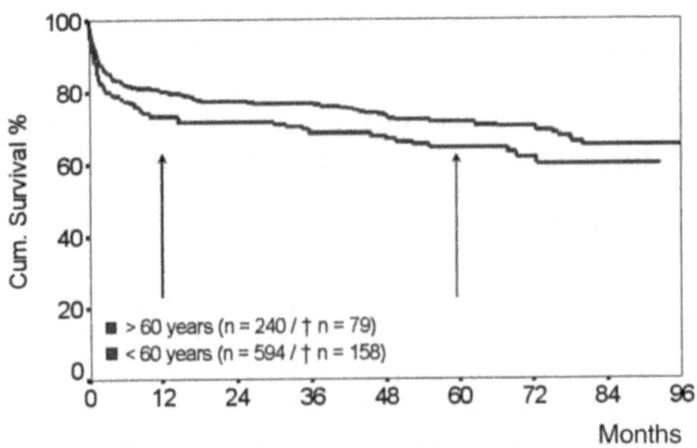

Fig. 8.3

Fig. 8.1. Current survival in female vs. male heart transplant recipients at the Heart Center Northrhine-Westphalia

Fig. 8.2. Current survival in pediatric (<16 years) heart transplant recipients (cardiomyopathy vs. congenital) at the Heart Center Northrhine-Westphalia

Fig. 8.3. Current survival in heart transplant recipients >60 years old vs. <60 years old at the Heart Center Northrhine-Westphalia

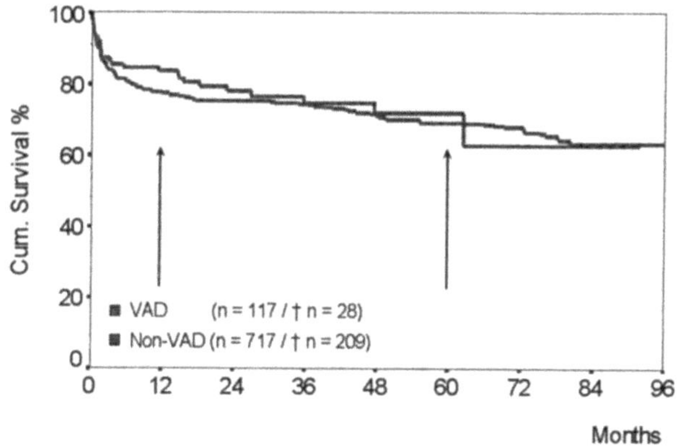

Fig. 8.4. Current survival of recipients with conventional HT vs. VAD prior to transplantation at the Heart Center Northrhine-Westphalia

Age/Gender (years)	*Diagnosis of Heart Disease*	*Cause of HTx Contraindication*	*VAD-System used*	*Duration of support*	*Outcome*
61 f	*DCM, NYHA IV*	*breast-cancer years ago, radiatio*	*LVAD Novacor*	*354*	*HTx 5/95 alive*
71 m	*IHD, NYHA IV*	*age, decision of the patient*	*LVAD Novacor*	*12*	*MOF expired*
63 m	*IHD, NYHA IV + IABP, +CVVH*	*age / multi-organfailure (MOF)*	*LVAD Novacor*	*5*	*MOF expired*
57 m	*DCM, NYHA IV 7 years post HTx*	*non-compliance*	*LVAD Novacor*	*74*	*apoplexia pneum. expired*
53 m	*DCM, non-Hodgkin chemotherapy*	*non-Hodgkin lymphoma*	*LVAD Novacor*	*5*	*gutperfor. expired*
66 m	*DCM*	*leukemia*	*LVAD Heart-Mate*	*160*	*alive*
5 m / 1 f	*4 DCM / 2 IHD*		*6 x LVAD*	*5-354 days (m: 101.7)*	*2 alive 4 expired*

Fig. 8.5. Permanent VAD support in patients with heart transplant contraindications at the Heart Center Northrhine-Westphalia

maintaining a small proportion of the functions of the own heart, have as yet been published. Our own results with a small number of cases bearing this diagnosis are not encouraging (see Fig. 5). Efforts to develop an implantable total artificial heart for long-term use are continuing without interruption, with no justifiable operation or alternative to HT currently being able to be offered to the affected patients (Refs. 22, 30).

8.5 Conclusion

HT represents the only currently available curative therapeutic option for terminal therapy-resistant cardiac insufficiency with a justifiable 5-year survival prognosis. With a view to the enormous number of pre-diagnosed/indicated patients currently being put forward for HT, ranging from infants to old age citizens, it is vital that attention continues to be paid to an appropriate, correct, differential therapeutic decision, which should always be an individual decision calculating the risks involved – relative to the possibilities and experience possessed by the physicians responsible. This form of therapy should, in our opinion, be reserved for a small number of specialist centers, and consolidation in this direction is to be attempted (Ref. 1).

8.6 Acknowledgments

The authors wish to thank Mrs Sarah L. Kirkby for her linguistic and technical assistance in preparing this article. Mr Stephan Wlost for preparing the graphs. Major support was given by the German Association of Organ Recipients (Reg. Assoc.).

References

1. Abraham WT, Bristow MR (1997) Specialized centers for heart failure management. Circulation 96:2755–2757
2. Bailey CL, Nehlsen-Cannarella SL, Conception W, Jolley WB (1985) Baboon-to-human cardiac xenotransplantation in a neonate. JAMA 254:3321–3329
3. Batista RJV, Santos JLV, Takeshita N, Bocchino Lise, Lima PN, Cunha MA (1996) Partial left ventriculectomy to improve left ventricular function in end-stage heart disease. J Card Surg 11:96–97
4. Brown G, Albers JJ, Fisher LD, et al. (1990) Regression of coronary artery disease as a result of intensive lipid-lowering therapy in men with high levels of apolipoprotein. N Engl J Med 323:1289–1298
5. Cazeau S, Ritter P, Bakdach S, Lazarus A, Limousin M (1994) Four chamber pacing in dilated cardiomyopathy. PACE 17:1974–1979
6. Chachques JC, Berrebi A, Hernigou A, Cohen-Solal A, Lavergne T, Marino J-P, D'Attellis N, Bensasson D, Carpentier A (1997) Study of muscular and ventricular function in dynamic cardiomyoplasty: A ten-year follow-up. J Heart Lung Transplant 16:854–868
7. Czaplicki J, Blonska B, Religa Z (1992) The lack of hyperacute xenogeneic heart transplant rejection in a human (letter). J Heart Lung Transplant 11:393–397
8. Dickstein ML, Spotnitz HM, Rose EA, Burkhoff D (1997) Heart reduction surgery: an analysis of the impact on cardiac function. J Thorac Cardiovasc Surg 113:1032–1040
9. Hardy JD, Chavez CM, Kurrus FD, Neely WA, Eraslan S, Turner MD, Fabian LW, Labecki TD (1964) Heart transplantation in man: Developmental studies and report of a case. JAMA 188:1132–1140
10. Hochleitner M, Hoertnagl H, Choi-Keung Ng, et al. (1990) Usefulness of physiological dual-chamber pacing in drug-resistant idiopathic dilated cardiomyopathy. Am J Cardiol 66:198–202
11. Horvath KA, Cohn LH, Cooley DA, Crew JR, Frazier OH, Griffith BP, Kadipasaoglu K, Lansing A, Mannting F, March R, Mirhoseini MR, Smith C (1997) Transmyocardial laser revascularization: results of a multicenter trial with transmyocardial laser revascularization used as sole therapy for end-stage coronary artery disease. J Thorac Cardiovasc Surg 113:645–654

12. Hosenpud JD, Novick RJ, Bennett LE, Keck BM, Fiol B, Daily OP (1996) The Registry of the International Society for Heart and Lung Transplantation: Thirteenth Official Report - 1996, J Heart Lung Transplant 15:655-674
13. Koerner MM, El Banayosy A, Posival H, Gromzik H, Koerfer R (1990) Ventricular assist device (VAD) systems combined with continuous high volume venous-venous hemofiltration (CVVH). Intensivbehandlung 15 Suppl.:A 104
14. Koerner MM, Tenderich G, Minami K, El-Banayosy A, Koertke H, Mannebach H, Baller D, Kleesiek K, Gleichmann U, Koerfer R (1996) Rare indication: heart transplantation in recipients aged 70 years and older. Cardiology in the Elderly 4:171-175
15. Koerner MM, Tenderich G, Mannebach H, Minami K, El-Banayosy A, Koertke H, Wlost S, Gromzik H, Kleesiek K, Meyer H, Gleichmann U, Koerfer R (1996) Heart transplantation at the Heart Center North Rhine-Westphalia in Bad Oeynhausen - 1995 Report. In Clinical Transplants 1995. Edited by Terasaki J, Cecka JM. Los Angeles: UCLA Tissue Typing Laboratory 137-144
16. Koerner MM, Tenderich G, Minami K, zu Knyphausen E, Mannebach H, Kleesiek K, Meyer H, Koerfer R (1997) Heart transplantation for end-stage heart failure caused by iron overload. B J Haematol 97:293-296
17. Koerner MM, Tenderich G, Minami K, Mannebach H, Koertke H, zu Knyphausen E, El-Banayosy A, Baller D, Kleesiek K, Gleichmann U, Meyer H, Koerfer R (1997) Results of heart transplantation in patients with preexisting malignancies. Am J Cardiol 79:988-991
18. Koerner MM, Tenderich G, Posival H, Minami K, Mannebach H, zu Knyphausen E, Thies WR, Kleesiek K, Gleichmann U, Meyer H, Koerfer R (1995) Rare indication and long-term results after heart transplantation, In: Current aspects and concepts of nursing, coordinating, bridging and rehabilitation in organ transplantation. Excerpta medica, Koerner MM, Koerfer R (eds) Elsevier Science B.V., Amsterdam, pp. 213-230
19. Koerner MM, Tenderich G, El-Banayosy A, Minami K, Mannebach H, Meyer H, Koerfer R (1996) Longterm results of heart transplantation after use of ventricular assist devices. J Heart Lung Transplant 15 (suppl):S 86
20. Leschke M, Schoebel FC, Mecklenbeck W, Stein D, Jax TW, Müller-Gärtner HW, Strauer BE (1996) Long-term intermittend urokinase therapy in patients with end-stage coronary artery disease and refractory angina pectoris: A randomized dose-response trial. J Am Coll Cardiol 27:575-584
21. McCarthy PM, Starling RC, Smedira NG, Buda TM, Scalia GM, Young JB (1997) Partial ventriculectomy with valve repair as an alternative to cardiac transplantation. J Heart Lung Transplant 16:A 41
22. Mehta SM, Aufiero TX, Pae WE Jr, Miller CA, Pierce WS (1995) Combined registry for the clinical use of mechanical ventricular assist pumps and the total artificial heart in conjunction with heart transplantation: sixth official report - 1994. J Heart Lung Transplant 14:584-593
23. Miller LW, Kubo SH, Young JB, Stevenson LW, Loh E, Costanzo MR (1995) Report of the Consensus Conference on Candidate Selection for Heart Transplantation - 1993. J Heart Lung Transplant 14:562-571
24. Mirhoseini M, Cayton MM (1981) Revascularization of the heart by laser. Microsurgery 2:253-260
25. Moosdorf R, Schoebel F-C, Hort W (1997) Transmyokardiale Laserrevaskularisation - morphologische, pathophysiologische und historische Grundlagen der indirekten Revaskularisation des Herzmuskels. Z Kardiol 86:149-164
26. Mudge GH, Goldstein S, Addonizio LJ, Caplan A, Mancini D, Levine TB, Ritsch ME, Stevenson LW (1993) Task Force 3: Recipient guidelines/Prioritization. JACC 22:1-64
27. Murphy FA (1996) The public health risk of animal organ and tissue transplantation into humans. Science 273:746-747
28. Novitzky D (1996) Selection and managment of cardiac allograft donors. Current Opinion in Cardiology 11:174-182
29. Patel HJ, Lankford EB, Polidori DJ, Pilla JJ, Plappert T, Sutton MStJ, Acker MA (1997) Dynamic cardiomyoplasty: its chronic and acute effects on the failing heart. J Thorac Cardiovasc Surg 114:169-178
30. Pierce WS, Sapirstein JS, Pae WE (1996) Total artificial heart: from bridge to transplantation to permanent use. Ann Thorac Sur 61:342-346
31. Rector TS, Benditt D, Chachques JC, Chiu R C-J, Delahaye F, Jessup M, Kirkorian G, Thiene G (1997) Titus J for the Worldwide Cardiomyoplasty Group, Retrospective analysis for early heart-related death after cardiomyoplasty. Heart Lung Transplant 16:1018-1025

32. Replogle RL, Kaiser GC (1997) Left ventricular reduction surgery (Society position paper). Ann Thorac Surg 63:909–910
33. Stoye J et al. (1997) Two sets of human-tropic pig retrovirus (letter), Nature 389:681–682
34. Sweeney MO, Ruskin JN, Garan H, McGovern BA, Guy ML, Torchiana DF, Vlahakes GJ, Newell JB, Semigran MJ, Dec GW (1995) Influence of the implantable cardioverter/defibrillator on sudden death and total mortality in patients evaluated for cardiac transplantation. Circulation 92:3273–3281
35. United Network for Organ Sharing (1996) Update: Listing Criteria Approved for Public Comment. Vol 12. Washington, DC: UNOS pp. 8
36. Vineberg A (1954) Clinical and experimental studies in the treatment of coronary artery insufficiency by internal mammary artery implant. J Int Coll Surg 22:503–518
37. Oosterga M, ten Vaarwerk IAM, DeJongste MJL, Staal MJ (1997) Spinal cord stimulation in refractory angina pectoris – Clinical results and mechanisms. Z Kardiol 86:107–113

PART III

Laser Techniques

CHAPTER 9

The History of Transmyocardial Revascularization

J.C. FISHER

9.1 Early Attempts at TMR

In 1933, J.T. Wearn [1] reported the discovery of natural channels connecting the left ventricular chamber to the myocardial interspaces of the human heart. The transmyocardial channels were confirmed microscopically by gelatin filling of these tiny clusters of "arteries". They connected distally to other channels woven into the fabric of the muscular fibers; these distal channels were termed *myocardial sinusoids*. Earlier, in 1708, Adam Christian Thebesius (1686–1732), a German physician, had described connections of the coronary veins with the myocardium, which were named *thebesian* veins in recognition of his discovery. In 1898 the American physiologist F.H. Pratt perfused oxygenated blood through the left ventricular wall in a cat and kept it alive for more than an hour with this myocardial blood supply alone. In 1926, R.T. Grant reported that a congenitally deformed child had cardiac sinusoids connecting with the surrounding veins and arteries. In 1935, Claude Beck [2] reported in the *Annals of Surgery* his development of a new means of supplying blood to the myocardium. This external source of blood from the epicardial surface, which he called "myocardial neocapillary formation", was produced by iatrogenic, traumatic scarring of the myocardium, combined with omentopexy and myopexy.

The Vineberg procedure [3], reported experimentally in 1954, used as its blood source the internal mammary artery, which was implanted in a mechanically created tunnel from the epicardial surface into the myocardium. This operation is still used occasionally as a procedure of last resort, but its efficacy is limited by closure of the myocardial tunnels from scar formation. In 1957, Massimo and Boffi [4] described the creation of new perfusing channels in the myocardium by implantation of plastic tubes with side-wall holes to let blood flow into the sinusoids. Goldman et al. [5] in 1956, Sen et al. [6] in 1965, and Khazei et al. [7] in 1968 each described the technique of mechanical acupuncture of the myocardium to create channels through which oxygenated blood from the left ventricle could flow directly into the myocardium. In 1971, Walter et al. [8] also reported this technique. However, Pifarre and co-workers [9] denied that transmyocardial acupuncture was effective, and they reported that experimental channels created by mechanical means closed due to fibrosis within 6 weeks postoperatively. They argued, incorrectly, that the intramyocardial pressure would always exceed the end-diastolic pressure within the left-ventricular blood pool, and would therefore prevent flow of blood from the ventricle into the transmyocardial channels. The theoretical conclusion drawn by Pifarre et al. ignored the experimentally demonstrated fact that 70% or more of myocardial blood flow in reptilian hearts is supplied through natural transmyocardial channels, in systole.

In 1971, in Wausau, Wis., S.M. Mirhoseini [10] pioneered the first successful attempt to create artificial transmyocardial channels atraumatically in beating canine hearts, using a 400-watt CO_2 laser manufactured by the American Optical Corporation in Southbridge, Mass. for industrial uses. This laser had a resonator some 4.27 m long. It was equipped with an articulated arm and a focusing handpiece for delivery of the beam to the target. It fired single pulses of 100 ms in duration and 400 watts in power, equivalent to 40 J of energy in each pulse. The laser was synchronized to fire each shot just after the crest of the R-wave on the animal's electrocardiogram, so as to bore a hole while the ventricular wall was relatively stationary and to avoid the fibrillation which resulted if the laser beam vaporized myocardium during the T-wave. A collection of 24 medium-sized dogs (each weighing at least 23 kg) was divided into four groups of six dogs each.

In group 1, the LAD coronary was ligated above the first diagonal, and 5–10 min later the whole area perfused by the LAD was perforated by laser channels (2–3/cm^2). Brisk bleeding was noted *in systole* from these channels; it stopped after a few minutes of light tamponade. Two dogs in group I survived for several years postoperatively, with no coronary perfusion to the left-ventricular myocardium. One animal died during application of the laser, perhaps from laser damage to part of the conduction system.

In group 2, the LAD was ligated above the first diagonal. After stabilization of each animal, the laser perforated only 1 cm^2 of the area perfused by the LAD with several channels, which bled briskly in systole. Four animals of this group fibrillated within 30 min and died after attempts at resucitation had failed. Two dogs survived and were killed at 1.5 months postoperatively; microscopic inspection showed patent laser channels, but with some scarring around them.

In group 3, the whole myocardium perfused by the LAD was perforated with 2–3 laser channels per square centimeter, and the LAD was then ligated above the first diagonal. Their myocardia showed no visible evidence of ischemia, and all of these dogs survived with no morbidity. They were killed sequentially at intervals from 4 weeks to 5.5 months postoperatively. Microscopic sections of their hearts showed patent channels with no scarring.

In group 4, the LAD was ligated above the first diagonal, but no laser channels were made. All six of these dogs fibrillated and died within 20 min.

9.2 Developments Since 1978

I first met Dr. Mirhoseini in San Francisco in 1978, at a meeting of the International Society for Microsurgery, where Mirhoseini originally presented the results of his canine experiments with TMR. From 1978 until 1987, I had frequent meetings and conversations with him in efforts, mostly unsuccessful, to promote the concept of TMR among cardiovascular surgeons at large. In October of 1984, I was invited by Dr. Jean-Pierre Bex to bring Mirhoseini to the Clinique de la Residence du Parc in Marseille, France, to demonstrate

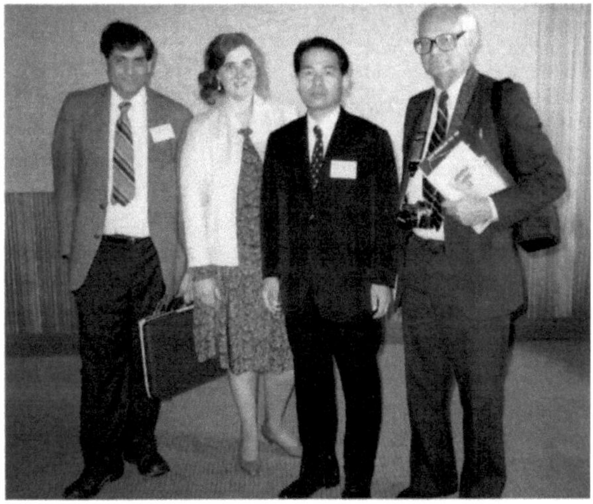

Fig. 9.1. Photograph taken at Cardio-Techno Meeting in Marseille, France, October 12, 1984. *From left*: Dr S.M. Mirhoseini, Mary M. Cayton, Dr. Masayoshi Okada (of Kobe, Japan), and the author. The meeting was held at the Hotel Concorde Palm Beach, Promenade de la Plage, Marseille. Drs. Mirhoseini, Okada, and Fisher were speakers on the program

TMR as an adjunct to saphenous-vein bypass of obstructed coronaries, a procedure which Mirhoseini had first performed late in 1983 on an elderly male patient at St. Luke's Medical Center in Milwaukee, Wis. The first patient in Marseille was a 55-year-old man from Italy, who received several vein grafts, followed by TMR of his cardioplegic heart with a 100-watt CO_2 laser that I had obtained from Cilas in Paris. The surgery went well, without complica tions, and the patient was taken to the intensive care unit. Dr. Mirhoseini, Mary Cayton (Mirhoseini's surgical nurse), and I offered to spend the night with the patient in the ICU, but this was refused by Dr. Bex. Early the next morning, I received a phone call from Bex, who stated, with evident chagrin, that the patient had died during the night in the ICU. Investigation of the incident by Dr. Mirhoseini, Ms. Cayton, and me showed unequivocally that the patient had died of cardiac arrest following deflation of the cuff of his endotracheal tube, inhalation of the tube down his right main-stem bronchus, and subsequent atelectasis of the right lung, leading to irreversible hypoxia. This unfortunate sequence of events had occurred while the resident physician, supposedly on duty in the ICU, was moonlighting at another hospital. Despite the fact that the death was due to negligence on the part of the clinic staff, Bex refused to allow adjunctive TMR on two other patients who had been scheduled for the next day.

When Mirhoseini and I returned to Milwaukee, the Institutional Review Board of St. Luke's Medical Center finally withdrew its former prohibition and permitted Mirhoseini to perform adjunctive TMR on a series of 12 patients who were chosen according to a set of criteria which included functional, ischemic myocardium not totally reperfusible by saphenous-vein bypass alone. Over the next 4 years, Mirhoseini performed adjunctive TMR on some 20 patients, all of whom showed marked, sustained improvement in their cardiac function, including better perfusion in the laser-drilled areas than anywhere else in the myocardium, as indicated by postoperative scintigraphy with thallium 201. In 1989, 4 years postoperatively, the fourth patient

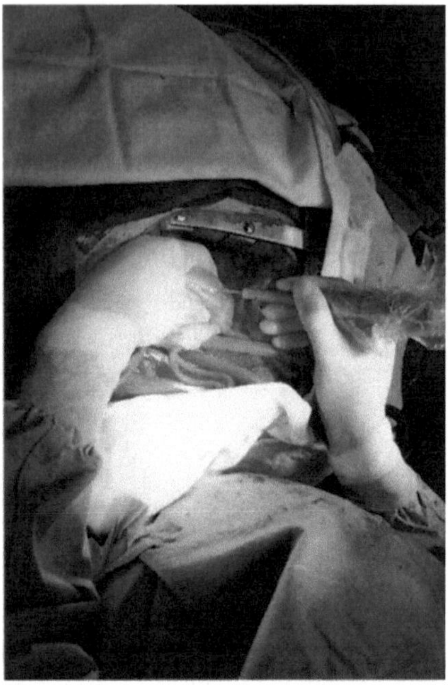

Fig. 9.2. Dr. S.M. Mirhoseini performing adjunctive TMR on the cardioplegic heart of a patient at St. Luke's Medical Center in Milwaukee, Wis. in the spring of 1985. The patient has been placed on extracorporeal heart-lung circulation. In Mirhoseini's *right hand* is the handpiece of a Sharplan Model 743, 80-watt CO_2 laser. His *left hand* holds the patient's still, chilled heart, while he is ready to fire the laser. The heart is exposed through a sternotomy and the chest is held open with a retractor, visible on the *left side*. The laser channels were bored where CABG could not provide adequate revascularization. (Photograph taken by the author)

in the series died of unrelated causes, and his family donated his heart to St. Luke's Medical Center, where Mirhoseini sectioned and microscopically examined it. The laser channels were all patent over their entire length, except for the outer 2 mm, and had developed normal endothelial linings.

In May of 1987, I was engaged as a staff consultant by St. Luke's Medical Center in Milwaukee, where I spent the next 5 years on a part-time basis attempting to expand and improve the institution's activities in laser surgery in all specialties. In the autumn of 1987, while I was attempting to raise funding from the St. Luke's Foundation to procure a powerful CO_2 laser for TMR on beating hearts, so as to demonstrate conclusively that the improvements in cardiac function following adjunctive TMR were caused by the laser channels and not by the vein grafts, Mirhoseini alleged that he was being forced into activities for which he was not ready. Because a condition of such funding was that he collaborate with the other cardiovascular surgeons on the staff, who had been openly critical of his activities and politically active to suppress them, he opposed my efforts to obtain financing and locate a manufacturer to build a prototype laser that could deliver 50 J of energy in a tenth of a second.

In December of 1987, I received a telephone call from Dr. John R. Crew, a surgeon at Seton Medical Center in Daly City, Calif., who had heard me speak about TMR at several vascular meetings in the United States. Crew said that Seton wanted to start a program in TMR on beating human hearts, and asked me to come to Daly City to teach the technique and its technology to the staff there. The day after Christmas in 1987, I met with Crew and key members of the Seton staff to start the program.

The first task was to find a manufacturer who could construct a CO_2 laser capable of delivering 50 J of energy within 100 ms. After brief consideration of Laser Industries in Israel, which was rejected because of its remoteness from California, I chose Laser Engineering in Milford, Mass. I met with Dr. Robert Rudko (President) and Mr. Francis Martin (Vice President for Marketing) of this firm at the airport in Fort Lauderdale, Fla., in the spring of 1988 to discuss the project. Shortly thereafter I drafted a contract between Seton Medical Center and Laser Engineering that provided for Seton to pay \$250000 in installments, contingent upon Laser Engineering's adherence to a timetable for the development of the laser. I supervised the design and construction of this protoptype Heart Laser, which was delivered to Seton in December 1989. It failed to meet the specification of 50 J in 0.1 s, but I accepted it in order to begin TMR on patients, and start the learning process while Laser Engineering began a second design to replace it, at no additional charge to Seton.

In January of 1990, following two failed saphenous-vein bypass operations and maximum medical therapy, an 82-year-old man with incapacitating angina pectoris was the first patient to receive TMR on his beating heart. Five days later he performed 8 min of exercise on a treadmill without angina of cardiac origin, although he reported pain from the left-side thoracotomy used to expose his heart for TMR, and he has survived to this day without further cardiac surgery, in good Karnofsky performance status. Between January of 1990 and the present, more than 25 patients have undergone beating-heart TMR at Seton Medical Center, some as qualifying candidates under the

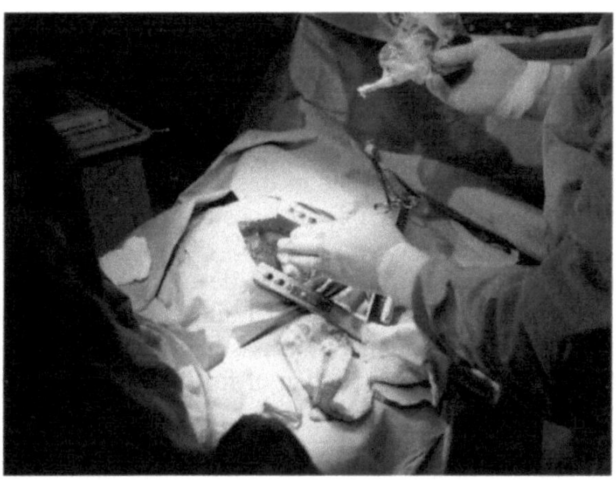

Fig. 9.3. The beating heart of Errol Taylor, aged 82, exposed through a left-side thoracotomy at Seton Medical Center, Daly City, Calif. on January 31, 1990. In his *right hand*, Dr. John R. Crew holds the handpiece of the prototype Heart Laser. This procedure required about 50 min, from skin to skin. The patient, who had been completely incapacitated by excruciating angina before the operation, underwent a thallium-201 stress test for 8 min on a treadmill 5 days postoperatively without cardiac pain. The thallium scintigraphy showed a significant improvement in his myocardial perfusion, although most of the patients who receive beating-heart TMR do not show increased perfusion until several months postoperatively. (Photograph taken by the author)

Investigational Device Exemption granted to Laser Engineering by the U.S. Food and Drug Administration, and a few as exceptions treated on a compassionate basis to save their lives.

In 1992, Laser Engineering, which by then had formed a separate corporation for TMR devices, PLC Systems, delivered a second model of the CO_2 Heart Laser that was capable of producing 80 J of energy in 0.1 s, with pulses synchronized to the R-wave of the electrocardiogram. This laser was able to penetrate even a heart having a left-ventricular wall thickness of 4 cm. The technique of TMR was refined by the addition of transesophageal ultrasound to show a trail of vapor bubbles in the left ventricle each time the laser beam penetrated the heart wall into that chamber. A dual endotracheal tube was used to allow deflation of the left lung, to aid in obtaining adequate access to the heart while dissecting dense adhesions from prior surgeries. A special laser handpiece with a distal flange like the mouth of a lamprey eel was devised to avoid the paroxysmal tachycardia that resulted from touching the epicardium with the narrow barrel of the first handpiece.

From the second patient onward, it was discovered that single-photon-emmision computed tomography using thallium 201, usually considered to be the gold standard of techniques for measuring myocardial perfusion, frequently did not show improved blood supply to the laser-drilled myocardium, even though most TMR patients experienced an immediate decrease in the intensity of angina pectoris. To this day, the unreliability of thallium-201 scintigraphy in demonstrating improved perfusion after TMR has led many newcomers to the TMR clinical investigations to theorize that the channels drilled by the Heart Laser do not improve myocardial perfusion, that they destroy neural tissue in the heart and thereby reduce angina, or that they somehow stimulate neoangiogenesis in the myocardium. Persistent skeptics, notably Hardy et al. [11] and Landreneau et al. [12], have published criticisms of TMR based upon poorly conceived and designed experiments, with immature dogs on extracorporeal heart-lung machines, that do not replicate the conditions of Mirhoseini's canine studies of 1971–1973. A fundamental principle of empirical science is that, in order to verify or disprove the results of a given experiment which is in question, that experiment must be duplicated in its entirety. Because the protocol of any experiment has at least some influence on the results, it is crucial to design the experiment in such a way that primary effects are revealed, and higher-order, less important phenomena do not obscure the evidence that is sought. One cannot measure the acceleration of gravity by emptying a bag of feathers from the top of a tower in a windstorm.

In the years from 1990 to 1995, I tried to persuade Robert Rudko to undertake the development of a NAD-NADH fluorimeter, using the designs, patents, and knowledge of Guy Renault [13] in Paris, who demonstrated that his laser-based fluorimeter could show, within seconds, changes of myocardial metabolism resulting from changes of perfusion, both positive and negative. I corresponded with Renault and arranged a meeting with Rudko, who persistently refused to consider the project. Rudko's stubborn refusal to develop an intraoperative laser fluorimeter led directly to the present state of confusion, among the cardiac surgeons performing TMR, about the exact

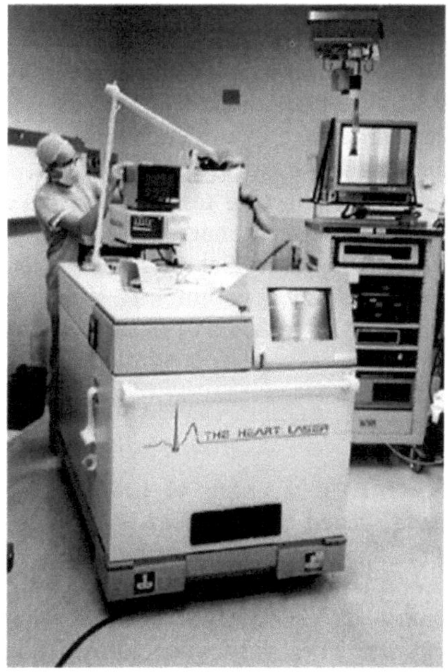

Fig. 9.4. The first unit of the second-generation design of the Heart Laser, shown in the operating room at Seton Medical Center, Daly City, Calif., in August 1991. This laser was capable of delivering about 80 J in a pulse of 0.1-s duration. It had a radio-frequency-excited, folded resonator tube with flowing gas at Mach 1. The control panel shown on the *right side* of the console is a touch-screen video monitor, which allows the operator to select energy per pulse, pulse duration, and firing delay after the crest of the R-wave on the patient's electrocardiogram. (Photograph taken by the author)

mechanism by which it reduces angina and improves Karnofsky status of former cardiac invalids. PET scanning, an expensive technique available only in a few wealthy research centers, does reliably show improved perfusion after TMR. In many cases, computed tomography using technetium sestamibi does the same. However, there is now no universally accepted technique for assessing the improvement in myocardial perfusion following beating-heart TMR.

After the early TMR procedures at Seton Medical Center, the U.S. Food and Drug Administration granted Laser Engineering (by then PLC Systems) permission to expand its clinical studies of TMR to other centers in the United States, Europe, and the Middle East. This expansion has proved to be of mixed value, because it has brought into the TMR studies a host of newcomers, mostly inexperienced in laser surgery, largely skeptical of any new techniques, and so wedded to traditional concepts of cardiology that they concoct all sorts of complex explanations for the clinically evident post-TMR improvements in angina and performance status. Among the few clinical investigators who understood the means by which TMR improves cardiac function was Keith Horvath [14], then at Brigham & Women's Hospital in Boston, who built his own NAD-NADH fluorimeter, which he used intraoperatively while performing TMR on the beating hearts of sheep. He found that an immediate increase in metabolic activity of the ovine myocardium occurred after TMR with the Heart Laser.

In 1996, in collaboration with David Knighton at the University of Minnesota in Minneapolis, John Crew used the donated heart of one of his Seton TMR patients, who died of cancer a few years after the procedure, to form a plastic cast of the intracardiac vascular "tree" by injecting the ventricles and coronaries with a liquid monomer and catalyst which quickly polymerized (John R. Crew, personal communication, May 1997). Dissolution of the myostructural parts of the heart in a special reagent then exposed the vascular tree, which showed all the laser channels patent from just below the epicardial surface to the endocardial, connecting with the myocardial sinusoids and the intramyocardial coronaries, subdividing into the small coronary arterioles connecting to the thebesian meshwork and ultimately to the coronary veins and coronary sinus. Despite this and other compelling evidence of improved myocardial perfusion through laser-drilled channels, much of the medical-surgical community stubbornly refuses to believe the true means by which TMR causes its cardiac benefits.

9.3 Recent Events

Since 1991, a group of cardiac surgeons, entrepreneurs, and opportunists have started a movement to develop a means of performing TMR from inside the left ventricle rather than from the epicardial surface inward. This group was undoubtedly inspired by the use of certain lasers to perform coronary angioplasty, notably the xenon-chloride excimer at a wavelength of 308 nm. They are fascinated by the concept of introducing a fiber through a catheter inserted into the common femoral artery, guided up through the iliac to the aorta, over the arch, and down into the left ventricle. The alleged advantage of this technique over outside-in TMR is the avoidance of the invasive left-side thoracotomy required by traditional TMR with the CO_2 laser. It presents another set of serious problems, however: guidance of the distal tip of the fiber to the desired spot on the endocardial surface, holding it there during drilling, avoidance of perforation through the epicardium of the left ventricle with possible puncture of a great vessel in the closed thorax, and lack of a laser with sufficient energy per pulse to make a complete channel in a single heartbeat.

The ideal laser for percutaneous, inside-out TMR is one that is fiber transmissible and has an absorption coefficient high enough and a scattering coefficient low enough to permit boring of myocardial channels with minimal damage to surrounding tissue, so as to avoid subsequent closure of the channels from cicatrization. The laser types that have been tried experimentally for fiber-delivered TMR are the xenon-chloride and the holmium:YAG. Since neither has sufficient energy per pulse to make a complete channel in one shot, multiple pulses are required. The divergence of the beam beyond a plane-ended distal fiber tip requires either that a focusing termination of the fiber be used, or that the tip of the fiber be mechanically advanced into the hole as boring progresses over several heart cycles. During the period from 1988 to 1990, Mirhoseini used both a xenon-chloride excimer and a holmium:YAG laser in his dog laboratory at the Veterans' Administration Hospital in Wood, Wis. to bore transmyocardial channels in the beating hearts of mongrel dogs (S.M. Mirhoseini, personal communication, 1989). He found that each of these channels closed from scarring within a period of days to weeks. He concluded that the mechanical trauma of pushing the fiber into the myocardium was responsible for the closure. This is the same phenomenon that thwarted the attempts of Sen and others who used mechanical devices to create transmyocardial channels.

Within the past 4 years, two newly founded companies in the United States, Cardiogenesis and Eclipse Surgical Technologies, both of Sunnyvale, Calif., have together accumulated more than 100 million investors' dollars with public offerings of stock based upon their optimistic expectations that the holmium:YAG laser will successfully create durable partial-thickness channels in the left-ventricular myocardium of human hearts, from the endocardial surface outward. Both companies expect that the process of clinical trials and pre-market approval of their laser systems for unrestricted human TMR will require several years and entail substantial costs. Furthermore, there are reports of several animal studies, such as those of Weng et al. [15] and Kadipasaoglu et al. [16], which indicate that myocardial channels made by the HO:YAG laser do not remain patent, and that the surrounding tissue shows both thermal and mechanical damage.

As of this writing, a third company, Trimedyne in Irvine, Calif., is engaged in the development of a HO:YAG laser system for inside-out TMR. All three of these companies, and their investors, are motivated more by hope than by reason, and their presence in the field of TMR has attracted dozens of clinicians inexperienced in laser surgery, who have no understanding of the biophysics of laser light in living tissue. The clinical trials of the Heart Laser of PLC Medical Systems have treated far more human patients (approximately 3000) to date than those of Cardiogenesis and Eclipse combined, yet in July 1997, the US FDA refused to grant pre-market approval to PLC for the Heart Laser, citing an insufficient number of clinical cases with long-term follow-up to demonstrate the safety and efficacy of TMR. In its refusal to grant pre-market approval for the PLC Heart Laser, the FDA stated (F. Martin, personal communication, July 1997) that it would accept relief of angina pectoris as an indication of efficacy, without requiring that PLC demonstrate improved myocardial perfusion as well. In this decision, the expert panel of the FDA was prudent, because Braunwald [17] defines angina as "a discomfort in the chest or adjacent areas, *which is caused by myocardial ischemia* [my italics] and is associated with a disturbance of myocardial function but without myocardial necrosis." He goes on to say: "In typical angina, the pain is related to an increase in myocardial oxygen demand... in the presence of a fixed and limited oxygen supply." Therefore, if myocardial ischemia is diminished or eliminated, angina will decrease or disappear. The speculative opinions that are being offered by some newcomers to TMR who doubt that its benefits result from increased myocardial perfusion through the laser channels include, most frequently, a presumption that the myocardium and/or the coronary vasculature has been denervated by the laser beam. It is preposterous to assume that 30 or 40 small (1-mm) channels in the myocardium (dozens of square centimeters in area) could cut so many of the unmyelinated sympathetic nerve filaments which lie between cardiac muscle fibers and around coronary vessels, and whose end-plates are sensitive to ischemia-triggered substances such as adenosine, bradykinin, histamine, and serotonin, that angina could be nearly or totally eliminated.

9.4 Predictions for the Future

The practice of coronary artery bypass grafting (CABG) will probably continue unabated for at least another decade in the developed countries of the world, for two reasons: (a) it is now so extensively accepted by cardiac surgeons, who show a dedication to preservation of the status quo; (b) it is a large source of revenue for hospitals and physicians. However, it is a procedure based solely upon anecdotal evidence from many millions of cases; there has never been a controlled study to demonstrate that CABG is a safe, effective means of treating myocardial ischemia resulting from atherosclerosis of coronary arteries. In fact, it has a number of distinct disadvantages: very significant morbidity and mortality; a half-life of patency for the vein grafts that is less than a decade and is very dependent upon the technique of harvesting, preserving, and installing the saphenous vein segments; and a disturbing incidence of mental changes attributable to partial obstruction of cranial microcirculation by free hemoglobin, resulting from hemolysis of erythrocytes by extracorporeal heart-lung machines. The search for a better surgical procedure to replace the 30-year-old CABG will continue.

TMR performed with holmium:YAG lasers will prove to be of temporary benefit at best. The Ho:YAG is essentially unsuited for TMR. Its absorption coefficient in water is only 30/cm and its scattering coefficient is about 8/cm. Its absorption density (fluence multiplied by absorption coefficient) is low, and its zone of inevitable thermal damage around the laser channel is comparable in width to the diameter of the channel itself. Furthermore, it is inherently a pulsed laser at room temperature, with a pulse width on the order of 300–500 μs and a peak power on the order of several kilowatts. Pulses of this sort cause explosive effects which tear muscle tissue. Ripping and heating of the myocardium around the laser channel are responsible for the documented [15] short duration of channel patency.

The xenon-chloride excimer laser at 308 nm in wavelength will be a better choice in terms of minimizing thermal damage around the channels. The absorption coefficient in skin (probably comparable to that for myocardium) is about 1900/cm [18], and the threshold fluence for ablation (0.66 J/cm^2) [18] is lower than for the Ho:YAG. The photochemical lysis of complex organic molecules requires about 7 J/mm^3 at 193 nm and is probably comparable at 308 nm. This is higher than the 3 J/mm^3 needed for photothermal vaporization of myocardium at 10600 nm, but not so high as to present an insurmountable problem. Inside-out TMR (designated by Cardiogenesis as PMR, for *percutaneous transmyocardial revascularization)* with the xenon-chloride laser beam, delivered through a quartz optical fiber, is optically and mechanically feasible with present-day technology.

If excimer-bored myocardial channels extending from the endocardial surface to a depth of 50% of the ventricular wall thickness remain patent for 2 years, the PMR procedure will offer benefits comparable to those of coronary angioplasty with the argon-fluoride excimer at 193 nm, but without the necessity of boring through calcified plaque and the risk of arterial perforation. If excimer PMR has no adverse, irreversible sequelae, it could become a viable alternative to excimer laser coronary angioplasty (ELCA) or replace it altogether.

References

1. Wearn JT, Mettier SR, Klump TG, Zschiesche LJ (1933) The nature of vascular connections between the coronary arteries and the chambers of the heart. Am Heart J 9:143–164
2. Beck CS (1935) The development of a new blood supply to the heart by operation. Ann Surg 102:801–813
3. Vineberg A (1954) Clinical and experimental studies in the treatment of coronary artery insufficiency by internal mammary implant. J Int Coll Surg 22:503–518
4. Massimo C, Boffi L (1957) Myocardial revascularization by a new method of carrying blood directly from the left ventricular cavity directly into the coronary circulation. J Thorac Surg 34:257–264
5. Goldman A, Greenstone Preuss FS, Strauss SH, Chang E-S (1956) Experimental methods for producing a collateral circulation to the heart directly from the left ventricle. J Thorac Surg 6:163–171
6. Sen PK, Udwadia TE, Kinare SG, Sen MS, Udwadia MS Parulker GB, Darel MS (1965) Transmyocardial acupuncture: a new approach to myocardial revascularization. J Thorac Cardiovasc Surg 5:50, 181–189
7. Khazei AH, Kime WP, Papadopoulos C, Cowley RA (1968) Myocardial canalization: a new method of myocardial revascularization. Ann Thorac Surg 6:163–171
8. Walter P, Hundeschagen H, Borst HG (1971) Treatment of acute myocardial infarction by transmural blood supply from the ventricular cavity. Eur Surg Res 3:130–138
9. Pifarre R, Jasuja ML, Lynch RD, Neville WE (1969) Myocardial revascularization by transmyocardial acupuncture: a physiological impossibility. J Thorac Cardiovasc Surg 58:424–431
10. Mirhoseini M, Cayton M (1981) Revascularization of the heart by Laser J Microsurg 2:253–260
11. Hardy RI, Bove KE, James FW, Kaplan S, Goldman L (1987) A histologic study of laser-induced transmyocardial channels. Lasers Surg Med 6:563–573
12. Landreneau R, Nawarawong W, Laughlin H, Ripperger J, Brown O, McDaniel W, McKnown D, Curtis J (1991) Direct CO_2 laser "revascularization" of the myocardium. Lasers Surg Med 11:35–42
13. Renault G, Sine M, Muffat-Joly M, Cornillault J, Pocidalo JJ (1985) In situ monitoring of myocardial metabolism by laser fluorimetry: relevance of a test of local ischemia. Lasers Surg Med 5:111–122
14. Horvath KA, Smith WJ, Laurence RG, Schoen FJ, Appleyard RF, Cohn LH (1995) J Am Coll Cardiol 25:258–263
15. Weng G, Williamson WA, Aretz HT, et al (1993) The effect of holmium:YAG laser-mediated transmyocardial channels on left ventricular contractility in an acute ischemic model. Lasers Surg Med [Suppl] 5:13
16. Kadipasaoglu KA, Cihan HB, Clubb FJ jr, et al (1997) Arrhythmogenic and histologic properties of three laser modalities [CO_2, Ho:YAG, & XeCl] for transmyocardial laser revascularization (TMLR). Lasers Surg Med [Suppl] 9:12
17. Braunwald E (ed) (1992) Heart disease: a textbook of cardiovascular medicine, vol 2, 4th edn. Saunders, Philadelphia, pp 1293–1294
18. Kaufmann R, Hibst R (1989) Pulsed ER:YAG and 308 nm UV-excimer laser: an in vitro and in vivo study of skin-ablative effects. Lasers Surg Med 9:132–140

CHAPTER 10

Transmyocardial Laser Revascularisation: A Matter of the Right Wavelength?

G. J. Müller · K. Dörschel · B. Schaldach

10.1 Introduction

The first clinical transmyocardial revascularisation (TMR) trials were performed in the 1950s, using mechanical puncturing devices such as needles and trocars. The underlying concept, which is still being discussed by most of the groups active today, is the finding that the human heart is a long-term result of biological evolution, starting with the reptile heart, which shows very few, slightly developed, coronaries but has extensive radial flaps into the ventricle; thus, the oxygen and metabolic uptake is performed by diffusion through the surface of these intraventricular flaps. The human heart has residual so-called sinusoidal gaps which are thought to be inflated by intracardial blood through the TMR channels. So far, non of the histological findings have been able to prove this concept, although the sinusoidal gaps can be identified.

Another hypothesis under discussion argues that the channels obtained by transmyocardial laser revascularisation (TMLR) open a number of vessels for the microcirculation, which then is shunted through the channels to the ventricle. Hence, oxygen support of the myocardium is enhanced. This hypothesis, too, is questionable for several reasons.

1. The intravascular pressure of the microcirculation in the myocardium is higher than the pressure of the ventricle. Therefore, a retrograde filling is unlikely.
2. The histological findings following TMLR procedures have shown that only a very small number of channels stay open for a considerable length of time. Taking into account that up to 40 punctures are made during a TMLR procedure, and that by now 2000 patients have been treated worldwide, fewer than 100 channels have been reported by all groups to stay patent [1].

Besides the early studies in the 1950s and 1960s, which used only needles and scalpels, an extended study was prepared in 1971 by a German cardiac surgeon, P. Walter, who used specially designed cannulas and trocars and varied the diameter of the puncture hole systematically. He was able to show that with these mechanically drilled holes, the perfusion of the myocardium is enhanced by only 15% during the first hours and up to several days [2].

In the early 1980s, Mirhoseini began the first continuous-wave (cw) CO_2 laser-based procedures in canine hearts, but he failed to show any beneficial effects. It was not until the late 1980s/early 1990s when, using a high-power pulsed CO_2 laser, Mirhoseini was able to show positive results [3–5].

Unfortunately, none of the investigators have restricted themselves to a well-defined indication, with regard neither to sex and age of the patients, to the staging of the actual disease, or to side effects, nor to pre-, intra- and postoperative medication. According to the literature, regardless of their sex and age, most of the patients treated suffered from severe diffuse angina pectoris; in most cases they had already had one or more coronary artery bypass grafts (CABGs) and were receiving intensive pharmaceutical treatment.

The data reported so far show that the average mortality for TMLR is as high as 10%! Research groups that have restricted themselves to a very limited indication only report a mortality which is still in the order of 5%. This has to be compared with the mortality of normal CABGs, which is less than 2% at major centres.

Regarding the most frequent indication for TMLR, namely the group of patients with therapy-resistant long-term diffuse angina pectoris, there are two different results: One is the patient's subjective feeling postoperatively in the short and the long term, the other is the objective finding. While 60–80% of these patients reported a subjective feeling of relief from their severe pain, the objective findings of left ventricular ejection fraction (LVEF) were not considerably improved, and single-photon emission computed tomography (SPECT) investigations showed acute improvements only up to several weeks postoperatively.

In a limited group of patients the subjective pain is reported to be improved by one or two angina classes better, although objective findings are not convincing. After 1 year, more than 70% of the patients treated reported a recurrence of their original disease. A few of these patients were treated a second time, with almost the same postoperative scenario [6].

Indeed, the results reported from current experience are not ideal. A major reason for this seems to be that the pathological mechanism of TMLR is not yet understood. One of the most limiting factors is that the staging of diffuse angina pectoris is more or less only clinical, because there is no objective method of describing and defining the number and the extent of the ischaemic islands within the myocardium. Some histological findings indicate that the success of TMLR procedures is limited to those patients in whom the ischaemic islands are not extensively developed and who still have extended bridging of vital myocardium. Therefore, there is a need for a monitoring method to identify the ischaemic islands and to quantify the amount of still vital but hibernating myocardium.

10.2 What Difference Does the Laser Make in TMR?

The laser is the only device that has shown some intermediate and, within a small group, also patent effectiveness of TMR procedures, although no one has been able to explain this success. Surprisingly enough, four different laser systems are in use, namely high-power pulsed CO_2 lasers, which need an articulated arm for delivery and can be employed in open-heart surgery only, excimer lasers, and holmium:YAG and neodymium:YAG lasers, which can be applied with fiber delivery systems, both transcutaneously and intraoperatively. All these lasers are pulsed systems, and they vary considerably in pulse length, repetition rate, peak power and beam quality.

In comparison to mechanical puncturing, these laser systems produce two additional major effects inside the myocardium besides drilling a channel: shock waves and thermal injury. As discussed already, just punching or drilling channels does not result in effective TMR. Therefore, either one or both of the additional modalities provided by pulsed lasers are important. These modalities are the pressure amplitude of the shock waves induced during tissue ablation and the thermal necrosis zone at the channel margins.

On the other hand, these two effects of a laser, shock wave and thermal injury, can be administered alternatively, since shock waves can be generated by small interstitial defibrillators, while thermal injury can be applied by bipolar rf-needles. Holes may be drilled in combination with these by mechanical devices or by some modified cavitation ultrasound surgical aspirator (CUSA) technique.

10.3 Laser-induced Shock Waves

The pressure amplitude of laser-induced shock waves may have three different effects. It is not yet understood whether all three, only two, one or even none of them contribute to the positive effects reported in TMR. There is still a chance that these effects might have an adverse influence. These three effects can be described as follows:

1. The shock waves rupture the channel wall and hence might open sinusoidal gaps for intermediate perfusion or might open the microcirculatory vessels to provide better shunt effectiveness to the channel.
2. The shock waves stimulate vascular spasm, the subsequent counterreaction is enhanced vasomotoric activity and, hence, better perfusion.
3. The shock waves most likely do have a third effect which can be explained as follows: The pathophysiology of the affected myocardium can be described by the dendritic (fingerlike) structure of ischaemic islands within a still vital but hibernating myocardium which does not inervate synchronously with the remaining part of the myocardium. The ischaemic islands can best be described as endangered or injured tissue, and it is well known that at the margin of injuries inside the myocardium they will cause so-called re-entry cycles which may interrupt the synchronous inervation induced by the signal coming from the AV node. As mentioned, there are a number of ischaemic islands, which therefore most likely have resulted in numerous chaotically firing re-entry cycles, all of which interfere with each other. Due to this interference, the remaining vital myocardium within the diseased ventricle is stumbled and hence can no longer be synchronously inervated. This is called 'hibernating'. The shock waves induced by the laser might break this interference completely, or at least in part, and give the hibernating myocardium a chance to inervate again synchronously; this in turn could result in improved perfusion because the vasomotoric activity will also be stimulated, due to the synchronous iner-

vation. This hypothesis is supported by recent results of pre- and postoperative ECG-mapping analysis by Krabatsch et al. (this volume).

These three laser-induced effects are most likely responsible for the immediate positive results of TMLR reported. The third effect seems to be most important; this means that a laser must be found that induces sufficiently strong shock waves. The physical laser parameters relevant for variation and optimisation of the pressure amplitude of the shock waves are the pulse length, the pulse energy and the effective optical penetration depth, which is a function of wavelength.

The effectiveness of the procedure is expected to improve if the ischaemic islands are small in both size and number. As ischaemia advances and the possibility of activating the hibernating myocardium declines, the result becomes increasingly inefficient.

10.4 Laser-Induced Thermal Injury

The second modality of lasers is the introduction of thermal necrosis at the channel margin. The channel diameter can be influenced by the following laser parameters: beam waist, fiber diameter (or applicator diameter) and feeding speed. The heat-affected margin of the channel can be adjusted by choosing an appropriate optical penetration depth, pulse length and the repetition rate (i.e. average power) (Fig. 10.1a, b). This thermal necrosis is nothing other than tubular burn scars. It is well known that size-limited burn scars will induce neoangiogenesis due to the resulting hypoxia.

Furthermore, this thermally induced necrosis of the channel walls will act as a morphological guiding structure for stimulation of new vessel growth. This effect takes time and might help to explain the positive long-term results. It has been proven, meanwhile, that after several months there is indeed vascularisation along the channel walls and even within the thrombotic closed channels, which gives support to this hypothesis.

It also has been shown that the injection of angiogenic factors only will result in new chaotically twisted angiogenesis. It has been proven, too, that local hypoxia stimulates the release of angiogenic factors. Combined, these findings support the idea of a morphological guiding structure which organises the filaments of newly growing vessels (Fig. 10.2).

In Table 10.1, laser systems which have thus far been used for TMR are compared in terms both of their shock wave pressure amplitude induced inside bulk myocardium and of their thermal necrosis thickness. It can be clearly seen that these most important parameters vary widely. Thus, the appropriate laser device must be chosen in terms of an optimised thermal necrosis to induce local hypoxia. Unfortunately, no data are yet available regarding the optimal necrosis.

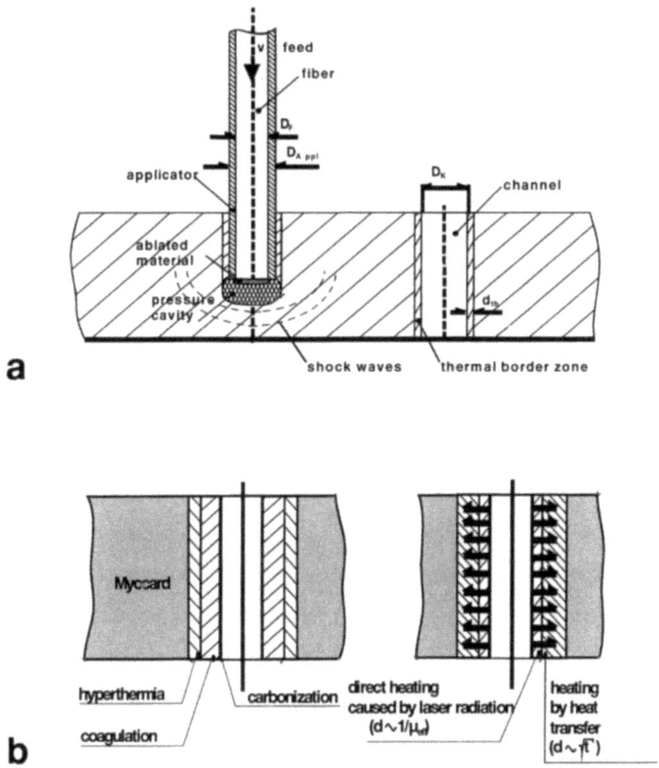

Fig. 10.1 a, b. Formation of a myocardial channel with fiber optic applicator defining relevant parameters

Fig. 10.2. The local hypoxia (thermal stimulus) induces angiogenesis, and the marginal necrosis of the thrombotic closed channel works as a morphological guiding structure

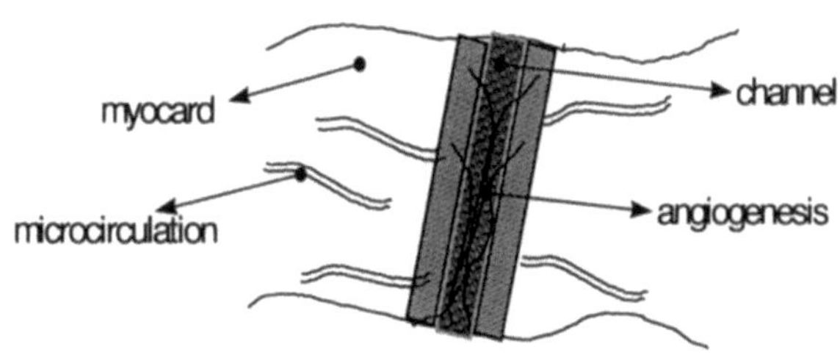

10.5 Conclusion and Outlook

The hypothesis presented is based on an analysis of the differences between transmyocardial channels drilled by pulsed lasers and others drilled mechanically. It is most likely that two different modalities, namely the shock wave-induced barytrauma and the thermal injury at the channel margin, contribute to the positive results of TMLR.

Table 10.1. Lasers used in TMR

Type	Wave length	Pulse length	Thermal damage	Shock wave pressure	Pulse energy, average power	Repetition rate	Channel diameter	Time per channel
Excimer	308 nm	150 ns	<50 μm	~500 bar	20 mJ/5 J 0.8 W/25 W	<40 Hz	0.5 mm	6 s
Nd:YAG	1.44 μm	600 μs	<350 μm	~10 bar	2 J/40 J 10 W/800 W	5 Hz	1 mm	4 s
Ho:YAG	2.08 μm	100–500 μs	<300 μm	~10 bar	2 J/40 J 10 W/800 W	5 Hz	1 mm	4 s
CO_2	10.6 μm	50 ms	<200 μm	~3 bar	40 J/40 J 800 W/800 W	one shot	1 mm	50 ms

Both modalities of a laser can be optimised independently by variation of the appropriate parameters. This means that effective TMLR is not restricted to a single wavelength or laser but can be performed using any pulsed laser system with a sufficiently high energy density at the tissue to be operated within the so-called photoablation domain [7, 8].

The results presented open up completely new prospects for the performance of TMR using much simpler devices, e.g. a fibre optic-based ultrasonic transducer [9-11]. The capacity of such a transducer for drilling holes into the myocardium is similar to that of a laser. Suitable for operation at up to 80 kHz, it is capable of delivering exactly the thermal energy required to induce thermal injury at the channel margin and also of transmitting, for example, q-switched pulses of a small neodymium:YAG laser that can be cost-favourably designed to administer the appropriate shock wave amplitudes. The cost of such a dual modality (ultrasound drilling and laser-induced shock waves) applicator device will be less than 10% that of the currently most widely distributed pulsed CO_2 laser system. First trials with such a device have recently begun, and the results will be reported elsewhere.

References

1. Müller GJ, Berlien HP (serial eds), Krabatsch T, Hetzer R (eds) (1996) Transmyokardiale Laserrevaskularisation: Stand und Ausblicke; Symposium Deutsches Herzzentrum Berlin, Fortschritte in der Lasermedizin 11, ecomed verlagsgesellschaft AG & Co.KG, ISBN 3-609-62830-8
2. Walter P, Hundeshagen H, Borst HG (1971) Treatment of acute myocardial infarction by transmural blood supply from the left ventricular cavity. Eur Surg Res 3:130-138
3. Mirhoseini M, Cayton MM (1981) Revascularization of the heart by laser. J Mircrosurg 2:253-260
4. Mirhoseini M et al (1982) Transventricular revascularization by laser. Lasers Surg Med 2:187-198
5. Mirhoseini M, Cayton M (1985) Use of cardioplegia for laser revascularization of myocardium. Lasers Surg Med 5:169
6. Krabatsch T et al (1996) Die transmyokardiale Laserrevaskularisation in der Therapie der diffusen koronaren Herzerkrankung. Z Herz-, Thorax-, Gefäßchir 10:19-26
7. Mueller G, Berlien H-P (1986) Lasers in medicine - technical state and prospects. Lasers Cardiovasc Dis. 1st Int Symposium, Baden/Vienna, June 26-28, 1986, ISBN 3-924016-06-2
8. Müller G, Harnoss BM, Kar H, Doerschel K, Berlien H-P (1988) Photoablation a question of wavelength? Laser Technol Ophthalmol, Verlag Kugler und Ghedini, ISBN 90-6299-040-1
9. Tschepe J, Desinger K, Stein T, Müller G (1996) Simultaneous transmission of laser radiation and ultrasound via silica glass fibers. Laser Optoelektronik 28:44 ff
10. Desinger K, Helfmann J, Stein T, Müller G (1996) Ein neues Konzept zur Kombinationsanwendung von Laser und Ultraschall für die minimal invasive Medizin. Krankenhaus 9:463 ff
11. Desinger K, Stein T, Tschepe J, Müller G (1996) Laser ultrasound surgical therapy (LUST). Minimal Invasive Med 7:123-127

CHAPTER 11

Basic Scientific Considerations in TMR – In Vitro and In Vivo Studies*

W. Grundfest · T. Papaiannou · W. Shi · R. Shehada · M. Fishbein · B. Schwortz · C. Ruppe · T. Pacala

11.1 Introduction

Transmyocardial revascularization (TMR), as originally proposed by Dr. Mirhoseini, attempted to provide blood flow to ischemic myocardium by drilling channels into the muscle of the left ventricle. The idea was to create a reptilian heart, in which blood from the left ventricle perfuses into the myocardium by a series of channels, or sinusoids. Using a specially designed CO_2 laser, the channels were drilled from the epicardial to the endocardial surface. Although epicardial bleeding stops within a few minutes of drilling the holes, several investigators believed that the holes remained patent and that blood perfused the myocardium directly from the ventricle. Extensive attempts to demonstrate this flow have met with equivocal results in both animal and clinical settings. Many investigators have found that the majority of holes close relatively quickly and believe that other mechanisms must be responsible for the observed clinical improvement, as evidenced by decreased intensity and frequency of angina, a reduction in the need for antianginal medications, and improved work capacity. However, to date no randomized control studies have demonstrated a physiologic improvement from the TMR procedure, and SPECT data have been equivocal.

Dr. Mirhoseini's choice of a CO_2 laser for this procedure was based on two considerations. First, he felt that a straight, regular channel through the myocardium was essential to maintain patency. " In order to prevent cardiac motion from making the channel irregular the laser pulse had to penetrate the myocardium in a single pulse of less than 100 ms. Second, he chose a pulsed laser to minimize thermal damage to adjacent tissue. However, the large CO_2 laser has several major drawbacks for clinical use. First, the laser occupies a 4 ft×8 ft space in the operating room and requires an articulated arm for energy delivery. This makes it cumbersome to use and precludes percutaneous transcatheter applications. Second, the ventricle must be full of blood to prevent perforation of the posterior wall. The blood serves a "beam stop" for the laser energy, but the absorbed energy creates a plume of gas bubbles and thermally damaged blood. The clinical significance of these effects is not known. Further, the need for a full ventricle places constraints on the use of this system in patients undergoing bypass surgery; the procedure cannot be done on an arrested heart with an empty ventricle. Third, the CO_2 laser en-

---

Presented at "Stellenwert der TMLR im Endstadium der koronaren Herzerkrankung" on May 16, 1997.
* Supported in part by a grant from United States Surgical Corporation

ergy can cut through the chordae tendineae, causing unsuspected mitral valve incompetence. The inability to precisely control the deposition of laser energy is a significant limitation of CO_2-based TMR.

Data from the literature and our own previous investigations revealed that the CO_2 laser produced thermal damage zones of 0.5–1.5 mm surrounding a 1-mm hole drilled by the PLC CO_2 laser under clinical conditions. Interestingly, damage was greater along the axis of the myocardial fibres. Holes drilled with this laser appear elliptical in shape. One axis parallel to the fibres is much longer than the axis perpendicular to the fibres. A 1-mm spot size produces a hole of approximately 1 mm in the long axis but only 0.5 mm in the short axis.

Given the technical limitations described above and the thermal damage zone produced by CO_2 laser ablation of myocardium, we investigated the possibility of alternative energy sources which could be delivered by fibre optics. The goal of this paper is to identify an energy source and delivery system which would produce a transmyocardial hole with minimal thermal damage and precise control.

Clinical evidence to date suggests that the original hypothesis of the reptilian heart may not be correct, and that TMR may provide its benefits (if any) through other mechanisms. Several investigators have shown that other laser sources can easily drill holes in the myocardium with differing effects. Any effort to rationalize choice of a laser source for TMR must be based on an understanding of how TMR works. Since the mechanism of action of TMR is currently not known, the alternative is to choose a laser based on a hypothetical mechanism of action and one which produces the desired effects.

This paper will focus on selection of the optimal laser/tissue interactions. "Optimal" can be defined in several ways and depends upon the desired tissue effects. These tissue effects can then be matched to one or more of the several mechanisms by which TMR produces its observed clinical effects. The critical issue - how does TMR work? - cannot be directly addressed in this paper. However, the choice of laser can be based on an examination of the hypotheses for the mechanism of action of TMR. The following hypotheses have been espoused by various investigators:

- Hypothesis 1: Laser-drilled channels reendothelialize, remain patent, and permit blood flow from the ventricle directly into the myocardium.
- Hypothesis 2: Laser-drilled channels close, but as clot lysis occurs, interconnections are formed between various capillary beds (sinusoids). Release of growth factors, due to cellular injury and the presence of platelets and thrombus in a confined space, induce angiogenesis, which increases vascular interconnections.
- Hypothesis 3: Laser-drilled channels close, produce small scars, and improve the compliance of the ventricular wall, allowing the heart to operate more efficiently.
- Hypothesis 4: Laser-drilled channels and surrounding damage zones denervate the myocardium, reducing anginal symptoms and improving work capacity.

- Hypothesis 5: Laser-drilled channels change the conduction characteristics of ischemic myocardium and improve myocardial contractility and ventricular function.
- Hypothesis 6: The observed clinical improvements may bear no relationship to the laser-drilled holes but may be a response to other factors, including optimization of and adherence to medication regimens, improved diet, appropriate rest and exercise, and placebo effects.

A combination of mechanisms may be responsible for the observed clinical improvements. The inability to define the physiologic basis for TMR makes optimization difficult. However, for each of the above mechanisms, parameters could be optimized to choose the desired tissue effects. Past experience with lasers in cardiovascular applications suggests that the less thermal and shock-wave injury, the better. Thermal injury leads to intense collagen deposition and scarring. If producing small scars in the myocardial wall is the mechanism of action, then lasers are not required, since this can easily be accomplished using heated needles. Similarly, the concept of denervating the myocardium and thus reducing anginal symptoms seems counterproductive, since inducing ischemia may produce undesirable consequences, such as arrhythmias and muscle damage.

This paper examines the various laser choices in TMR with emphasis on optimizing parameters of a 308 nm xenon-chloride excimer laser and delivery system. In order to identify optimal parameters, a broad range of experimental techniques were employed. These techniques were used to identify the delivery systems, energy settings, and environmental considerations that produce the most uniform tissue ablation with the least thermal and shock-wave damage.

11.2 Methods and Materials

11.2.1 Lasers and Delivery Systems

Three 308 nm xenon-chloride excimer lasers were used:
1. Custom-built (JPL) excimer laser, pulse duration of 135 ns
2. Spectranetics CVX300, pulse duration of 140 ns
3. AIS Dymer 200, pulse duration of 200 ns

Repetition rates were continuously variable, from 1 to 80 Hz.

A broad range of fibre-delivery systems were used, all of which were made from ultrapure silica fibreoptics obtained from Polymicro (Phoenix, Ariz.) or Spectranetics (Boulder, Colo.). Single fibres ranged in diameter from 400 to 1000 µm. Multiple fibre bundles used 100-µm or 50-µm catheters. Single fibres were used for the in vitro studies, while in vivo studies were performed using 1.4-mm diameter bundles.

For excimer lasers, all energies are expressed in mJ/mm^2. Energies from 10 to 80 mJ/mm^2 were used.

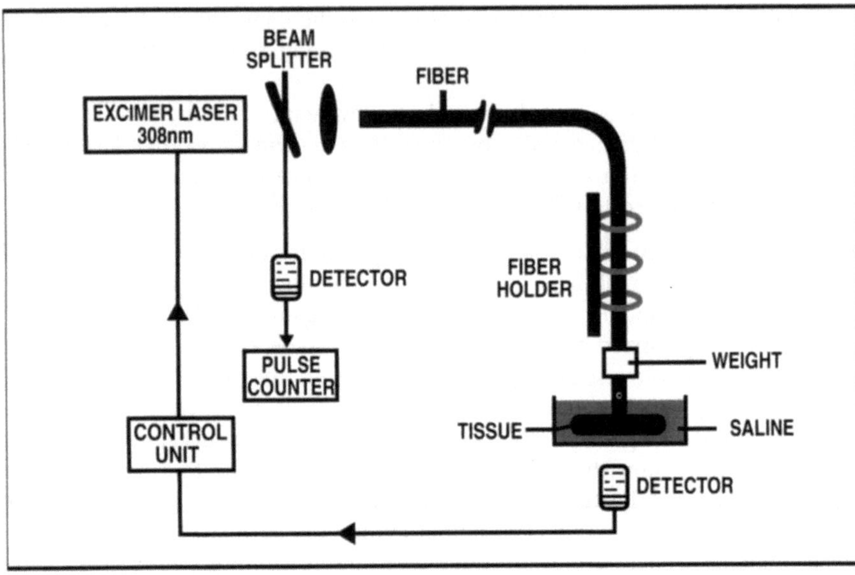

Fig. 11.1. Excimer laser (308 nm) ablation with fibreoptics: experimental setup

11.2.2
Apparatus for Determining Ablation Efficiency as a Function of Fluence and Repetition Rate

In order to define the optimal setting for ablation of myocardium the 308 nm excimer laser is coupled through a beam splitter and lens into a fibre optic element (single fibre or bundle; see Fig. 11.1). The beam splitter sends light to a detector and pulse counter. The fibreoptic array is mounted vertically in a holder, and a weight of known mass is attached to the fibre. The fibre is brought into contact with tissue surrounded by water, saline, or blood. The bottom of the cell holding the tissue has a transparent window, and the tissue is placed on top of this window and fixed in place. A detector below the window triggers a control unit to stop the laser when it measures two thirds of the energy of the ablative pulse. The thickness of the tissue is known and the number of pulses is precisely measured by the counter. The energy of each pulse is also measured and recorded so that variations from pulse to pulse can be included in the calculations. Data are then recorded at various repetition rates (5–60 Hz) and fluencies of 15–50 mJ/mm^2.

11.2.3
Apparatus for Controlling Fibre Advancement

As a prelude to clinical application, a mechanism for controlling fibre advancement into the myocardium was developed. This mechanism advances the fibre out of the tip of a hand-held probe at a constant rate. The rate can be set from 0.01 mm/s to 10 mm/s.

11.2.4
Holmium YAG Operating at 2.014 μm

A Schwartz ElectroOptics 123 holmium:YAG laser operating at 2.014 μm was used. The pulse duration of this laser is 1.5 μs. Analysis of the pulse shows spiking substructure within the pulse. The repetition rate was from 2 to 10 Hz.

Low OH fibres, ranging in diameter from 400 to 1000 μm, were specially designed to efficiently transmit this wavelength. Single fibres as well as fibres with expanded tips were used to simulate clinical applications. Bundles of fibres were not employed for this study. Energies for the holmium:YAG study are expressed in joules/pulse. Energies from 0.2 to 2 J were used.

11.2.5
CO_2 Operating at 10.600 μm

A PLC CO_2 laser operating at 10.600 μm was used. A single pulse is used to penetrate the myocardium. Clinical settings for this laser are pulse duration of 50 ms at 45 J/pulse. However, the laser can be operated at pulse durations of 40–99 ms, at energies of 25–80 J, with a spot size of 1 mm, for a fluency of 20–63 J/mm^2.

At the intensities and pulse durations used for this study, CO_2 laser light cannot be delivered through fibreoptics. The delivery system is an articulated arm consisting of a series of lenses and mirrors which guide the laser light to the target. A zinc-selenide lens with a focal length of 300 mm was used to provide a long beam waist.

11.2.6
Tissue Specimens

Segments of bovine myocardium, including pericardium, were obtained from a local meat-processing plant within 12 h of harvest. Segments of porcine and canine myocardium were obtained from the Cedars-Sinai vivarium within 24 h of harvest. Postmortem human myocardial specimens were obtained within 24 h of autopsy.

11.2.7
Animal Protocols

All experiments were performed according to protocols approved by the Institutional Animal Care and Use Committee for TMR experiments. Acute porcine experiments were performed on farmer pigs weighing 30–50 kg, after a minimum 5-day quarantine. Porcine models were pretreated with bretylium 7–10 mg/kg, lidocaine 2–3 mg/kg, and propanolol 0.025–0.03 mg/kg.

Two surgical approaches were used: a midline median sternotomy or an intercostal approach between the third and fourth ribs. Once the pericardial sac was identified, it was opened and exposure of the anterior lateral wall was easily accomplished. Animals were killed within 12 h of the procedure and always maintained under deep anesthesia. After TMR holes had been drilled, the heart was excised and each hole was placed in its own container of formalin solution for fixation. A map of the heart and a grid of the TMR holes was made to assure that the settings for each hole were clearly defined and properly marked on each specimen bottle.

11.2.8 Histology

All specimens were fixed in 10% formalin for more than 48 h prior to embedding. Sectioning for light microscopy was performed, and the tissues were stained with hematoxalin and eosin.

Slides were initially viewed under transmitted light on an Olympus microscope. Polarized light microscopy was performed with an Olympus microscope (BH-2 multi-port at 12.5 x or 40 x objective lenses). Each slide is imaged twice using a color video camera (Hitachi KP-C553 CCD, 722×492 pixels under normal and polarized light). The polarized light is generated by using a sub-stage polarizer and first-order red filters. A magnification reference grid was digitally superimposed to ensure uniform measurements. Microscopic images were stored digitally in a 486-based personal computer using a matrox frame grabber (Illuminator Pro CCIR-601–720×486). Loss of birefringence was marked using a wireless pen of a digitizing tablet (Wacom SD420 E 12×12 digitizing tablet). The boundaries of the hole were also outlined on the digital image. This outline represents the inner boundary of the thermally damaged region. The outer boundary, the edge of loss of birefringence, represents the outer marker for computer analysis.

The outlined 720×486 image is converted into a 648×486 VGA format and stored as a new file for further analysis using Matrox lnspector Version 1.7. The areas of the hole were segmented in white and areas of thermal damage were segmented in black. Following this segmentation, the software measured the areas of the TMR hole and surrounding thermal damage. The software was calibrated to real-world dimensions using the previously described 0.5 mm scale superimposed on the image. Validation studies showed the ability to resolve 0.002 mm on the 0.5-mm grid system. Computer software was used to count the number of pixels of the hole and the area of thermal damage as defined by loss of birefringence. The image processor received the data without knowing the original source in order to eliminate bias from the histology data.

A total of 2453 tissue specimens were imaged and analyzed as described above: 1600 specimens were obtained from excimer-irradiated myocardial specimens, 430 specimens were obtained from holmium:YAG-irradiated tissue, and 423 were obtained from CO_2-irradiated tissue.

11.2.9 Thermographic Imaging

Temperature measurements at the ablated surface were made using an Agema 782 Thermovision Infrared Camera with Agema software which permits measurement of temperatures. Spatial resolution of greater than 0.5 mm and thermal resolution of ±1°C was achieved using an 80-mm lens with extension rings. Images were captured digitally and on videotape.

11.2.10 Pressure Measurements

Pressure measurements were obtained in water- or blood-filled chambers during tissue ablation. Calibrated PDVF2 transducers were used to measure pressure transients for the excimer and holmium lasers, and the output was displayed on a digitizing oscilloscope. The transducers were placed 1 mm away from the catheter tip at 45° to the fibreoptic element and the tissue.

11.3 Results

11.3.1 Determination of Optimal Ablation Parameters In Vitro

Using the setup described above, a fluency of 35 mJ/mm^2 at a repetition rate of 20–30 Hz produced the optimal ablation efficiency. The highest ablation efficiency measured was 0.87 mm^3/J at a repetition rate of 20 Hz and a fluency of 34.5 mJ/mm^2. However, slightly higher energies and repetition rates gave values of 0.81 mm^3/J or 0.83 mm^3/J (see Tables 11.1 and 11.2 and Fig. 11.2 and 11.3).

Histology from initial in vivo studies revealed wide variations in hole size, thermal damage zones, and shock-wave effects. Analysis of the data showed that this wide variation was due largely to motion of the operator and the beating heart. When fibre advancement was too slow, large thermal damage zones of 0.5 to 1.0 mm were observed. When fibre advancement was too rap-

Table 11.1. Ablation rate (μm/pulse) vs. fluency and repetition rate

Fluence (mJ/mm^2)					
Rep rate (Hz)	17	22.5	28	34.5	39
5	2.5±0.3	8.2±1.5	14.2±1.3	21.1±2.6	27.9±3.5
20	7.3±1.5	13.0±1.3	20.4±2.9	28.8±2.2	32.6±4.1
35	7.8±1.0	15.8±1.5	22.0±1.9	26.9±2.6	28.8±2.6

Table 11.2. Ablation efficiency (mm^3/J) vs. fluency and repetition rate

Fluence (mJ/mm^2)					
Rep rate (Hz)	17	22.5	28	34.5	39
5	0.15	0.38	0.52	0.64	0.73
20	0.45	0.60	0.75	0.87	0.83
35	0.47	0.73	0.81	0.81	0.75

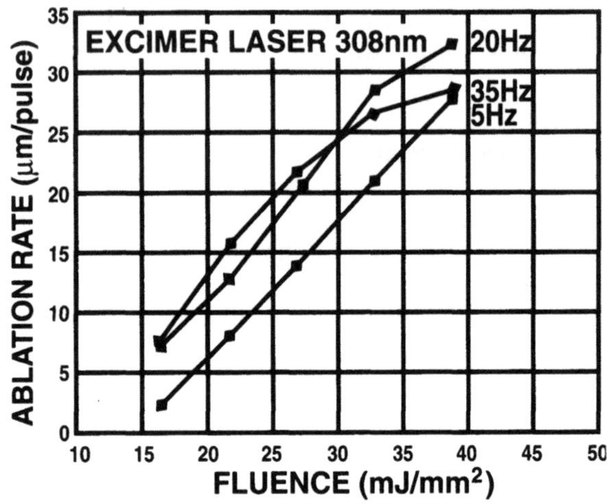

Fig. 11.2. Ablation rate vs. fluency and repetition rate

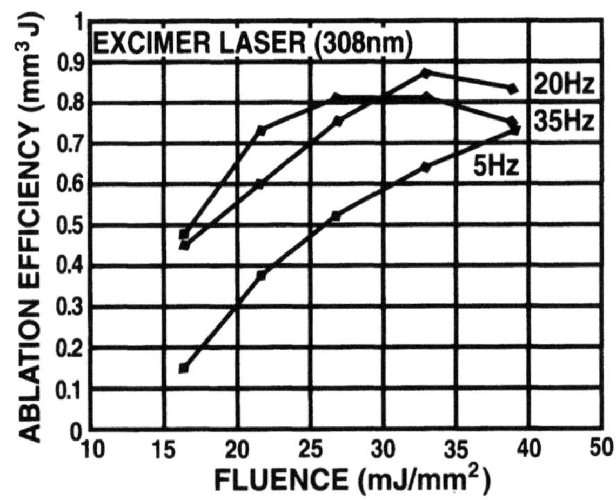

Fig. 11.3. Ablation efficiency vs. fluency and repetition rate

id, holes of only 0.5–0.6 mm in the long axis were observed; however, there was minimal if any thermal damage associated with these holes. In order to minimize motion effects, a constant advancement rate mechanism was developed to control the motion of the fibre. This control system permitted us to define the optimal advancement rate, which is a trade-off between hole size and thermal damage. Since each pulse ablates approximately 40 μm of tissue, it was determined that when the advancement rate exceeds the ablation rate for a given repetition rate only small holes are drilled. In contrast, when the advancement rate is too slow, the ablation rate exceeds the advancement rate, and thermal damage and blast injury become greater. We determined that the optimal hole size is best obtained when the advancement rate is slightly slower (90–95%) of the ablation rate. If minimal thermal damage is desired an advancement rate greater than the ablation rate can be employed; however, only small holes will be generated.

11.3.2
In Vitro Ablation By Holmium:YAG Laser Energy

The holmium:YAG laser produced holes of approximately 3.0–6.0 mm/pulse depending upon the fluency. Fibre diameters of 400, 600, and 1000 μm were used at energies of 0.5–2 J/pulse. At an energy of 0.5 J/pulse with a 400-μm fibre, crater depth varied from 1.1 to 3.3 mm with ragged walls and substantial evidence of thermal injury (tissue coagulation). However, hole size was smaller than the fibre diameter (0.3–0.4 mm). At 1.0 J/pulse, 600-μm fibre, the depth of the hole varied from 2.2 to 4.8 mm. Shredding of tissue and thermal coagulation extended 1–3 mm from the wall of the crater, and crater diameter ranged from 0.4 to 1.2 mm in diameter. At 2 J/pulse with a 1-mm diameter fibre, depth of ablation per pulse was approximately 3.0–5.0 mm/pulse. There were wide variations in hole depth and thermal damage. Thermal damage ranged from 0.6 to 2.2 mm in diameter.

The CO_2 laser showed substantial variation in thermal damage zones and hole size as a function of alignment with the myocardial fibres. Damage zones along the axis of the fibres ranged from 0.2 to 1.5 mm, while damage zones perpendicular to the axis of the fibres ranged from 0.1 to 0.8 mm. Examination of the ablated channels generally displayed elliptical holes, although some were round. Interestingly, hole morphology changed as a function of the layer of the myocardium. In some areas a channel might be circular and in other areas dramatically eccentric or elliptical. Holes ranged from almost perfectly circular to ones which were 1 mm in the long axis and 0.2 mm in the short axis.

11.3.3
Comparison of Three Laser Systems In Vivo

TMR was performed in porcine models using the CO_2, holmium:YAG, and excimer systems as described above. Fibreoptically delivered laser energy is easier to apply to the surface of the heart and removes the need for the cumbersome articulated arm. The PLC laser system and the holmium:YAG laser system were ECG triggered; the excimer laser was not synchronized to the ECG. During drilling of holmium:YAG holes intermittent episodes of ventricular tachycardia occurred in one third of the procedures. These resolved spontaneously at the end of the ablation process (in 3–5 s). During drilling of excimer holes ventricular tachycardia occurred in approximately one third of the procedures. Interestingly, the ventricular tachycardia resolved after ablation ceased even if the catheter was in the ventricle.

All three systems effectively drilled holes into the myocardium. CO_2 laser holes were surrounded by a small ring of blanched tissue approximately 0.2 mm in diameter (thermal denaturation). Holmium:YAG holes showed a larger zone of blanching which varied from 0.4 to 0.8 mm in diameter, depending upon the energy setting used. The excimer laser-drilled holes showed a 0.1- to 0.3-mm zone of blanching depending upon the energy setting used.

CO_2 ablation is accompanied by ejection of a plume of steam. Hole size varied from 1 to 0.8 mm. The presence of the fibre in the holmium and excimer systems forces ejection of gas and cellular debris around the fibre. At high repetition rates (60–80 Hz) for the excimer laser, tissue fissuring was observed on the myocardial surface. At repetition rates of 20–40 Hz the excimer ablation process proceeded with minimal damage to adjacent tissue. Hole size was always equal to or slightly less than the diameter of the drilling probe. Drilling channels with the holmium:YAG laser required only 3–5 pulses per hole. However, the holes created at 1 or 2 J/pulse were often irregular owing to tissue rupturing from escaping gas, and hole size varied widely (1.0–0.3 mm). Holmium:YAG holes drilled at 0.5 J/pulse were always less than 0.6 mm in diameter.

Thermographic measurements reveal that the CO_2 ablation process produces a plume of hot gas (steam) which is always above 135°C. The crater walls often reached temperatures in excess of this. In vivo, the zone of thermal damage (tissue blanching) creates an area 1.5–2.5 mm in diameter. This zone corresponds to the area of tissue heated to 60°C or higher, as measured by the thermal camera. The holmium:YAG ablation also drives peak temperatures above 100°C (75° above baseline) and produces a larger zone of thermally injured tissue (above 60°C) 2–3 mm in diameter. Because the holmium:YAG holes are smaller, with larger zones of thermal damage, the result is a substantially greater volume of necrotic tissue than seen with the CO_2 and excimer lasers. Temperatures measured with the excimer laser show a rise over baseline of 24–28°C. When the heart was irradiated at 37°C and a repetition rate of 40 Hz, the surface temperature was 61–65°C. If the heart was cooled to 28°C, temperatures did not exceed 56°C. Thermal damage zones (temperatures above 60°C) for noncooled hearts were 0.1–0.4 mm in diameter, resulting in substantially smaller volumes of necrotic tissue around excimer drilled holes.

11.3.4 Analysis of Pressure Transients

Measurements of pressure transients during ablation in tissue showed peak pressures of 80–100 bar for holmium:YAG at 100 J/cm^2 and peak pressures of 10–14 bar for excimer ablation in tissue at 80 mJ/mm^2. Under clinical conditions of 1 J/mm^2, holmium:YAG pressure transients exceeded 100 bar with tissue in blood and for an excimer operating at 35 mJ/mm^2 with tissue in blood pressure transients reached 72 bar. When the blood was removed, holmium:YAG pressure transients remained at 100 bar, while excimer transients dropped to 15 bar.

11.3.5 Histologic Analysis of In Vivo Studies

Histologic analysis revealed wide variations in hole shapes and sizes and thermal damage zones for all three lasers, even at the same energy setting for a given laser. This variability is the reason for conducting an analysis of this large number of slides to produce statistically valid data. Analysis of CO_2-drilled holes showed wide variation in hole shapes and sizes and thermal damage zones. Hole sizes ranged from 0.2–1.6 mm in the long axis to 0.1–0.8 mm in the short axis. Almost all the holes (greater than 90%) were eccentric. Of particular note is the presence of extended zones of thermally denatured tissue which follow small capillaries away from the crater center. These finger-like projections appear to be the result of steam being driven into the small capillaries during the ablation process. In some cases the damage zones extended 3 mm from the crater.

Analysis of holmium:YAG-irradiated tissue shows irregularly shaped holes with ragged edges due to tissue tearing and thermal coagulation. Hole size ranges from 0.2 mm in the short axis to 0.9 mm in the long axis. The zones of thermal injury range from 0.4 mm on the short axis to 3.0 mm on the long axis. Pronounced tissue tearing, as evidenced by fissures of 1–4 mm in length, were prominent particularly at higher energies. At lower energies hole sizes were dramatically reduced (0.2–0.4 mm in diameter). Parameter optimization for the holmium:YAG laser is difficult, since there is a substantial trade-off between hole size and thermal injury. At energies required to ablate a channel with a diameter of 0.8 mm or greater, substantial thermal damage results. At these same energies, tissue fissuring is pronounced.

Analysis of excimer-irradiated tissue clearly demonstrates the need to carefully select operating parameters. At high energies and high repetition rates hole sizes range from 0.6 mm in the short axis to 1.4 mm in the long axis, but these holes were accompanied by thermal damage zones of 1.0 mm in the short axis and 2.5 mm in the long axis. The energy levels were set at 35 mJ/mm^2 for further parameter optimization. The combination of controlled fibre advancement and use of repetition rates from 20 to 60 Hz allowed us to identify optimal settings. An analysis of hole size verses thermal damage defines the optimal operating parameters as being 25–40 Hz at an energy of 35 mJ/mm^2. Fibre advancement speeds are optimal when the ablation rate is slightly greater than the advancement rate. This produces the largest possible hole with a thermal damage area approximately 0.3 mm in diameter. Faster advancement speeds produce smaller holes with even less thermal damage; slower advancement speeds produce large holes but with substantially greater (0.6–1.0 mm in diameter) thermal damage.

11.4 Discussion

We have examined three different lasers and their applicability for drilling holes in the myocardium for the TMR procedure. All three lasers will drill holes, but each has its advantages and disadvantages. The CO_2 laser drills a hole in one pulse; however, evidence to date does not show this to be an advantage. This laser occupies a large space in the operating room, requires an articulated arm for energy delivery, and requires a ventricle full of blood for safe operation. It produces smooth-channeled holes with a wide range of thermal damage zones. Steam escaping from the channel is driven out through the capillaries, producing substantial thermal injury along the vascular channels. It is precisely these channels which theoretically connect to improve blood flow. Therefore, the thermal injury and the accompanying scarring and collagen deposition are probably not desirable.

The holmium:YAG laser is small, easy to operate, and can be delivered fibreoptically. It easily drills a channel in the myocardium, but these holes are accompanied by substantial thermal injury to adjacent tissue. Each pulse creates a crater 2–5 mm in depth with thermal damage zones of 1 mm or greater beyond the channel edge. The tissue fissuring (tearing) could, in theory, open new channels to adjacent blood vessels, but the thermal coagulation (burn) which accompanies these fissures is a strong stimulus for collagen deposition and scar formation.

The excimer laser can be operated over a broad range of energies and repetition rates. This flexibility requires determination of the optimal operative settings for clinical use. The laser is small, and its energy can be delivered through fibreoptics. Each pulse ablates only 30–50 μm; however, if the laser energy is deposited in one spot for too long, thermal damage occurs. If the fibre is advanced too quickly only a small hole is made. In order to insure operation at the optimal advancement rate and provide the operator substantial control of the channel-drilling process, an automated fibre feed system was developed. This system dramatically reduces the wide variation in histology seen with hand-drilled channels. The principle advantages of the excimer laser are its ability to drill holes of uniform size with small zones of thermal damage without danger to adjacent tissue.

Based on histologic, thermographic, and pressure measurements from both in vivo and in vitro experiments, the excimer laser provides the surgeon with a precise method of creating channels in the myocardium with minimal damage to adjacent tissue. While the mechanism of action of TMR remains unknown, 308 nm laser light provides a method of hole drilling that is compatible with either open-chest or percutaneous techniques. The flexibility of the delivery system and the control afforded by ablation in the ultraviolet (308 nm) will permit development of a safe percutaneous PMR technique.

CHAPTER 12

Working Mechanism of Pulsed CO_2, Holmium and Excimer Laser Systems with Regard to Transmyocardial Revascularisation (TMR): In Vivo Implications

R. Verdaasdonk · A. Sachinopoulou · P. Gründeman · J. Beek

12.1 Introduction

The use of lasers to create transmyocardial channels in hibernating myocardium is being considered as an alternative for patients who cannot be treated with ordinary bypass surgery. The physiological mechanism behind the therapy is not yet understood and is still hard to prove in studies. Although the idea of transmyocardial revascularisation (TMR) started with the perfusion concept of a reptile heart [1], the functioning might also be ascribed to neoplastic revascularisation of the hibernating myocardium [2]. At the basis of the biological response is the creation mechanism of the channel. Therefore, it is beneficial to study and understand the working mechanism of the creation of channels by the various lasers currently being use [3]. With this knowledge it is possible to control the characteristics of the channels, depending on the laser parameters. Based on earlier experience [4], it is believed that the channels for transmyocardial laser recanalisation (TMLR) should meet the following conditions: the channels for 'reperfusion' should be about 15–25 mm long and 1 mm in diameter. For minimal invasive treatment, the channels should be created on a beating heart within the diastolic phase (<100 ms) or on an arrested heart using multiple pulses. Long-term patency is expected when the walls of the channels have minimal thermal damage.

Thousands of patients worldwide have been treated using mainly an 800-W continuous-wave (cw) CO_2 laser (Heart Laser, PLC) capable of creating channels with the characteristics described above. On average, the patients improved by two classes in the angina symptom score [5, 6]. Besides, the high-power cw laser, other laser systems are under investigation for TMR treatment. In this study three pulsed lasers systems were compared with regard to their working mechanism of tissue ablation and to their capability and efficiency in creating channels in myocardium in vitro and in vivo.

12.2 Materials and Methods

12.2.1 Laser Systems

The three pulsed laser systems investigated in this study were:

1. A pulsed CO_2 laser (Coherent Ultrapulse 5000, Palo Alto, Calif., USA) with a wavelength of 10.6 µm. This wavelength is strongly absorbed by the

water contents of the tissue. The system produces 600 W at a duration of up to 1 ms. The resulting pulse energy of 250 mJ can be repeated at 400 Hz, so the average power is 100 W. The beam is delivered through an articulated arm focused by a lens to a 1-mm spot. There is no fibre delivery system available yet for the CO_2 laser.

2. A holmium laser (Coherent Versapulse, Palo Alto, Calif., USA) with a wavelength of 2.1 μm. This wavelength also is mainly absorbed by water, but the initial penetration depth is 500 μm compared with 50 μm for the CO_2 laser. Laser energy of 350–1000 mJ is produced in 350 μs at a maximum repetition frequency of 25 Hz, resulting in an average power of 25 W. The beam is coupled to a 300-μm fibre delivery device with a 1-mm spot at the tip.
3. A xenon-chloride excimer laser (Medolas, Munich, Germany) with a wavelength of 308 nm. In contrast to the other lasers, the proteins in the tissue, like the cell membranes, absorb the light. Consequently, energy transfer from the membranes heats the cell water content. The energy of only 10–50 mJ is produced within 120 ns at a maximum frequency of 40 Hz, resulting in an average power of only 2 W. However, the peak power during the pulse is over 25000 W. The beam is coupled to a 1000-μm fibre delivery device.

12.2.2
In Vitro Experiments

12.2.2.1
Visualisation of the Ablation Process in Liquid and Tissue

High-speed photography was used to visualise phenomena during and after the laser pulse with a resolution of 1–40 μs. A flashlight was triggered with a preset delay from the start of the laser pulse. The delay time could be varied from 1 μs to 10 ms covering the whole time frame of the tissue ablation mechanism. The close-up images show a field of 10×15 mm with a resolution of 20 μm. The experiments were performed in clear media such as saline and polyacrylamide gel.

12.2.2.2
Visualisation of the Thermal Effects in Tissue

An imaging method based on colour Schlieren techniques was used to visualise the temperature gradient in a phantom tissue [7]. Minor changes in the density of a medium induced by temperature differences are optically colour coded and recorded in real time on video. The images show a close-up field of 10×15 mm with a resolution of 20 μm.

12.2.2.3
Measurement of the Ablation Speed of the Focused CO_2 Beam

The setup for visualisation of the ablation process was also used to determine the ablation speed of the CO_2 laser. From images captured at increas-

Table 12.1. Laser parameters and conditions

	CO_2	Ho:YAG	XeCl Excimer
Energy per pulse (mJ)	250, 500	350, 750	25
Exposure window (s)	0.05, 0.10, 0.20		0.2
Repetition frequency (Hz)	Single, 1, 3	5	20, 40
Spot/fiber tip diameter (μm)	500, 1000	1000	1000
Weight (g)		10, 25, 35	50, 60, 70, 80

ing delays, the depth of the ablation crater was measured and the speed of ablation was calculated.

12.2.2.4
Measurement of the Penetration Speed of Fibre Delivery Systems in Myocardium

The displacement of the fibre delivery system into tissue was measured during activation of the excimer and holmium laser in a 'penetration' tower set-up [8]. During tissue penetration the output of displacement sensors was recorded by a personal computer. The penetration speed was determined from the displacement per series of pulses in time.

12.2.2.5
Laser Parameters and Conditions

The speed of crater formation was determined in relation to the parameters shown in Table 12.1. The experiments were performed in saline and a polyacrylamide gel to provide a transparent medium with absorption characteristics similar to tissue for the CO_2 and holmium laser. In case of the excimer laser a chromaphore was added to simulate the absorption of tissue. It is assumed that the thermal characteristics and the mechanical characteristics of the gel are comparable with those of tissue. For the fiber penetration measurements bovine myocardium was used.

In Vivo Experiments

In a pig model, the feasibility of creating channels in the myocardium of a beating heart was tested for the three laser systems. Channels were created using an ECG-triggered train of laser pulses while the beating heart was locally immobilised using the 'Utrecht Octopus' device [9]. The pulses were delivered within the relaxation phase of the cardiac cycle and were repeated each cycle until perforation was achieved. Following the procedure the animals were sacrificed and tissue samples were processed for histology.

12.3
Results

12.3.1
Mechanism of Tissue Ablation

The mechanism of tissue ablation can be divided into three phases:
1. Laser pulse: during the length of the laser pulse explosive vapour is formed, creating an expanding vapour bubble.
2. Bubble: at the end of the laser pulse the water vapour starts cooling and the vapour bubble collapses while transferring the energy released during condensation to the environment.
3. Thermal relaxation: the direct environment of the original vapour bubble is heated and the energy is conducted to surrounding tissue while it is cooling to ambient temperatures.

These three phases are depicted in Fig. 12.1 along a time scale of the ablation mechanism for the three lasers investigated. Pictures representative for the various phases are incorporated in the figure. The phases are discussed in more detail below.

12.3.1.1
Mechanical Effects: Explosive Vapour Expansion

Using high-speed photography, the formation of explosive expanding vapour bubbles was captured as illustrated in the inserts of Fig. 12.1 for all three lasers. Due to the high power density, tissue water is instantly turned to vapour during exposure. The vapour expands to ambient pressure, increasing to around 1600 times its original volume in a time frame of 50 μs–1 ms (Fig. 12.1, frames A, D, G). The expansion of the vapour follows the path of least resistance. At the tissue surface, this will be towards the surrounding air or water interface. Deeper into the tissue, however, the vapour goes into fissures alongside the channel wall (Fig. 12.1, frames B, E, H).

In case of the holmium and the CO_2 lasers, the tissue ablation continues during the vapour expansion since the pulse length overlaps the lifetime of the vapour expansion period. The vapour bubble creates a channel through which the laser light can reach tissue at deeper layers. If the laser pulse is powerful and sufficiently long, a transmural channel can be formed during a single exposure. This is performed with the Heart CO_2 laser system with a pulse length up to 20 ms. In case of the excimer laser, the vapour is still expanding to ambient pressures 'long' after the laser pulse of only 120 ns. Compared with the holmium and CO_2 lasers, the volume of vapour created per pulse is much less.

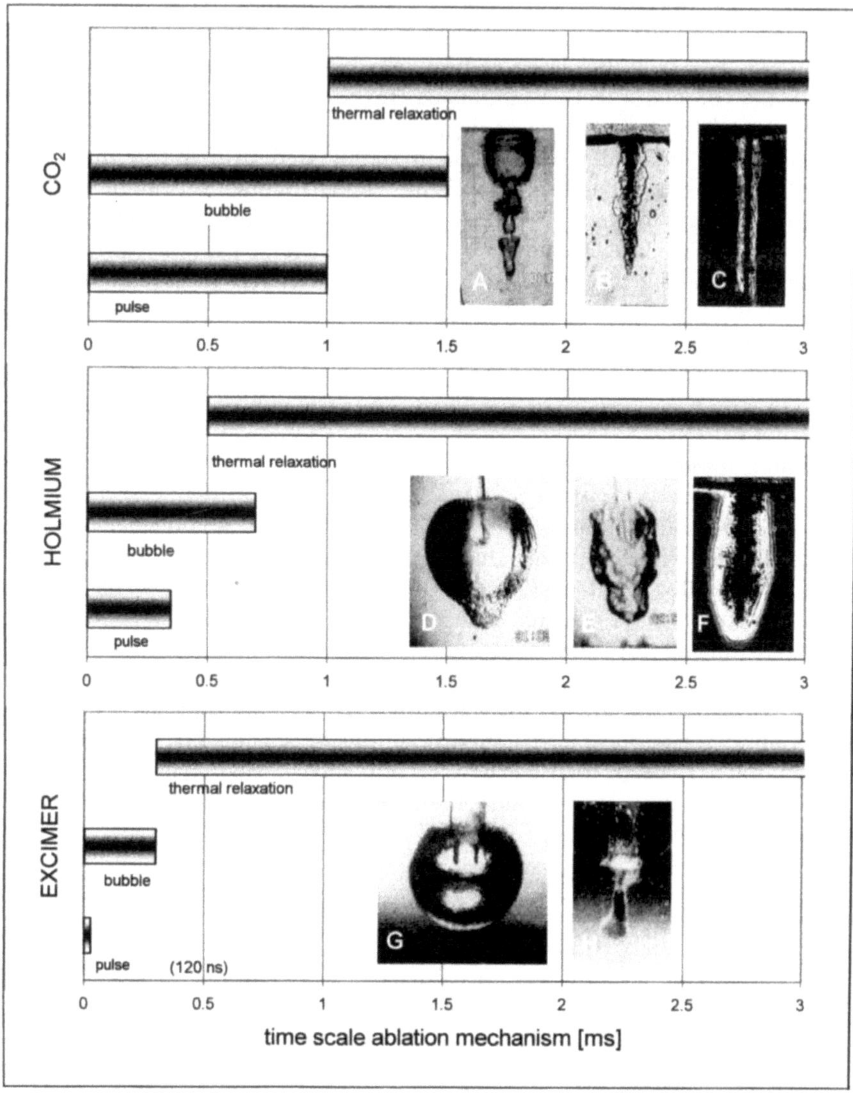

Fig. 12.1. The three phases of the ablation mechanism (*pulse, bubble, thermal relaxation*) for the three lasers investigated are depicted along a time scale of milliseconds. The *inserts* show representative frames of the phases obtained with either high-speed or thermal imaging in water or transparent tissue. The phases are discussed in detail in the text

12.3.1.2
Thermal Effects: Vapour Condensation

During expansion the vapour cools and condenses, reversing the process to implosion. The latent heat of vaporisation is released during condensation, heating the tissue. After each laser pulse, the thermal energy is conducted into the surrounding tissue. The temperature gradient along the wall of the ablation crater was visualised using an optical method based on Schlieren techniques. Frames C and F in Fig. 12.1 show the extent of thermal effects for the CO_2 and holmium laser, respectively. When a series of pulses was delivered, the thermal effects accumulated in the surrounding tissue. Both the CO_2 laser and the holmium laser deliver a considerable amount of energy in each pulse (on the order of 500–750 mJ) compared with the excimer laser (only 25 mJ). Thus, after relaxation of the vapour bubble, this amount of energy locally heats the tissue. The thermal images captured for CO_2 and holmium lasers (Fig. 12.1, frames C and F, respectively) show a clear area of thermal effect along the crater wall. The thermal effects in case of the excimer laser were hardly visible, although due to the high repetition rate of the laser pulses (40 Hz), the thermal effect accumulated and still caused a local temperature increase.

12.3.2 Penetration Speed

In case of the holmium and the excimer laser, the light was delivered with a fibre in contact with the tissue. During the tissue vaporisation, the fibre penetrated the created channel. Owing to the presence of the fibre, the vapour cannot escape to the air at the surface. Instead, it forces its way through the tissue, creating fissures and contributing to the mechanical ablation mechanism. The fibre penetration was measured in relation to the exerted force during exposure of bovine myocardium. The results showed penetration speeds up to 1 mm/pulse at the energy settings presented (Fig. 12.2). In comparison, the CO_2 beam focused on a 0.5 mm spot created channels of 2 mm/pulse. In focus (spot size 0.1 mm), the length of the channel increased up to 30 mm for a single pulse.

12.3.3 Penetration Efficiency

The results of the tissue penetration experiments of the three laser systems are summarised for comparison in Fig. 12.2. For each laser two settings are presented at the highest performance with regard to pulse energy, pulse frequency and spot size.

The penetration efficiency is evaluated from different perspectives:

1. *Penetration per pulse*: this criterion is important if only a limited time is available to create the channel, e.g. the time of relaxation of a beating heart. The CO_2 laser creates the longest channel with just one pulse.
2. *Penetration per second*: this criterion is important when multiple pulses are applied shortly after one another. Obviously, it is closely related to the penetration per pulse and the repetition frequency of the laser system. Again, the CO_2 laser is the fastest in relation to the other two.
3. *Penetration per Joule*: this criterion shows how efficient the laser energy is used in the ablation mechanism to displace tissue. The excimer laser is the most efficient. Indirectly, it indicates that the other two lasers waste more energy as thermal energy.

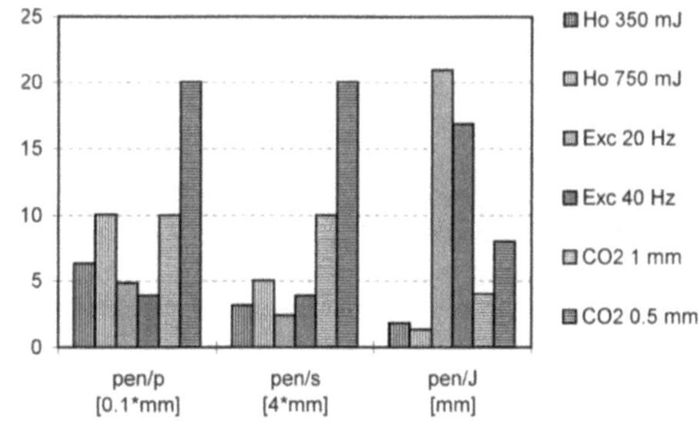

Fig. 12.2. Penetration efficiency of the holmium (*Ho*), excimer (*Exc*) and CO_2 (CO_2) laser at two settings each. Compared are: penetration per pulse (*pen/p*), penetration speed (*pen/s*) and penetration per unit of energy (*pen/J*). The scale is adapted by the factor presented in the units

12.3.4
In Vivo Study

The three lasers were successfully applied in vivo using the 'Utrecht Octopus' device [9] for local immobilisation of the area where the channels were created. The device enabled multiple pulse trains during several heart cycles to create one channel without problems in directing the beam or the fibre. In several cases TMLR was even performed thoracoscopically on the beating porcine heart [10]. During penetration of the left ventricle wall, no major changes in the ECG signal were observed, nor did arrhythmias occur, in contrast to earlier experience without ECG-triggered pulses. Arrhythmias occurred in particular when the holmium laser was used untriggered, and a total collapse in cardiac output was observed, which fortunately recovered after a short time.

Macroscopic and microscopic evaluation of the tissue samples obtained directly after the animals were killed, showed that the fibre-based delivery devices created irregular channels, with ruptures to the sides, and that thermal damage was most prominent with the holmium laser. The CO_2 laser created smooth channels with substantial thermal damage.

12.4
Discussion

The in vitro experiments show that channels are formed in the myocardium using pulsed laser as a combination of mechanical and thermal effects. The explosive vapour formation induces ruptures in the tissue while the vapour seeks the path of least resistance. Especially, a fibre delivery device will occlude the opening to the surface, resulting in ruptures along the channel wall. Since the vapour is not able to escape, the heat of condensation is also released in the tissue, contributing to thermal damage in the surrounding tissue as observed with thermal imaging in vitro and by histological examination of tissue obtained from the in vivo study. However, it has not been determined to what extent the mechanical and thermal effects contribute to the biological response and clinical outcome of the TMLR procedures. Therefore, the physiology of TMR needs to be understood. If, according to the original hypothesis, the channels provide a direct perfusion of the myocardium by oxygen-rich blood from the ventricle, the channels should stay open and the fissures might act as a microvasculature. However, the associated thermal damage might induce clot formation and closure of the channel [11]. Only a few studies support this theory. In most cases, more than half of the channels created are reported to be occluded within a few days after the procedure [12–14]. However, thousands of patients have been treated, and most clinical trials show a significant decrease in patients' symptomatic complaints [2].

Another hypothesis concerning the mechanism of action of TMLR treatment is that the heart muscle provoked by laser channels reacts by forming a neo-microvascular structure [2, 13, 15]. Therefore, the channels do not need to be transmural or to remain open. It is not clear what length and diameter these lesions should have, or what extent of thermal damage is required to stimulate this response.

Currently, all three laser types investigated in this study are being used in clinical trails. The fibre-delivered laser systems are being developed to perform a TMLR procedure percutaneously [16]. The initial clinical results are comparable, independent of the laser system used. This suggests that the shape of the channels does not really have a bearing on the clinical outcome.

12.5 Conclusions

In combination with optimised delivery systems and dosimetry, pulsed CO_2, holmium and excimer laser systems can be used to create transmyocardial channels thoracscopically on the beating heart within a few cardiac cycles. The contribution of mechanical effects in the creation of the ablation channels is substantial. Since the physiology of TMLR still needs to be understood, it is not clear what channels have the best potential to induce reperfusion of the myocardium.

References

1. Kohmoto T, Argenziano M, Yamamoto N, Vliet KA, Gu A, Derosa CM, Fisher PE, Spotnitz HM, Burkhoff D, Smith CR (1997) Assessment of transmyocardial perfusion in alligator hearts. Circulation 95:1585–1591
2. Whittaker P, Rakusan K, Kloner RA (1996) Transmural channels can protect ischemic tissue assessment of long-term myocardial response to laser-made and needle-made channels. Circulation 93:143–152
3. Jansen ED, Frenz M, Kadipasaoglu KA, Pfefer TJ, Altermatt HJ, Motamedi M, Welch AJ (1997) Laser-tissue interaction during transmyocardial laser revascularization. Ann. Thorac Surg 63:640–647
4. Sachinopoulou A, Beek JF, Tukkie R, Meijer DW, Gründeman PF, de Mol BAJM, Bannenberg J, Verdaasdonk RM, van Gement MJC (1996) Transmyocardial Revascularisation Lasers Med Sci 10:83–91
5. Moosdorf R, Maisch B, Hoffken H (1996) Transmyocardial laser revascularization – limits and possibilities. Z Kardiol 85 [Suppl 6]:281–285
6. Horvath KA, Cohn LH, Cooley DA, Crew JR, Frazier OH, Griffith BP, Kadipasaoglu K, Lansing A, Mannting F, March R, Mirhoseini MR, Smith C (1997) Transmyocardial laser revascularization: results of a multicenter trial with transmyocardial laser revascularization used as sole therapy for end-stage coronary artery disease. J Thorac Cardiovasc Surg 113:645–653

7. Verdaasdonk R (1995) Imaging laser induced thermal fields and effects. In: Jacques (ed) Laser-tissue interaction. VI. Bellingham. SPIE proc. vol. 2391, pp 165–175
8. Verdaasdonk RM, Jansen ED, Holstege FC, Borst C (1991) Mechanism of CW Nd:YAG laser recanalization with modified fiber tips: influence of temperature and axial force on tissue penetration in vitro. Lasers Surg Med 11:204–212
9. Borst C, Jansen EW, Tulleken CA, Gründeman PF, Mansvelt Beck HJ, van Dongen JW, Hodde KC, Bredee JJ (1996) Coronary artery bypass grafting without cardiopulmonary bypass and without interruption of native coronary flow using a novel anastomosis site restraining device ("Octopus"). J Am Coll Cardiol 27:1356–1364
10. Gründeman PF, van Leeuwen TG, Verdaasdonk RM, Jansen EWL, Mansvelt Beck H, Borst C (1996) Thoracoscopic creation of transmural laser channels in the beating porcine heart using conventional lasers: closed chest application of the 'Octopus' cardiac immobilization method. [Abstract] Circulation 94:(I)477
11. Krabatsch T, Schaper F, Leder C, Tulsner J, Thalmann U, Hetzer R (1996) Histological findings after transmyocardial laser revascularization. J Card Surg 11:326–331
12. Gassler N, Wintzer HO, Stubbe HM, Wullbrand A, Helmchen U (1997) Transmyocardial laser revascularization. Histological features in human nonresponder myocardium. Circulation 95:371–375
13. Kohmoto T, Fisher PE, Gu A, Zhu SM, Derosa CM, Smith CR, Burkhoff D (1997) Physiology, histology, and 2-week morphology of acute transmyocardial channels made with a CO_2 laser. Ann Thorac Surg 63:1275–1283
14. Kohmoto T, Fisher PE, Gu A, Zhu SM, Yano OJ, Spotnitz HM, Smith CR, Burkhoff D (1996) Does blood flow through holmium YAG transmyocardial laser channels? Ann Thorac Surg 61:861–868
15. Fleischer KJ, Goldschmidt Clermont PJ, Fonger JD, Hutchins GM, Hruban RH, Baumgartner WA (1996) One-month histologic response of transmyocardial laser channels with molecular intervention. Ann Thorac Surg 62:1051–1058
16. Kim CB, Kesten R, Javier M, Hayase M, Walton AS, Billingham ME, Kernoff R, Oesterle SN (1997) Percutaneous method of laser transmyocardial revascularization. Cathet Cardiovasc Diagn 40:223–228

CHAPTER 13

Transmyocardial Laser Revascularisation: Are New Approaches with New Lasers Possible?

M. M. Ivanenko · P. Hering · M. Klein · E. Gams

13.1 Introduction

The purpose of this article is to briefly describe the main physical mechanisms of laser ablation of biological tissues and to analyse the prospects of new laser systems for transmyocardial laser revascularisation (TMLR).

From a physicist's point of view, the TMLR procedure is generally based on the ability to concentrate laser light in a thin beam of very high intensity, which effectively ablates soft biological tissues. For a surgeon, TMLR is a nontrivial and elegant way to help patients with coronary artery disease. Throughout the world, many investigators have utilised and further developed this procedure (see, e.g. [1–5]) as it may, hopefully, complement or in some cases even substitute for traditional angioplasty and complicated heart-bypass surgery. However, further research and clinical data are needed to explain the mechanisms involved. The discussion is focused particularly on (a) how long the created transmyocardial channels can stay open; (b) how these channels affect the electrical conductivity of the perforated region; and (c) how extensive is/are the thermal damage, shock waves and mechanical disruptions caused in the myocardium. Today, a *prior* optimisation of laser parameters and even the selection of the best laser type for TMLR is difficult. Instead, one can try different operating modes and different lasers, which should meet several basic requirements:

1. The laser must be able to 'drill' the transmyocardial channel with a diameter $d \approx 1$–1.5 mm.
2. Thermal damage to surrounding tissue must be acceptable.
3. The laser should be suitable for application in an operating theatre, i.e. reliable, simple to manipulate, relatively compact, with no electrical interference, etc.

Using laser light, three general approaches to heart perforation are possible: creation of the transmyocardial channel with (a) a single powerful laser shot, (b) a burst of quickly successive short laser pulses, and (c) multiple weak laser pulses, not synchronised with the heart rhythm.

The parameters of the laser systems that have been evaluated with respect to TMLR have been summarised in Table 13.1, together with the results published so far. Where possible, the important ablation parameters such as peak intensity I (W/cm^2), pulse energy density Φ (J/cm^2) and specific ablation energy w_{abl} (J/mm^3) have been recalculated on the basis of those publications. Following is a brief account of the essential properties of each laser type and a discussion of the results obtained.

Table 13.1. Laser systems for TMLR

Laser:	CO_2 quasi-cw	CO_2 ultrapulsed	CO_2 Q-switch	Ho:YAG			Nd:YAG	XeCl		
Wavelength, λ	10.6 μm			2.1 μm			1.44 μm	308 nm		
Pulse energy, E	15–40 J	0.5 J	0.02–0.05 J	1–2 J	0.75 J	2 J	1–2 J	20–40 mJ	20 mJ	21 mJ
Pulse duration, τ	20–50 ms	1.4 ms	250–350 ns	100–500 μs		~ 350 μs	600 μs	150 ns	120 ns	
Repetition rate, f	Single shot	200 Hz	200–20000 Hz	5–20 Hz	5 Hz	3 pulses per diastole	5–20 Hz	40 Hz	40 Hz	40 Hz
Average power, P	(800 W cw)	100 W	10–400 W	5–10 W	3.75 W		5–10 W	0.8–1.6 W	0.8 W	0.82 W
Beam delivery	Articulated mirror arm			Silica (quartz) fibre of 0.3- to 1-mm core diameter or fibre bundle						
Channel diameter, d	1 mm	0.5 mm	1 mm	1 mm	1 mm	1.75 mm	1 mm	0.5–1 mm	0.5 mm	(≤ ?) 1 mm
Peak intensity, I	0.1 MW/cm^2	0.2 MW/cm^2	~ 10 MW/cm^2	1.2–0.5 MW/cm^2		0.24 MW/cm^2	0.2–0.4 MW/cm^2	70–30 MW/cm^2	~ 80 MW/cm^2	
Time per channel	20–50 ms	200 ms		4–8 s	4 s	~5 s	4–8 s	3–6 s	10 s	<1 s
Pulses per channel	1	40		40–80	20	12/8 mm	40–80	120–240	400	30
Pulse energy density, Φ	2000–5000	250 J/cm^2		130–250 J/cm^2	100 J/cm^2	85 J/cm^2	130–250 J/cm^2	10–5 J/cm^2	10 J/cm^2	2.7 J/cm^2
Specific ablation energy, w_{abl}	2–5 J/mm^3	~ 5 J/mm^3	Reduced ?	~ 5 J/mm^3	~ 1 J/mm^3	1.25 J/mm^3	~ 5 J/mm^3	~ 2 J/mm^3	~ 4 J/mm^3	≥0.04 J/mm^3
Thermal damage	>200 μm		Reduced ?	~ 300 μm		~ 75 μm	~ 350 μm	10–50 μm	30 μm	
Shock wave pressure	~ 3 bar			~ 10 bar			~ 10 bar	~ 500 bar		
Geometry	Smooth channels			Irregular channels with ruptures to the side						
Specimen	Beating heart	In vitro, bovine m. 2 cm thick		In vitro	In vitro, bovine m. 2 cm thick	Beating dog heart	In vitro		In vitro	In vitro, bovine m. 2 cm thick
Additional conditions	ECG triggering		Proposal, HHU Düsseldorf		35 g pushing force	ECG triggering				80 g pushing force
Reference	[6–8]	[9]		[6, 7]	[9]	[10]	[6, 7]	[6]	[7]	[9]

m., myocardium

13.2 CO_2 Lasers for TMLR

The CO_2 laser emits invisible infrared (IR) light at a wavelength $\lambda = 10.6$ µm. The laser is widely used in surgery because of the high tissue absorption at this wavelength, good beam focusability, high power, high efficiency and reliability of the system. The light is generated in a mixture of the inert gases $CO_2/N_2/He$, usually excited by means of radio-frequency (RF) or direct-current (DC) electrical discharge. In so-called superpulsed or ultrapulsed systems the RF discharge can be pulsed with a periodicity of up to several kilohertz. Here, instead of continuous oscillation (cw), pulses of several hundred microseconds or several milliseconds in duration are emitted with a peak power exceeding the cw level by several times. Much shorter (100 ns–1 µs) and more powerful pulses are generated by transversely excited atmospheric gas pressure (TEA) CO_2 lasers. The TEA systems are less reliable and more cumbersome, however, due to very powerful electrical discharge circuits. The cw power level of medical CO_2 lasers normally varies between 10 and 200 watt. The overall electrical efficiency η ("from plug") is 3–6%, and thus considerably higher than that of most other lasers. An essential disadvantage of the system is not associated with the laser himself, but arises from the absence of thin and flexible light-guides for middle IR.

Compared with other medical applications, a much higher laser power is required in order to create a transmyocardial channel with a single shot. Until now, 800-watt, quasi-cw (long pulse) CO_2 lasers, produced by PLC Systems Inc., USA, have been employed for this purpose. The laser light is delivered to the beating heart through an intercostal incision 15–25 cm long using an articulated mirror arm and a long focusing optic. New specialised thoracoscopic applicators also permit surgery through several small (2-cm) incisions [11].

The CO_2 laser pulse duration, and thus the total energy applied, is typically adjusted to between 20 and 90 ms, depending on the thickness of the myocardium and fat layer. The ECG-triggered pulse is applied at the end of a diastole and does not disturb the heart operation. The entire ventricle perforation procedure requires minimal time ($\sim$2 min for 30–50 holes). The observed thermally altered zone in the channel is typically about 200–300 µm thick. The measured damage thickness depends, however, on various experimental conditions and the evaluation method applied. Sensitive methods such as birefringence microscopy reveal an extended thermally damaged zone: for a 10-ms pulse duration, Jansen et al. [5] report a damage zone of 100 µm in the direction along myofibrils and of 550 µm across them, whilst 300 µm and 650 µm, respectively, are reported for a pulse duration of 50 ms.

Also an in vitro attempt has been made using a burst of millisecond pulses generated by an 'ultrapulsed' CO_2 laser [9]. The laser system used (UltraPulse 5000, Coherent) emitted 0.5-J pulses of 1.4 ms duration at a repetition rate $f = 200$ Hz. To compensate for less average power and to deliver the ablation energy needed ($\sim$5 J/mm^3), the beam must be more tightly focused ($d = 0.5$ mm) and the burst duration has to be increased up to 0.2 s. However, it remains to be proven whether this procedure is suitable for TMLR on a beating heart.

13.3 XeCl, Nd:YAG and Ho:YAG Lasers

In the next approach, low (1–10 W) average power pulsed laser systems were used for TMLR. Experiments with Ho:YAG (2.1 μm) [4, 6, 7, 9, 10], Nd:YAG (1.44 μm) [6, 7] and XeCl (308 nm) [6, 7, 9] lasers have been reported (Table 13.1). The small single-pulse energies of these systems are compensated for by a short pulse duration, so that the peak light intensities are higher or even much higher than those of the quasi-cw CO_2 laser. This results in strong overpressure of the ablation products and the formation of irregular channels with wall ruptures at the sides. The effect is particularly pronounced for the XeCl laser ($\tau = 120$–150 ns, $I = 30$–80 MW/cm^2, $\Delta p \sim 500$ bar). Several tens or even hundreds of laser pulses are necessary to 'drill' the channel using low pulse energy. This also adds to the irregularity of the channel geometry.

The long 'drilling' duration encountered with the low average power laser systems requires surgery to be carried out on a nonbeating heart. Otherwise, a light-guide fibre and/or a special contact applicator must be used to fix the direction of 'drilling'.

A complicated TMLR operation on a nonbeating heart with open chest and use of a heart-lung machine is reasonable only when combined with bypass surgery. In the contrast, the use of a highly flexible and thin (0.3–1 mm) quartz light-guide fibre or a bundle of 50- to 100-μm fibres with a total diameter of up to 1.5 mm provides the advantages of minimally invasive surgery. The fibre may be directed to the myocardium through a very small incision or even percutaneously [4] through the femoral artery, as in balloon angioplasty. TMLR from the inner endocardial side would likely provide some additional advantages, e.g. no outward bleeding if the TMLR channel end is close to the outer epicardial heart layer. The direction of the TMLR channels can also be easily regulated using a fibre.

The availability of thin, flexible low-loss silica (quartz) fibres for the spectral region of 0.2–2.3 μm was one of the main reasons for trying Ho:YAG, Nd:YAG and XeCl lasers. The specific ablation energy values given for each of these systems (see Table 13.1) are only estimated, because a precise geometry of the ablation channels (ablated volume) was not reported in the referred publications. The specific energy found typically varies between 2 and 5 J/mm^3. The value of 2 J/mm^3 represents just the energy needed to heat up and evaporate the tissue water.

13.3.1 XeCl Lasers

XeCl lasers belong to the family of excimer lasers. They are very similar in construction to TEA CO_2 lasers, but they use a gas mixture of Xe/Cl_2/He(Ne) as the active medium. The excited atoms in the discharge form an XeCl dimer (excimer), which dissociates very fast, emitting short (10–200 ns) ultraviolet (UV) light pulses at $\lambda = 308$ nm. The typical 'surgical' XeCl laser is relatively compact and emits several tens of millijoules with $f < 100$ Hz in a rather nonuniform beam profile, which may contain undesirable 'hot spots' (local intensity peaks). Its overall 'plug' efficiency is $\eta < 1\%$. In addition, the corrosive and toxic laser gas mixture must be exchanged after several million shots, and other technical servicing also becomes necessary every few months.

An extremely small specific ablation energy, $w_{abl} = 0.04$ J/mm^3 at $\Phi = 2.7$ J/cm^2, and a short 'drilling' time (<1 s) was reported for XeCl lasers by Sachinopoulou et al. [9]. From other publications [6, 7] a 'normal' w_{abl} value of 2–4 J/mm^3 at $\Phi = 5$–10 J/cm^2 was recalculated. The difference most probably relates to an artefact. According to Sachinopoulou et al. [9], a 950-μm fibre was pushed into the myocardium with a static force of 0.8 N (80 g). Thus we suppose it was rather 'laser-assisted' mechanical perforation than ablation in that case. If such a mechanical effect is predominant, the final channel may be smaller than the diameter of the fibre (applicator) because of the myocardium's elasticity. In this situation, the thermal damage would be minimal. In any case, according to some reports [6, 7], the excimer lasers provide for the smallest area of thermal damage, i.e. less than 50 μm. It has already been reported [6] that operations on a beating heart using an XeCl laser at $f = 20$–40 Hz and no ECG triggering are well tolerated.

13.3.2 Nd:YAG Lasers

Nd:YAG lasers are solid-state lasers (1–2% of Nd ions in the yttrium-aluminium-garnet crystal matrix) with a main emission wavelength of 1.064 μm in the near-IR region. The crystal rod is excited using flash-lamps (the lamps must be exchanged after $\sim 10^6$ shots; poor laser beam quality, $\eta < 3\%$) or laser diodes (nearly perfect Gaussian output beam, η is up to 10%). Nd-laser light causes energetic blood and tissue coagulation and is less effective with respect to ablation when compared with the other laser systems described.

The Nd:YAG laser used as reported in the literature [6, 7] was especially adjusted to $\lambda = 1.44$ μm (at the expense of laser efficiency), where muscle tissue absorbs better than at the normal wavelength of 1.06 μm. However, the absorption at 1.44 μm is still lower than at longer IR wavelengths or in the UV region, so that the specific ablation energy amounts to 5 J/mm^3, causing greater thermal damage than the other systems. To our knowledge, there are no reports on any in vivo TMLR attempts with this laser.

13.3.3 Ho:YAG Lasers

Like the Nd laser, Ho:YAG lasers use a YAG crystal matrix doped with Ho and additionally with Cr and Tm ions. The pulse duration usually varies between 100 and 600–800 μs; the pulse energy amounts to a few joules; repetition rate $f < 40$ Hz; efficiency $\eta < 1\%$.

The absorption of soft biological tissues increases in the IR region. The Ho:YAG laser (2.1 μm) emits the longest wavelength, which can still be guided by silica fibre. Commercial Ho:YAG laser systems are now being marketed that are equipped with special TMLR fibres (e.g. from CardioGenesis Corp., USA). Interesting results of in vivo studies on canine subjects have been published, indicating that both epicardial [10] and percutaneous endocardial TMLR [4] are well tolerated when fibre-equipped Ho:YAG lasers are used and do not lead to any ventricular dysfunction.

The preceding review of the data in the literature and of different laser systems does not yet permit a decision on the best alternative to high-power CO_2 TMLR lasers. To evaluate the prospects of new systems an analysis of the main physical mechanisms of laser-tissue interaction is required.

13.4 Basic Physical Mechanisms of Laser Tissue Ablation

Laser light can be absorbed, scattered and partially reflected by tissue. The amount reflected by muscles and blood is small. However, scattering is a significant factor, particularly in the near-IR ($0.76<\lambda<2.5$ µm), visible (400–760 nm) and near-UV region, where it even dominates absorption for most tissues (see Table 13.2). In that region, the wavelength is comparable to the size of numerous intercellular elements. Thus, the so-called Mie scattering is very effective, preferentially in a forward direction (anisotropy factor $g>0.8$). In the UV spectral range (λ <400 nm), Rayleigh scattering (scattering coefficient $\mu_s \sim 1/\lambda^4$) is considerably large as well.

Absorption in the IR region is associated with vibrational excitation of molecules. Because of the high water content (70–85%), the absorption coefficient μ_a for soft biological tissues is very close to the μ_a value for H_2O at λ >1.5 µm. An especially strong H_2O absorption band at 3 µm practically coincides with the wavelength of the Er:YAG laser. High absorption is also observed in the UV region due to electronic absorption bands of proteins. In the visible and near-IR region hundreds of chromophores (e.g. hemoglobin) contribute to the absorption, but it is much weaker than in the IR or UV region.

The absorbed energy can induce ablation in different ways. Two mechanisms are most important for soft biological tissues: thermal ablation (vaporisation) and direct photoablation. If high-energy UV photons are applied, molecules can be excited in highly lying repulsive electronic states. The excitation is followed by 'immediate' molecular dissociation and ejection of fragments. Such direct photoablation is characterised by very clean ablation craters. Only a minor part of the laser pulse energy remains in the tissue in the form of heat, so that the inherent thermal damage is very small. This efficient direct photoablation is observed with an ArF laser (193 nm), with a photon energy (6.4 eV, Table 13.2) just great enough to break the strong double C=C chemical bond. The 193-nm laser light, however, cannot be satisfactorily transmitted through light-guide fibres. Another excimer system, the KrF laser (248 nm, 5 eV), is suspected to cause mutagenic effects in the cells and is therefore not used in medicine. The photon energy of the XeCl laser (4 eV) is high enough to break only single chemical bonds in organic molecules, so that the thermal mechanism competes with photoablation at this wavelength.

With thermal ablation the tissue water evaporates very fast. The energy, initially deposited into the molecular internal motion, is transformed into heat on a picosecond time scale. The following explosion-like expansion of vapour causes a precise removal of the affected tissue. The vapour carries

Table 13.2. Optical and ablation characteristics of some human tissues at different wavelengths

	Laser:	CO_2	Er:YAG	Ho:YAG	Nd:YAG	Nd:YAG	XeCl	KrF	ArF
	Wavelength, λ	10.6 µm	2.94 µm	2.1 µm	1.44 µm	1.064 µm	308 nm	248 nm	193 nm
	Photon energy, eV	0.1	0.4	0.6	0.9	1.2	4.0	5.0	6.4
Coefficients of absorption, μ_a/ scattering, μ_s, cm^{-1} (ref.: [13–15])	Blood:	$\approx \mu_a(H_2O)$	$\approx \mu_a(H_2O)$	27.91/203.5	34.35/359.4	9.77/508.6	250–260		
	Muscle:	$\approx \mu_a(H_2O)$	$\approx \mu_a(H_2O)$			2/215			
	Myocardium:	$\approx \mu_a(H_2O)$	$\approx \mu_a(H_2O)$						
H_2O μ_a, cm^{-1} [12]		860	12000	36	11	0.61	0.0058	0.018	0.1
Absorption length l_a		15 µm	1 µm	~200 µm	~300 µm	≥1300 µm	6 µm ?		
Threshold ablation energy density Φ^o		3 J/cm^2	0.2 J/cm^2	~40 J/cm^2	~60 J/cm^2	≥250 J/cm^2	1 J/cm^2		

away not only the cell debris but also most of the absorbed energy. The specific ablation energy w^o_{abl} (J/mm^3) can be roughly estimated as the energy needed to heat the tissue from 37°C up to 100°C and to evaporate it:

$$w^o_{abl} = \rho(c \cdot \Delta T + L) \approx 2\,\mathrm{J/mm^3} \tag{1}$$

with the myocardium density $\rho = 1.06$–1.08 g/cm^3, the heat capacity $c = 3.55$–3.72 J/g/K, the latent evaporation heat $L \approx 1800$ J/g and $\Delta T = 63$ K. Any additional loss due to heat transfer into the surrounding tissue, as well as partial light absorption by the ablation debris, etc., has not been accounted for.

The calculated 'internal' specific ablation energy w^o_{abl} does not depend on laser parameters. On the contrary, a light energy density of Φ^o (J/cm^2), which should be delivered to the tissue for ablation, depends on the absorption (μ_a) and scattering (μ_s), and thus on the laser wavelength. The laser light intensity in tissue quickly (~exponentially) drops with the depth. About two thirds of the energy is lost after an effective absorption length

$$l_a = 1/\mu_a\,, \qquad \text{at } \mu_a \gg \mu_s\,, \text{ or}$$

$$l_a = 1/\sqrt{3\mu_a(\mu_a + \mu_s(1-g))}, \quad \text{in case of a strong scattering.} \tag{2}$$

To vaporise the layer of the depth l_a one needs obviously at least an energy density of

$$\Phi^o = w^o_{abl} \times l_a\,. \tag{3}$$

The calculation of the l_a and Φ^o values for different laser types is given in Table 13.2. The smallest Φ^o values are achieved with the Er:YAG ($\Phi^o = 0.2$ J/cm^2), followed closely by the CO_2 laser. For the XeCl laser, Müller and Dörschel [7] report a value l_a of only 6 µm, which leads to $\Phi^o = 1.2$ J/cm^2. Other sources [12–15] reported considerably higher values for biological tissues (e.g. $l_a \approx 100$ µm for aorta wall). Ho:YAG and Nd:YAG lasers demonstrate much poorer ablation characteristics because of weak absorption and strong scattering at their wavelengths.

Efficient ablation is always accompanied by minimal thermal damage of the affected tissue. The following rules can be set up:

1. The absorbed laser energy has to be concentrated in a minimal volume (easily achievable for tissue with high μ_a and low μ_s). The residual light, which penetrates deeper into the tissue (beyond the ablation volume) does not generate enough heat for evaporation, but induces thermal damage.
2. At a fixed pulse energy a shorter, and thus more intensive laser pulse induces faster evaporation than a longer low-intensity pulse. At a sufficiently high intensity I, the evaporation front moves into the tissue much faster than heat could do. The energy loss to the surrounding tissue is then minimal and the thermal damage zone at the bottom of the ablation channel is approximately l_a. As a criterion, one could compare the characteristic ablation time $\tau_{abl} = \Phi^o/I$ to the thermal relaxation time $\tau_T = l_a^2/4\delta$ (thermal conductivity $\delta = 0.0012$–0.0015 cm^2/s for myocardium). The thermal relaxation time shows how fast the heat deposited in a thin absorption layer l_a is transferred to the deeper tissue. The value of τ_T is only 2 µs for the Er:YAG laser but 3.5 s for the Nd:YAG laser. Nevertheless, at

their typical pulse duration and intensity (see Table 13.1) all lasers included in Table 13.2 meet the criterion $\tau_{abl} \ll \tau_T$. We would like to stress that the often-used comparison of the thermal relaxation time τ_T with laser pulse duration is actually meaningless, since the thermal relaxation occurs independent of the laser pulse width. A short ($\tau \ll \tau_T$) but not sufficiently intensive ($\tau_{abl} > \tau_T$) pulse produces massive thermal damage.

3. Edges and walls of the ablation channel reveal extensive thermal damage due to interaction with the low-intensity wings of the laser beam profile (heating only) and because they are affected by multiple laser pulses. This damage could be reduced by applying a 'hat' intensity profile of the laser beam.
4. Short sub-μs laser pulses cause an additional photomechanical ablation effect due to a very high overpressure of the evaporated liquid. Induced microexplosion is able to mechanically obliterate some extra tissue volume. Such an ablation is characterised by less thermal damage and by a certain number of mechanical ruptures. Experiments with 100-ns-pulses of TEA CO_2 lasers confirm this suggestion [16–18]. The threshold of 0.7 J/cm^2 reported by Müller and Berlien [16] is more than four times lower than the Φ^o value for 10.6 μm.

13.5 New Lasers for TMLR?

The information above indicates that the Er:YAG laser is an excellent ablation instrument. This is why Er:YAG systems have been so intensively developed over the past few years (see e.g. [19]).

13.5.1 Er:YAG Laser

The Er:YAG laser (2.94 μm) is similar to the Nd:YAG or the Ho:YAG laser. A modern Er:YAG system delivers up to several hundred millijoules with $f \approx 100$ Hz, or even several joules at smaller repetition rates. The pulse duration is $\tau = 100$–800 μs; the overall efficiency is $\eta \approx 1\%$.

The Er laser pulse energy achieved is not high enough to 'drill' a transmyocardial channel with one shot. Use of a light-guiding fibre is impossible owing to the lack of appropriate mid-IR fibres. The most advanced zirconium-fluoride fibre is brittle and hygroscopic. Other existing mid-IR light guides manifest high losses or some other drawbacks. However, further rapid progress in the development of mid-IR light guides is expected. For instance, there are interesting reports about hollow glass light guides with inner metallic/dielectric layers [20, 21], and liquid-core light guides have recently been developed by our group [22–24].

13.5.2 Q-Switch CO_2 Laser

In our opinion, the use of short sub-μs pulses generated by a CO_2 laser could be very promising for TMLR applications. Such pulses could provide the al-

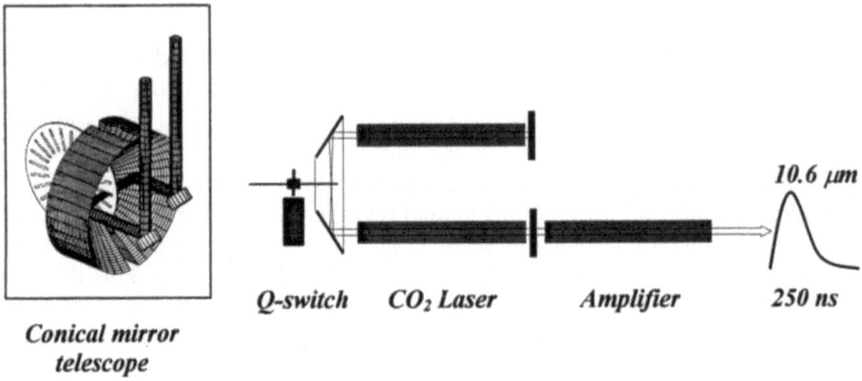

Fig. 13.1. Mechanically Q-switched high-repetition-rate CO_2 laser-amplifier system with conical mirror telescope

ready mentioned advantages of a smaller ablation threshold, higher efficiency and less thermal damage. However, the use of CO_2 lasers prevents the application of flexible light-fibres, and the light must be delivered to the myocardium in a single burst of many pulses with an optimal pulse energy and peak intensity. The total burst duration can be very short due to the high pulse repetition rate. We recommend the use of a 'Q-switched' high-repetition-rate CO_2 laser (see Fig. 13.1) as a new source of sub-μs IR pulses.

Q-switching permits time-controlled laser oscillation and is widely used in laser technology. Blocking the laser action within the cavity by some means, the usual population inversion in the laser-active medium can largely be increased. Then, with an appropriately fast switching method the quality Q of the cavity can be brought back to a large value, resulting in a very short and intensive emission of laser light.

Our laser system was originally developed for photochemical laser enrichment of stable isotopes [25]. It is based on a fast mechanical Q-switch and provides a convenient way of generating short and powerful pulses at a high repetition rate. Commercially available cw or super(ultra)pulsed CO_2 laser systems can be up-graded with this Q-switch technology. For this, one has to install an additional optical telescope and a fast-rotating chopper disk which interrupts the beam in the telescope focus plane into the laser cavity. The result is that very short (100–500 ns) laser pulses are generated at a peak power that is several hundred or even several thousand times higher than the cw laser power level. The pulse repetition rate can be adjusted to between 100 Hz and 100 kHz. At a high repetition rate (tens of kilohertz) the average output power of the optimised Q-switched laser is not far from the cw power level.

The parameters of our research Q-switch CO_2 laser system are summarised in Table 13.1. The duration of a single pulse is 250–350 ns. The pulse energy amounts to 50 mJ at 200 Hz and 20 mJ at 10 kHz, resulting in an average power of up to 400 watts. Focused down to a diameter of 1 mm, the beam yields a peak intensity $I \geq 10$ MW/cm^2. Our preliminary experiments have shown that at such intensity the ablation was distinctly promoted by additional photomechanical effects, whilst at the same time undesired plasma formation was avoided. A relatively strong acoustic effect accompanies tissue incision. It can be easily monitored with a simple microphone and used for process control. A detailed investigation of the physical ablation parameters and thermal effects is currently in progress.

13.6 Conclusion

The high-power quasi-cw CO_2 laser has been tested in TMLR operations on beating hearts for several years. The main requirement for the development of this 'heart' CO_2 laser was the need to 'drill' the transmyocardial channel with only one shot. The new results show, however, that TMLR can also be successfully done with a thin light guide 'slowly' penetrating into the myocardium and transmitting multiple weak laser pulses to the tissue. Several disadvantages of the high-power CO_2 laser thus become evident. The system is cumbersome, and light delivery relies on an articulated-arm mirror system, which strictly limits the operating technique. Excess laser pulse energy is required in order to 'drill' the channel with certainty. This leads to evaporation of blood on the epicardial side and formation of gas bubbles in the ventricle. To control the procedure, a transoesophageal echocardiographic probe must be inserted into the gullet. The extent of the thermally damaged zone around the channel is at least 0.2–0.3 mm and can be considerably larger, according to some reports.

Less thermal damage and more efficient ablation could probably be attained with a burst of short sub-μs pulses of CO_2 laser. We have already demonstrated [26] that 300 ns pulses of a high-repetition-rate Q-switch CO_2 laser 'cleanly' ablate bone tissue. Current experiments with soft biological tissues are aimed at clarifying how much the ablation efficiency might be improved and the thermal damage reduced compared with the quasi-cw or superpulsed CO_2 laser system.

It is known that superficial ablation characteristics can be realised in the IR with an Er:YAG laser at $\lambda = 2.94$ μm. Unfortunately, the lack of suitable fibre light guides for $\lambda > 2.3$ μm still prevents the implementation of this system, which is otherwise very favourable for medical applications. Promoted by several companies, other IR medical systems such as the Ho:YAG laser (2.1 μm) work well with silica-glass fibres and are convenient to use. However, their ablation characteristics are much poorer than those of Er:YAG, CO_2 or excimer lasers.

Of all systems under evaluation, the XeCl laser so far causes the least thermal damage. The efficiency of the system in terms of ablation is ensured by extremely high photon energy and peak intensity of the laser pulses, as well as by the high tissue absorption in UV. The possibility of using a thin and flexible light-guide fibre greatly facilitates surgery and permits the application of the percutaneous technique. The low average power excimer laser is also much smaller and not as expensive as the 'heart' CO_2 laser. These features make the XeCl laser a very interesting alternative to the high-power CO_2 laser for TMLR.

References

1. Moosdorf R, Schoebel FC, Hort W (1997) Transmyokardiale Laserrevaskularisation – morphologische, pathophysiologische und historische Grundlagen der indirekten Revaskularisation des Herzmuskels. Z Kardiol 86:149–164
2. Nagele H, Kalmar P, Lubeck M, et al (1997) Transmyokardiale Laserrevaskularisation – Behandlungsoption der koronaren Herzerkrankung? Z Kardiol 86:171–178
3. Kohmoto T, Fisher PE, Gu A, et al (1997) Physiology, histology, and 2-week morphology of acute transmyocardial channels made with a CO_2 laser. Ann Thorac Surg 63:1275–1283
4. Kim CB, Kesten R, Javier M, et al (1997) Percutaneous method of laser transmyocardial revascularization. Cathet Cardiovasc Diagn 40:223–228
5. Jansen ED, Frenz M, Kadipasaoglu KA, et al (1997) Laser-tissue interaction during transmyocardial laser revascularization. Ann Thorac Surg 63:640–647
6. Müller G (1997) TMLR – eine Frage des richtigen Lichtes? Oral report at 1st Düsseldorfer TMLR-Symposium, May 16–17
7. Müller G, Dörschel K (1995) Grundlagen und Anwendungen der Photoablation am Herzmuskelgewebe. In: Krabatsch, Hetzer (eds) Transmyokardiale Laserrevaskularisation: Stand und Ausblicke. Symposium Deutsches Herzzentrum Berlin. Ecomed, Landsberg/Lech, pp 15–20
8. Maas D (1995) TMLR bei koronarer Herzkrankheit – Indikationen, operative Technik und Taktik, klinische Resultate bei 152 Patienten. In: Krabatsch, Hetzer (eds) Transmyokardiale Laserrevaskularisation: Stand und Ausblicke. Symposium Deutsches Herzzentrum Berlin. Ecomed, Landsberg/Lech, pp 21–42
9. Sachinopoulou A, Verdaasdonk R, Rudolf M, Beek J (1996) Comparison of ablation channels created by the ultrapulsed CO_2 laser, holmium laser, and 308-nm excimer laser in view of transmyocardial revascularization. Lasers in Surgery. Proc SPIE 2671:42–47
10. Kohmoto T, Uzun G, Gu A, et al (1997) Blood flow capacity via direct acute myocardial revascularization. Basic Res Cardiol 92:45–51
11. deGuzman BJ, Lautz DB, Chen FY, et al (1997) Thorascopic Transmyocardial Laser Revascularization. Ann Thorac Surg 64:171–174
12. Niemz MH (1996) Laser-tissue interactions. Springer, Berlin Heidelberg New York
13. Roggan A (1997) Dosimetrie thermischer Laseranwendungen in der Medizin. Fortschritte in der Lasermedizin, vol 16. Müller, Berlien (eds). Ecomed, Landsberg/Lech
14. Tuchin VV (1993) Lasers and fiber optics in biomedicine. Laser Physics 3:767–820
15. Cheong W-F (1995) Summary of optical properties. In: Welch AJ, vanGemert MJC (eds) Optical-thermal response of laser-irradiated tissue. Plenum, New York London, pp 275–303
16. Alimpiev SS, Artjushenko VG, Butvina LN, et al (1988) Polycrystalline IR fibers for laser scalpels. Proc SPIE 906:183–190
17. Kubo U, Hashishin Y, Okada K (1988) Optical beam guides for medical CO_2 and excimer lasers. Proc SPIE 906:214–219
18. Lademann J, Thieme W, Babucke H, Steffen H, Koch H (1992) Application of mini TEA CO_2 laser in neurosurgery. In: Waidelich, Wilhelm (eds) Laser in der Medizin: Vorträge des 10. Internationalen Kongresses Laser 91. Springer, Berlin, pp 206–209
19. Vogler K, Reidl M (1996) Improved erbium laser parameters for new medical applications. Biophotonics Int 6:40–47
20. Abel T, Hirsch J, Harrington J (1994) Hollow glass waveguides for broadband infrared transmission. Optics Letts 19:1034–1036
21. Osawa M, Kato Y, Watanabe T, et al (1995) Fabrication of fluorocarbon polymer-coated silver hollow-glass waveguides for the infrared by the liquid-phase coating method. Optics Laser Technol 27:393–396
22. Klein S, Meister J, Diemer S, Jung R, Fuß W, Hering P (1997) High-power laser waveguide with a circulating liquid core for IR applications. Proc SPIE 2977:155–163
23. Meister J, Diemer S, Jung R, Klein S, Haisch S, Fuß W, Hering P (1997) Liquid-core fused-silica capillary lightguides for applications in the UV/VIS and NIR spectral range. Proc SPIE 2977:58–66
24. Diemer S, Meister J, Jung R, Klein S, Haisch M, Fuß W, Hering P (1997) Liquid-core light guides for near-infrared applications. Appl Optics 36:9075–9082
25. Fuß W, Göthel J, Ivanenko M, Kompa KL, Schmid WE (1992) Multiwavelength Q-switched CO_2 laser with continuous discharge. Appl Phys [B] 55:65–70
26. Ivanenko MM, Hering P (1998) Wet bone ablation with mechanically Q-switched high-repetition-rate CO_2 laser. Appl Phys [B] (in press)

PART IV

Clinical Experience with TMLR

CHAPTER 14

Transmyocardial Laser Revascularisation with the CO_2 Laser

H.-M. STUBBE

14.1 Introduction

Over the past several years there has been a distinct increase in the numbers of second and third coronary operations performed. This increase is the result of demographic and medical developments. On the one hand, the age of the patients is rising, and on the other hand, the number of patients with complex accompanying illnesses which would have contraindicated operations with heart-lung machines some years ago is also on the rise. Due to these factors, the numbers of high-risk patients and of those who cannot undergo bypass surgery due to local inoperability are increasing.

For a small number of these people there is a chance of a heart transplantation. Slight variations in the course of the illness keep requiring hospitalisation or may even lead to death caused by infarctions [14].

With the agreement of the Ethics Committee of the General Medical Council (*Ärztekammer*) in Hamburg, we have begun a study to examine the new treatment transmyocardial laser revascularisation (TMR) concerning the perioperative risks and the long-term results. Here we present some of our own first experience as well as international results with this procedure.

14.2 Hemodynamic Basis

The idea underlying TMR is that if channels are created in the wall of the left ventricle, arterial blood can find its way from the left ventricle to the vessel system of the myocardium, primarily the sinusoid system. For many years attempts have been made to create such connections. The model for this is found in nature. The myocardial perfusion in reptiles (snakes, frogs) occurs via such ventricular-sinusoid connections, as reptiles have only a very rudimentary coronary vessel system.

In 1988, Mirrhoseini reported on the clinical use of the CO_2 laser [9]. Based on results of long-term animal experiments, he introduced a first clinical series of 12 patients. The advantage of his CO_2 laser is that due to high energy absorption the tissue is removed by vaporisation. Mirrhoseini himself had shown in animal experiments that the CO_2 laser could be used on beating hearts. The laser beam perforates the ventricle wall with minimal damage to the surrounding tissue, so that short-term bleeding is not a problem and the diameter of the channels can be well calibrated by means of optical systems.

Two years after these animal experiments the channels were open and endothelialised, and 83% of the animals survived a ligature of the ramus interventricularis anterior. No animal in the control group without laser treatment survived [6–8].

14.3 Technical Requirements and Operation Techniques

The "heart-laser" is an 800-watt CO_2 laser with an output of 5–80 joules. The impulse distance is 5–9 ms, the delay 1–999 ms. The wavelength is 10.6 μm. The target beam is a 5-milliwatt helium laser. The light transmission is carried out via an articulated arm with seven mirrors which transmit up to 97% of the energy. This type of laser measures 99×168×208 cm and the whole device weighs nearly 1000 kg. It is manufactured by PLC Medical Systems, Milford, Mass.

Surgery is performed:

1. *As a single operation.* In 90% of the cases we decided on laser therapy alone. Our goal was to prove that changes in the ischaemic status of the myocardium which were recorded at follow-up were due exclusively to the laser treatment. There are two medical advantages: the requirements of minimal-access surgery are met, and no extracorpereal circulation is required. In the right lateral position an anterolateral thoracotomy 8–10 cm long is made in the fourth or fifth intercostal space, the pericardium is opened up, the myocardium is exposed and the ischaemic areas on the beating heart are supplied with one channel/cm^2. After two or three of these channels have been made, digital compressing is carried out for 2 min, after which the bleeding stops. The operation takes less than 120 min, the blood loss is less than 300 ml, and no transfusions are necessary. The patient can be extubated 2–3 h after surgery, and mobilisation is started the following morning. Successful perforation of the ventricle wall can be demonstrated by transesophageal echocardiography. The gas which was produced by the tissue vaporisation is evidence that the ventricle cavum has been achieved. In blood the light beam is stopped after a few millimetres. With ECG triggering of the energy output, only end-diastolic 'shots' can be carried out, so that hardly any injuries of intraventricular structures can occur.
2. *As a combined operation:*
   a) In case of bypass-suited coronary vessels and simultaneous ischaemia, laser treatment can be carried out in unsupplied regions with missing connections at the end of the heart-lung machine-supported phase in bypass operations.
   b) Following large anterior myocardial infarctions with occlusion of the LAD and formation of an anterior myocardial aneurysm, the ventricle septum can be treated directly once the aneurysm has been resected.
   c) The chamber septum can also be reached via the right atrioventricular valve.
3. *As a minimally invasive operation.* In appropriate cases TMR can be carried out thoracoscopicially with simultaneous use of video.

14.4 Indications

More than 60 such heart lasers are being used at present worldwide. So far, approximately 2500 patients have been treated. The University Hospital Hamburg-Eppendorf was the third German hospital to use TMR. The first operation took place on April 6, 1995.

At the time of trial clinical use in the USA, strict regulations were issued by the Federal Drug Administration (FDA). In the USA, ten multicentred and FDA-controlled clinics examined these operating techniques. Results of these studiesare mentioned below [4].

We adopted these criteria and selected our patients accordingly. The preoperative examination protocol (Table 14.1) is as follows:

1. LV angiogram (Centerline method, pathological chords)
2. Positron-emission tomography (FDG uptake, mismatch)
3. ^{99m}Tc-MIBI protocol (resting and under dipyridamole stress)
4. Stress echocardiogram (resting and under dobutamine stress)
5. Right heart examination (resting and after 5 min, 50 watt)
6. Bicycle ergometry
7. Spiroergometry
8. Clinically (NYHA, infarctions, nitroglycerin consumption, cardiac incidents)
9. Pulmonary function diagnosis

To date, 152 patients have been entered into this protocol. Most of them came from other centers where the possibility of bypass operations had been ruled out.

Fifty-six patients were selected for TMR treatment alone; in eight cases the surgery was carried out as a combined bypass operation; in 61 cases we opted for nonsurgical therapy; eight patients were treated by further bypass operations; four patients were referred for balloon dilatation (PTCA); three patients were put on the waiting for list transplantation; six patients died during the preexamination phase; and six patients are currently being screened or are waiting for their operation. The criteria for TMR can be summarised as the diagnosis of "final-stage coronary heart disease". This means therapy-refractory, symptomatic coronary heart disease (CCS classification 3 and 4) in patients of both sexes with maximum antianginal therapy.

Table 14.1. Examination protocol

	Quality of life	Clinical data	Pulmonary function	LV-angiography	Tc-MIBI	Right heart cath.	Stress-ergom.	Stress-echo	PET
Pre-op	X	X	X	X	X	X	X	X	X
Hospital release	X	X							
6 months post-op	X	X			X	X	X	X	
12 months post-op	X	X	X	X	X	X	X	X	X

These are high-risk patients for conventional bypass operations (i.e. missing connecting vessels, complete calcification), or they suffer from diffuse coronary diseases and cannot undergo revascularisation by means of bypass operations or percutaneous transluminal coronary angioplasty. Of the 152 patients, 95% have had one or more previous operations. The average age is 64 years (47–82).

14.5 Results

When assessing the results gained so far, one must take into consideration the final stage of the disease with its long medical history. With this in mind, we compare our results with those of the American multicentre study [4].

The 56 patients in our study have been followed up for an average of 18.6 months. The intermediate follow-up for the 200 patients in the American study was carried out after 10.3 months. The very high mortality (Table 14.2) must be looked with a view to the criteria, which is a great disadvantage for everybody involved. It is clear that the mortality is related to when the study was entered. Mortality dropped from 15% in the first group of 40 patients to 5% in the current group of patients 121–160. There has not been a single perioperative death in the second group.

The fact that mortality decreases with increasing experience is not – or not only – related to the surgical learning curve. Everyone involved in the process of diagnostics, indications, anaesthesia, surgery, intensive care medicine and after-treatment with this group of patients is faced by new challenges and profits from earlier experience.

In the American group of patients a clear correlation between mortality and the age of the patients or left ventricular ejection fraction can be found. The most important risk factor is definitely the left ventricular ejection fraction. This can be seen at the international level as well as in our study. This is also reflected in the experience of conventional bypass surgery [12]. From our group of patients only one person died with an ejection fraction >50%.In Djiddah, Rafah has treated 90 patients primarily with the heart laser. In this (not negatively selected) group of patients mortality was 0%, although more than 90% were in CCS stage IV [11]. We also kept track of those patients who could not be treated with interventional therapy; the mortality in this group was 22.6%. Although these two groups are not randomised and have many clinical differences, they reflect the natural course of coronary heart disease in its final stage.

Table 14.2. Perioperative mortality

	UKE ($n=56$)	USA multicentre ($n=200$)
30 days	8.9% (5)	9.0% (18)
Follow-up	10.7% (6)	9.0% (18)

UKE, Universitäts Krankenhaus Eppendorf (Hamburg)

Table 14.3. Perioperative mortality

	UKE ($n=56$)	USA multicentre ($n=200$)
Rhythm disturbances	1.8% (1)	9.0% (18)
Infarctions	8.9% (5)	2.5% (5)
Rethoracotomy	3.6% (2)	1.0% (2)
IABP or assist device	1.8% (1)	4.0% (7)
Wound infections	8.9% (5)	0.5% (1)
Pneumonia	0.0%	2.5% (5)

UKE, Universitäts Krankenhaus Eppendorf (Hamburg)

14.6 Morbidity

Wound infection was the most frequently occurring perioperative complication (see Table 14.3). The rate of 8.9% ($n=5$) is distinctly higher than that for patients with bypass operations. We think this is due to the number of people in the operating theatre (visitors) as well as to traumatisation of the wound edges in the attempt to get good visibility when performing surgery on a preoperated patient.

Five patients suffered perioperative infarctions, defined as Q-wave infarctions. The enzymatic detection techniques, including troponin-T and troponin-I, proved to be unsuitable. Because of the intended ablation of myocardial tissue, there was a proven increase of classical infarction enzymes in almost all cases. One patient had a ventricular tachycardia on the second postoperative day, and two patients required a rethoracotomy due to secondary haemorrhages. In one case an intercostal artery was involved, in the other case LIMA was the cause. We had no pulmonary complications, and we attributed this to the renunciation of a selective intubation. As described by other centres, constant ventilation of the left lung also seems to prevent pulmonary complications. We observed no mental or neurological disorders.

14.7 Angina Classifications

The average CCS stage of 3.3 months preoperatively has gone down to 1.8 months postoperatively (see Fig. 14.1). We think this improvement is considerable, especially as all centres report similar results and the 200 FDA-controlled cases in the USA show almost identical courses. The result for the patient is much better quality of life. The subjective decrease of angina goes together with an objectively better performance.

Performance capacity, expressed as the time taken during bicycle ergometry, increased significantly. We started with 50 watt and increased by 25 watt every 30 s. Preoperatively, the patients were able to take a strain of 98 s; postoperatively they were able to take 122 s. Statistically this improvement is highly significant ($p<0.01$). It must also be pointed out that 25% of the patients were not in any condition to perform bicycle ergometry preoperatively.

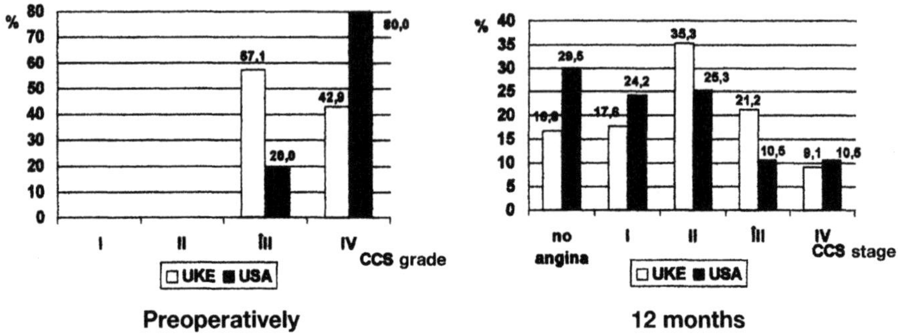

Fig. 14.1. Improvement in the clinical status after TMR (*UKE*, Universitätskrankenhaus Eppendorf)

14.8 Follow-Up Results

Examination of the right heart catheter shows an improvement of the heart performance at rest and under strain, although the results are not yet sufficient for statistical evaluation. In the USA results of the nuclear-medical perfusion study are available. They show that perfusion defects have been reduced by 50%. We have not been able to confirm this tendency.

In order to assign the marked glucose (Fig. 14.2) to the treated and untreated areas of the left ventricle, we use a model tried and tested in other studies which allows the individual segments of the left ventricle to be differentiated according to their anatomical position. Septal portions cannot be reached by the laser, so they should appear unchanged after TMR, apart from slight effects on the edges. This is not the case, however; changes below statistical significance are demonstrated in all segments.

Concerning the metabolic situation of the left-ventricular myocardium before and after TMR we were not able to show definite statistical improvements. Using a four-level score – score 1 = normal myocardium, score 2 = hi-

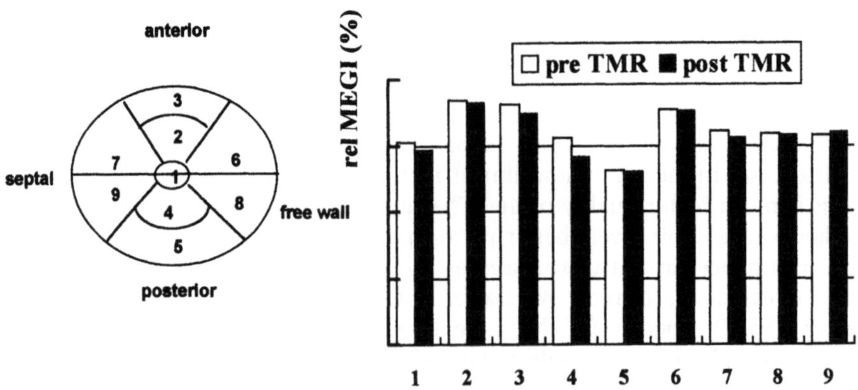

Fig. 14.2. Mean segmental glucose (FDG) uptake before and after TMR

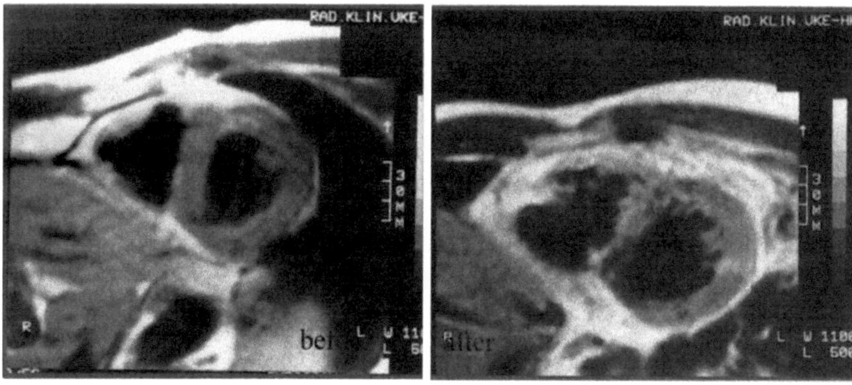

Fig. 14.3. Magnetic resonance imaging before and after TMR

bernating myocardium, score 3 = FDG low but provable, score 4 = scar – we calculated the percentage of segments assigned to each condition. We found less normal myocardium, more hibernating myocardium, less "remnant-vital" myocardium and more scarred myocardium. In our opinion, these results are not yet interpretable. The number of follow-up patients ($n=11$) as well as the interval of time after surgery should be increased. The American multicentre study was much more successful, particularly in this area. The situation in the septum was almost unchanged (as expected) and a drastic reduction in the reversible defects was found [4].

Magnetic resonance imaging might possibly be a method of proving the effects of TMR (see Fig. 14.3). We examined eight patients pre- as well as postoperatively. Gadolinium was used as a contrast medium. Five patients showed results that could be evaluated. These results were assessed by two independent radiologists. Additionally, a computer-supported test program was used. Clearly and visibly, a greater accumulation of contrast medium was attained.

With the aid of the new ACCUSON echocardiograph "Sequoia 512" we examined patients intraoperatively as well as up to 18 months postoperatively. With this apparatus it is possible to show some of the channels without contrast medium [10].

In the meantime this has been achieved in other TMR centres as well. Using Doppler sonography we were able to clearly show a systolic flow in the direction of the myocardium. It appears that the possibility of demonstrating channels correlates with the clinical condition; thus we were able to show the existence of channels in patients with perceptible clinical improvement after TMR. With therapy failures (two of 16 patients) this was not possible.

The trouble with presenting histologic findings in this field is that they naturally stem as a rule from therapy failures. Therefore, the literature (also from our group) contains predominantly reports of closed channels [3].

In Fig. 14.4 an open channel can be seen. It stems from a female patient who suffered sudden cardiac death 150 days after undergoing TMR. An open connection to the ventricular cavum can be seen. Of course, it is difficult to

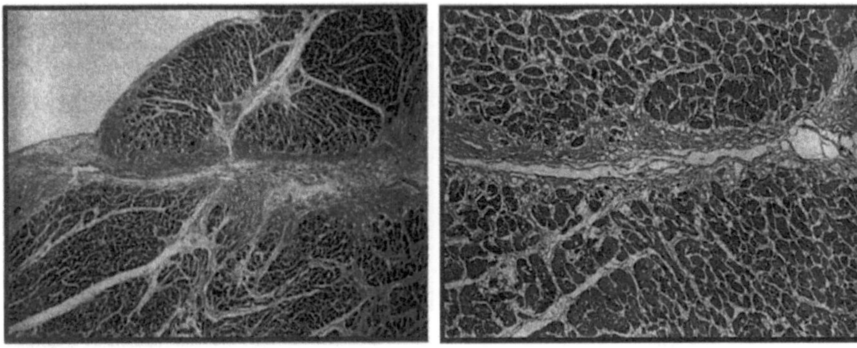

Fig. 14.4. Histological examination shows an open channel 150 days after TMR (Masson-Goldner stain)

present a complete 'ostium' in only one cross-section. In the intermediate third of the ventricular myocardium on open lumen lined with a single layer of immunohistochemically proven endothelium is visible. A collagen layer similar to that found in traumatised myocardium is also visible, however. Be that as it my, channels are open after 150 days!

In experiments we have examined how the extent of pericanalicular cell damage depends on the kind of laser used. In single-shot treatments with holmium, thulium or CO_2 lasers the zone of necrosis increases by a factor of 2 from laser to laser. Under our test conditions this meant a necrotic zone of 120 μm using the CO_2 laser, 250 μm with the thulium laser and 500 μm with the holmium laser. From our point of view it seems best to use the CO_2 laser [1]. The tissue ablation seems to be optimal in this configuration. The advantages of single-shot treatment are obvious. As producing an open channel takes an average of 40 ms, it is not a problem to work on the beating heart.

14.9 Possible Modes of Action

At present we can only speculate as to the modes of action of TMR. Here some arguments are presented to counter certain published hypotheses. (a) Placebo effect: The technical requirements, the mystery attached to the laser beam, the novelty of the method and, last but not least, the public response (here as well) suggested a placebo effect. Worldwide, 2500 patients have had surgery with the aid of the CO_2 laser so far. The increasing number of scientifically justified findings make such an explanation more and more unlikely. (b) Damage to nerve tissue: On average we created 30 channels. Considering that the diameter is only 1 mm, only very small areas of the inner surface of the left ventricle are affected. (c) Damage to ischaemic tissue: At most, only 1% of the myocardial mass is damaged. The postoperative scintigraphic and PET findings rule out such an effect. (d) Improved lymphatic drainage via the channels: In theory, such a mechanism is conceivable, although no proof has yet been found. (e) Effect of heat proteins: No proof exists. (f) Connection to the sinusoid system: This was the original working concept. The newly built channels gain access to the sinusoid system and in this way perfuse the ischaemic myocardium. Apart from accidential findings in our experimental work, we have not seen any indications for such connections. In principle, one must bear in mind that the sinusoid vessel system is much less developed in human beings than in reptiles. (g) Connection to the coronary vessel.system: This hypothesis is based on clinical as well as experimental experience. Echocardiographic and histologic findings hint that perfusion does occur in this way. (h) Angioneogenesis: Surely the attraction of using laser in pericanalicular repair processes points to angioneogenesis [2].

Our current working hypothesis follows from the above: The primary effect, i.e. being free of complaints immediately after surgery, can be explained (only) through connection of the channels to parts of the arterial capillary coronary system. In the clinical course, indications for slower recoveries are often found. Some patients require 8–12 weeks to be free of complaints; it would take about this time to build up a new capillary bed in the treated area.

14.10 Conclusions

Although we have no proof in our group so far as to the efficacy of long-term courses as well as objective measuring techniques, we can say the following:

1. With TMR a reduction of angina symptoms by at least two angina classes can be achieved for 80% of the patients with coronary heart disease and proven ischaemic or hibernating stage-IV myocardium.
2. Mortality, which is still rather high at present, can be reduced to approximately % (also by expanding the indications).
3. Perioperative morbidity is low (apart from a currently too high rate of infections in our group).
4. With regard to angina pectoris symptoms, the technique is clinically effective.
5. We were not able to show an improvement of left ventricular contractility.
6. Using standard nuclear imaging techniques, we were not able to show improved perfusion.
7. The optimistic magnetic resonance imaging findings need to be counterchecked using high-performance equipment.
8. Perfused channels can be verified echocardiographically without having to use contrast medium. This also seems to correlate with the clinical results.
9. A perioperative mortality of 5–10% must be expected in cases where the group of treated patients was selected had particularly negative health conditions.

Although the physiological basis of this technique is not completely clear, we think that the surprisingly good results concerning the symptoms as well as the performance of a group of patients who were previously refractory to therapy are reason enough to recommend this kind of therapy to patients with advanced coronary heart disease. Using TMR it seems possible to reduce natural mortality in the final stage of coronary heart disease by one third. TMR can be performed on patients in the final stage of coronary heart disease with an estimated risk.

References

1. Crew J (1991) Transmyocardial revascularization by CO_2-laser. Surg Technol Int 1:236–238
2. Frazier OH, Cooley DA, Kadipasaoglu KA, Pehlivanoglu S, Lindenmeier M, Barasch E, Conger JL, Wilansky S, Moore WH (1995) Myocardial revascularization with laser: preliminary findings. Circulation 92 [Suppl II]:II 65–II 85
3. Gassler N, Wintzer H-O, Stubbe H-M, Wullbrand A, Helmchen U (1997) Transmyocardial laser revascularization, histological features in human nonresponder myocardium. Circulation 95:371–375
4. Horvath KA, Cohn LH, Cooley DA, Crew JR, Frazier OH, Griffith BP, Kadipasaoglu K, Lansing A, Mannting F, March R, Mirrhoseini MR, Smith (1997) Transmyocardial laser revascularization: results of a multicenter trial with transmyocardial laser revascularization used as sole therapy for end-stage coronary heart disease. J Thorac Cardiovasc Surg 113:645–654
5. Khazai AH, Kime WP, Papadoupoulos C, Cowley RA (1968) Myocardial revascularzation: a new nethod of revascularzation. Ann Thorac Surg 6:163–171
6. Mirrhoseini M (1977) Revascularization of the myocardium with laser. In: Davila JC (ed) Second Henry Ford Hospital International Symposium on cardiac surgery. Appleton-Century-Crofts, New York, pp 595–597
7. Mirrhoseini M, Cayton MM (1981) Revascularzation of the heart by laser. J Microvasc Surg 2:253
8. Mirrhoseini M, Fisher JC, Cayton MM (1983) Myocardial revascularization by laser. Lasers Surg Med 3:241
9. Mirrhoseini M, Sheligikar S, Cayton M N(1988) New concepts in revascularzation of the myocardium. Ann Thorac Surg 45:415–420
10. Nägele H, Kalmar P, Rödiger W, Stubbe HM (1997) Farbdoppler-echokardiografischer Nachweis transmyokardialer Kanäle im Langzeitverlauf nach Laserrevaskularisation. Z Kardiol 86 [Suppl 2]:214
11. Rafah H (1995) TMR and virgin cases. Fifth International TMR Symposium, Paris
12. Risum O, Nitter-Hauge S, Abdelnoor M, Levorstad K, Arafa O, Svennevig JL (1996) Mortality and morbidity after coronary bypass surgery related to preoperative left ventricular ejection fraction: a follow-up study. Eur Heart J 17:874–879
13. Sen PK, Udwadia TE, Kinare SG, Parulkar G.B (1965) Transmyocardial accupuncture: a new approach to myocardial revascularization. J Thorac Cardiovasc Surg 50:181
14. Stubbe H-M, Kalmar P (1993) Zur Situation der herzchirurgischen Versorgung in Hamburg. Hamburger Arztebl 47:306–307

CHAPTER 15

Transmyocardial Laser Revascularisation in the Treatment of Severe Diffuse Coronary Artery Disease

TH. KRABATSCH · L. TAMBEUR · E. LIEBACK · F. SCHÄPER · R. HETZER

15.1 Introduction

For more than 60 years it has been known that in warm-blooded species the myocardium is perfused primarily via coronary arteries which provide a capillary network, but that there are direct connections between the ventricular chamber and the capillaries by thebesian veins and sinusoids [1].

Until coronary artery bypass grafting became the standard method for treating coronary disease, several surgical approaches were common that provided additional blood flow to the myocardium via extracoronary pathways. The Vineberg procedure was one of these, whereby the internal thoracic artery was implanted directly into the left ventricular myocardium without any vascular anastomoses [2]. To the end, this procedure remained controversial, even though there were indications of a measurable improvement of myocardial perfusion in some cases. Later, the implantation of perforated plastic tubes with one end reaching into the ventricular chamber for carrying blood from the left ventricular chamber into the myocardium was investigated [3, 4].

It was the German surgeon Paul Walter [5] who, based on reports in 1956 from the Indian surgeon Sen [6], created channels by simple needle puncture which connected the ventricular chamber with the intramyocardial vascular network. With the rise of CABG in the late 1960s, this method fell into disuse.

In the early 1980s, Mirhoseini and co-workers created transmyocardial channels for the first time with the help of a laser [7–10]. The use of a laser is presumed to ensure that the channels do not close within the early period after creation.

It was initially assumed that following transmyocardial laser revascularisation, during every contraction of the heart small amounts of blood are pressed through the channels into the intramyocardial vascular network, thus increasing the myocardial blood supply. Other theories have recently been debated, including angiogenesis, or destruction of free nerve endings or whole nerves conducting anginal pain signals.

The creation of transmyocardial channels on the beating heart is convenient using a laser that can release high energy within a short time. The majority of institutions performing transmyocardial revascularisation (TMR) use the Heart Laser, a carbon dioxide laser (wave length $\lambda = 10\,600$ nm) delivering invisible radiation with an energy output of 800 W. For the creation of one channel this laser requires about 40 ms.

In Germany more than 1000 TMR operations have been performed within the past 3 years. The first transmyocardial laser revascularisation in Germany was performed at the Deutsches Herzzentrum Berlin in the summer of 1994. This chapter summarizes the experience gained with TMR at our institution.

15.2 Materials and Methods

Within the period from July 1994 to August 1997, a total of 165 patients underwent TMR at the Deutsches Herzzentrum Berlin. In 20 patients TMR was an adjunct to coronary bypass grafting. For the remaining 145 patients the laser procedure was the only therapy. Anamnestic and clinical data from all 165 operated patients are shown in Table 15.1. Patient group 1 (isolated TMR) was investigated following a protocol consisting of echocardiography, thallium perfusion scan during physical exercise, and left heart catheterisation, as well as a special questionnaire on complaints and quality of life of the patients. Clinical assessments were made prior to discharge (echocardiography) and at 3, 6, 12 and 18 months postoperatively.

The patient had to meet the following criteria before we decided to perform a TMR:

- There is severe diffuse coronary artery disease present.
- The patient suffers from severe angina (or equivalents, CCS class 3 or 4) leading to marked deterioration in the quality of life.
- A maximum of antianginal therapy has been carried out.
- The patient is not a candidate for PTCA, CABG or heart transplantation.

We consider TMR not to be indicated when the patient's left ventricular contractility is severely diminished (LVEF<30%) due to one or more myocardial infarctions. The presence of ischaemic but viable myocardium should be a prerequisite for transmyocardial laser revascularisation. Informed consent was obtained from each patient treated.

Table 15.1. Characteristics of the 145 patients who underwent TMR

		Group 1 (TMR)	Group 2 (TMR + CABG)
n		145	20
Sex (m:f)		5.2:1	2.2:1
Age (years)		63.0±7.0	61.9±9.0
Previous CABG (%)		90.3	5.0
Patients with 3-vessel disease (%)		85.5	95.0
No. of infarcts per patient		1.5±0.7	1.0±0.3
No. of PTCA per patient		0.5	0.27±0.3
Maximum workload (Watts)		58.0±30.6	83.2±39.2
Left ventricular EF (%)		44.0±11.6	43.1±5.6
Angina class (CCS)		3.2±1.0	3.1±0.9
Lung function	FEV1 (%)	83.4±15.6	
	VC (%)	81.4±14.0	
Renal function	Creatinine (mg/dl)	1.3±0.7	
	Urea (mg/dl)	43.5±23.0	

Patients who received TMR as an adjunct to coronary bypass grafting were excluded from further investigation. We consider it impossible to differentiate between CABG effects and TMR effects in this patient group.

15.3 Results

The following results are based on the 125 patients who underwent TMR as the only therapy. Postoperatively, the absolute majority of patients reported a distinct decline in angina. These facts are depicted in Fig. 15.1. Seventy-two percent of our patients assessed that they had profited from the laser operation. Angina had diminished in 82.4% and dyspnoea was reduced in 67.2% of the patients who had reported these complaints preoperatively. A decline in complaints was defined as diminished frequency or intensity of angina or equivalents, or occurrence of them at a distinctly higher level of physical stress.

Pre- and postoperatively, all patients were classified, according to the suggestions of the Canadian Cardiovascular Society, into one of four angina classes. The results are summarised in Table 15.2.

In order to characterise the patients who profited from the TMR procedure compared with those who reported no changes, both subgroups were analyzed for significant differences with regard to 50 different anamnestic and clinical factors. These factors are specified in Table 15.3. Significant differences between both groups were found only in preoperative left ventricular ejection fraction. While more than 75% of the patients with a preoperative LVEF of 30% or more profited from TMR, only 34% of the remaining patients reported significantly diminished angina or dyspnoea ($p<0.05$).

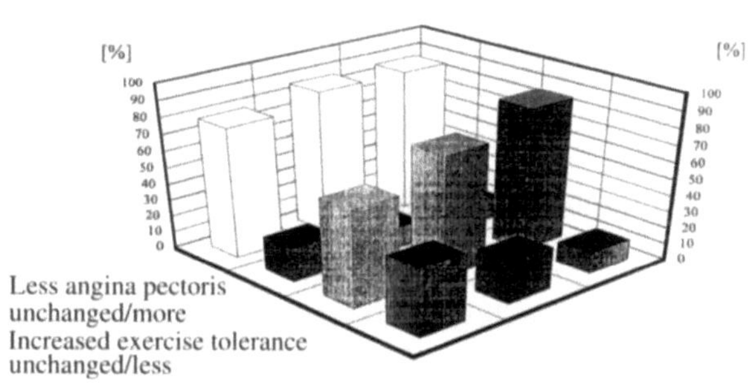

Fig. 15.1. Subjective findings following TMR

Table 15.2. Pre- and postoperative angina class (CCS)

Preoperatively	3 months postop.	6 months postop.	12 months postop.	18 months postop.
3.4±0.9	2.7±0.8	2.1±0.9	2.7±1.0	3.0±1.1

Table 15.3. Parameters analysed pre- and intraoperatively

	Anamnesis	Ventricular function	Lab/ diagnostics	TMR	
Sex	Type of CAD	LVEF	Creatinine, urea	TMR target area	Follow-up interval
Age	Previous infarctions	LVEDP	Lung function (FEV1, VC)	No. of channels	
Marital status	Previous CABG	Left ventricular wall thickness	QOL questionnaire	Overall energy delivered	
Medication	Previous PTCA	LVEDD		Energy per channel	
Blood group	NYHA class	LV contractility		Intraop. low cardiac output	
Height	CCS class	Maximum workload			
Weight	Hospital stays	Perfusion scan			
Preop. stay	Further diseases				
		ECG			

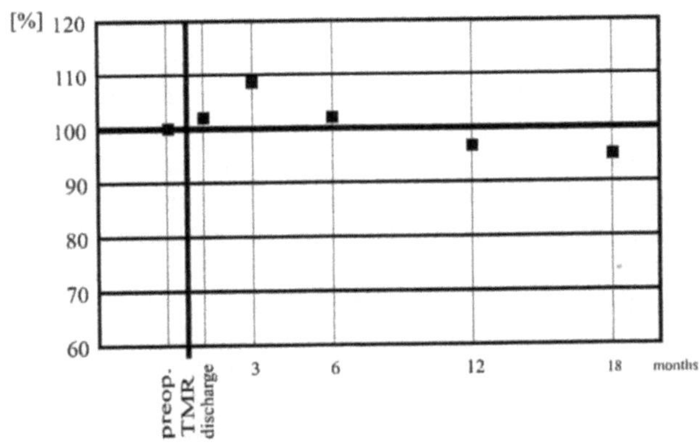

Fig. 15.2. Left ventricular ejection fraction (echocardiography): changes in the relative value compared with the preoperative LVEF

15.3.1 Left Ventricular Contractility

The ejection fraction of the left ventricle as an expression of global left ventricular contractility tended to increase postoperatively, but the difference did not reach statistical significance. The highest value was measured at 3 months after TMR. The average increase of LVEF to 109% of the initial value only barely missed the level of significance ($p=0.082$). These findings are visualised in Fig. 15.2.

For a detailed analysis of left ventricular wall motion we divided the left ventricle into 20 areas. For each area we determined the extent of wall motion disturbance. Based on this, we calculated a left ventricular wall motion disturbance index by summing up the values for the 20 areas. This index changed in accordance with the LVEF. Again, the difference did not reach statistical significance. However, in this global index the septal contractility is involved, even though we did not create laser channels in septal areas. A specific wall motion disturbance index, calculated only for treated areas, showed an improvement of myocardial contractility in the regions of interest in 68% of our patients 3 months postoperatively.

15.3.2 Thallium Perfusion Scan with Physical Endurance

The myocardial perfusion scan using thallium 201 revealed ischaemic areas in only 60% of the patients. In the remaining patients we found more or fewer scars in the left ventricle. Among the patients with preoperative evidence of myocardial ischaemia we found a reduced extent in 44% of the postoperative perfusion scans. In 42% we saw unchanged scans, and the remaining 14% of the patients presented with increased ischaemic perfusion defects. Among the patients with improved perfusion scans were five presenting with

Table 15.4. Ergometric endurance and reasons for cessation of the test pre- and post-TMR

	Preoperatively	Examination after			
		3 months	6 months	12 months	24 months
Medium workload (W)	58.0	73.3	77.1	79.2	94.0
Cessation because of:					
- angina pectoris (%)	49.4	29.4	27.0	0	
- changes in ECG (%)	12.3	7.8	7.7	0	
- dyspnoea (%)	42.0	45.1	65.4	100	

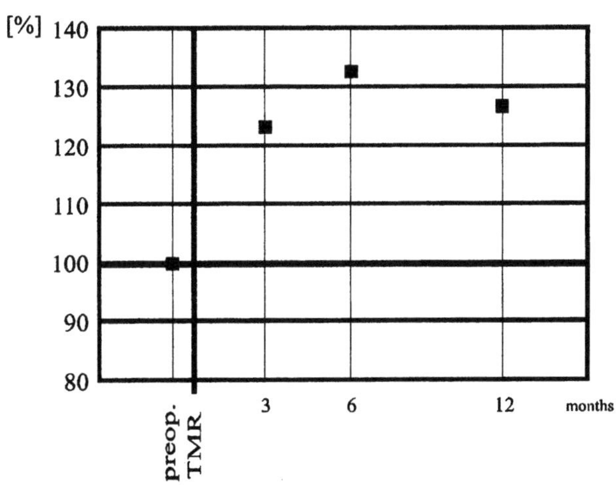

Fig. 15.3. Physical endurance: changes in the relative value compared with the preoperative workload

less ischaemia in the area of the septum, although the latter had not been treated in any of the cases.

During the thallium scan the patients underwent physical exercise testing with a bicycle ergometer. The maximum workload and the reasons for termination of the examination are summarised in Table 15.4. It becomes clear that the majority of patients had a significantly higher endurance postoperatively. Angina occurred less and less during the examination, with dyspnoea becoming the primary reason for stopping this physical stress test.

15.3.3
Perioperative Morbidity and Mortality

Twelve of the 165 operated patients died during the postoperative course; one of them had undergone a combined procedure (TMR + CABG) and 11 had received TMR as the only therapy. This results in a 7.6% mortality. We compared the 11 patients with a fatal outcome after TMR alone with the 134 survivors regarding the 50 factors listed in Table 15.2. However, we found no significant differences between the two subgroups.

In three of the 145 operated patients in the TMR only group we observed increasing mitral incompetence during the postoperative course. It was assumed that the laser beam had injured the chordae during the TMR operation. Some weeks later, chordal rupture occurred and mitral incompetence was established. However, during the routine echocardiographic examination prior to discharge there was no evidence of mitral regurgitation in any of the three patients. Thus, the mitral incompetence could have been of ischaemic origin.

15.3.4
Histological Findings

The relatives of eight of the 11 patients who died after TMR alone gave their consent to a postmortem examination. In cooperation with the Rudolf Virchow Hospital's Institute of Pathology, detailed histological analysis was performed on the hearts of these patients, in whom a total of 250 channels had been created. In the process, several hundred individual slides were prepared.

After being explanted, the heart as a whole was fixed in formalin for at least 3 weeks. The left ventricle was divided into pieces with a maximum length of 2 cm. Pieces with obvious TMR channels were cut longitudinally to the expected channel. Areas with no macroscopic evidence of TMR channels were cut into slices of 2–4 mm. Both sets of specimens were then embedded in paraffin and cut into slices of 6–8 μm and subsequently stained with hematoxylin-eosin (HE). Immunohistological staining using the avidin-biotin method was performed in addition. The analyses were performed with the DAKO ChemMate Detection Kit (Code No. K 5005) and the DAKO TechMate staining machine.

As primary antibodies we chose CD 68 (DAKO Clone KP1, dilution 1:4000) for reaction with macrophages, CD 31 (DAKO Clone JC/70 A, dilution 1:100) which reacts with endothelial cells, a polyclonal collagen type IV staining agent (MEDAC GmbH, Lot 013.05, dilution 1:400) for collagenic fibers, and MIB 1 (Dianova, Clone MIB 1, dilution 1:100) which reacts with the Ki-67 antigen, a proliferation-associated nuclear antigen. Morphometric analysis was performed with the LEICA Quantimed Q600 Morphometer.

We found the TMR channels created by a CO_2 laser surrounded by a zone of necrosis extending about 500 µm. In hearts from patients who died in the early postoperative period (1–7 days postop.) almost all channels were closed by fibrin clots, erythrocytes and macrophages. There were no obvious connections between the channels and the ventricular cavity.

In specimens from patients who died 2 or more weeks after the procedure, a granular tissue with high macrophage and monocyte activity was observed. Within this tissue we observed a developing network of capillaries. Otherwise, the tissue filling the channels did not substantially differ from scar tissue. We did not observe connections between the ventricular cavity and the new capillaries.

15.3.5 Comments

Up to now, transmyocardial laser revascularisation has remained an incomprehensible therapeutic procedure with regard to its functional principle. Frazier and co-workers were able to show that PET examinations after TMR indicated significant improvements in myocardial perfusion, at least in subendocardial areas [11]. However, these results can be explained by an altered relation between subendocardial and subepicardial perfusion, without any additional blood flow to the myocardium.

Using contrast-medium echocardiography, it was recently demonstrated that there seems to be a flow through some of the created channels from the left ventricular chamber into the myocardial wall 3 months after TMR [12]. Casuistic autopsy findings have indicated that transmyocardial channels created with a laser remain open for a month or even years [13, 14], yet to date, systematic examinations for proving the long-term patency of the channels are either lacking or encounter methodological problems. Histological results found by our team make it more likely that rapid channel closure occurs within the early postoperative phase.

The published experimental TMR data are inconsistent. Various groups have shown the positive effects of laser revascularisation in models of acute ischaemia in animal experiments [15, 16]. In contrast, other groups either cannot confirm this or doubt the possibility of improving myocardial circulation by transmyocardial channels in general [17, 18]. Particularly the inhomogeneity of the experimental data gives reason to doubt the concept that, following TMR, oxygenated blood is directed from the left ventricle into the myocardium, according to the principle of the amphibian heart.

These doubts are supported by findings from Whittaker and co-workers. They demonstrated that nontransmural laser channels offer almost the same possibility of protecting the myocardium against subsequent ischaemia [19].

In Table 15.5 we have summarised some of the theses currently under debate concerning the underlying principle of TMR. Even though there is no

Table 15.5. Mechanisms possibly responsible for the TMR effects

"Classical" perfusion theory (amphibian heart)	Blood flow from the left ventricular cavity to (a) sinusoids (b) native vasculature
Unspecified laser effect	Promotes angioneogenesis directly A consistently high concentration of angiogenic growth factors exists in the channel area due to monocyte and macrophage infiltration
Neurophysiological model	Perception of angina becomes impossible due to thermal injury to neural structures Initiation of neuronal inhibitory mechanisms by negative spinal feedback
Extensive thermal destruction of myocardial areas	Blood supply is now sufficient for the remaining myocardium Transformation of ischaemic areas into (indolent) scar tissue Less demand as a result of release of heat-shock proteins (ischaemic preconditioning) Less demand as a result of structural disorganisation of adjacent myocytes
Placebo effect	Laser perceived as a high-tech instrument
Equilibration of subendocardial and subepicardial perfusion	The perpendicular orientation of TMR channels filled with richly capillarised scar tissue leads to a balanced perfusion of the whole myocardium

consensus about the underlying functional principle, several groups have reported positive effects for patients who underwent transmyocardial laser revascularisation [20–22]. More than 80% of our patients had less angina and a significantly better quality of life postoperatively. This value is even higher in patients whose preoperative left ventricular contractility is not or only slightly restricted. The CCS classification can only poorly reflect this fact. Patients who report a significantly diminished frequency of angina at rest in the postoperative phase remain in CCS class 4, despite their having a markedly improved quality of life.

The global left ventricular contractility seems to be unchanged after TMR. Although we measured a 9% higher LVEF at 3 months after TMR, the values dropped to the preoperative value within the months that followed. However, when assessing the echocardiographically measured increase in left ventricular ejection fraction, one has to take into account that the possibility for improvement in contractility did not exist for patients with normal LVEF (approximately 10% of our patients). Furthermore, all of the remaining patients exhibited areas of scarred myocardium after infarction. After all, in the patients' anamneses we found an average of 1.5 infarctions per patient. Therefore, the extent of possible improvement in contractility is a priori restricted.

The majority of ^{201}thallium scans showed no improvement in myocardial perfusion. Only 37% of our patients had increased myocardial perfusion in laser-treated areas, but it must be kept in mind that only 60% of the preoperative perfusion scans revealed ischaemic myocardium. It is not possible to precisely quantify the circulation in individual areas with this method.

The maximum workload (bicycle ergometer) increased after TMR and remained stable at the higher value ($p<0.01$). Our practice of reducing antianginal medication rapidly to the lowest possible dose within the first 3 months after the operation has to be critically assessed. It can be assumed that the maximum workload would be even higher if the patients had remained at their preoperative level of medication. On the other hand, the perfusion scans probably would have shown fewer ischaemic areas under those circumstances.

Twelve of the 165 patients died postoperatively (mortality 7.3%.) The predominant cause of death was acute heart failure following myocardial infarction and severe ventricular arrythmias. We concluded that transmyocardial laser revascularisation carries a significant mortality; therefore, in our hands TMR remains an ultima ratio therapy.

We consider it necessary to further investigate the underlying principle of TMR. Unanswered are questions about the ideal type of laser or the optimal channel diameter or channel density. Perhaps other types of lasers (holmium, erbium, excimer) will produce better long-term effects. Furthermore, the patient group profiting from TMR has to be further characterised.

Experience is currently being gained in thoracoscopic laser revascularisation. This minimally invasive operation is performed with the aid of a laser thoracoscope. In the future it may be possible to carry out catheter-guided TMR from a percutaneous approach in the catheter laboratory.

References

1. Wearns JT, Mettier SR, Klump TG, Zschiesche AB (1933) The nature of the vascular communications between the coronary arteries and the chambers of the heart. Am Heart J 9:143–170
2. Vineberg AM (1967) Technical considerations for the combined operation of left internal mammary artery or right and left internal mammary implantations with epicardiectomy and free omental graft. J Thorac Cardiovasc Surg 53:837–847
3. Massimo C, Boffi R (1957) Myocardial revascularization by a new method of carrying blood directly from the left ventricular cavity into the coronary circulation. J Thorac Surg 34:257–264
4. Goldman A (1956) Experimental methods for producing a collateral circulation to the heart directly from the left ventricle. J Thorac Surg 31:364–374
5. Walter P, Hundeshagen H, Borst HG (1971) Treatment of acute myocardial infarction by transmural blood supply from the left ventricular cavity. Eur Surg Res 3:130–138
6. Sen PK (1965) Transmyocardial acupuncture – a new approach to myocardial revascularization. J Thorac Cardiovasc Surg 50:181–189
7. Mirhoseini M, Cayton M (1981) Revascularization of the heart by laser. J Microsurg 2:253–260
8. Mirhoseini M (1986) Laser myocardial revascularization. Lasers Surg Med 6:459–461
9. Mirhoseini M (1988) New concepts in revascularization of the myocardium. Ann Thorac Surg 45:415–420
10. Mirhoseini M, Shelgikar S, Cayton M (1988) Direct laser revascularization of the myocardium. Lasers Surg Med 8:150–151
11. Frazier OH, Cooley DA, Kadipasaoglu KA, et al (1995) Myocardial revascularization with laser. Preliminary findings. Circulation 92 [Suppl II]:II-58–II-65
12. Berwing K, Bauer R, Strasser R, Klövekorn WP, Bertschmann W (1996) Transmurale Laserrevaskularisation: erste Nachweise einer Perfusion über offene Laser-Kanäle. Kardiologie 85 [Suppl 2]:197
13. Mirhoseini M (1983) Myocardial revascularization by laser: a clinical report. Lasers Surg Med 3:241–245

14. Cooley DA, Frazier OH, Kadipasaoglu KA, Pehlivanoglu S (1994) Transmyocardial laser revascularization: anatomic evidence of long-term channel patency. Tex Heart J 21:220–224
15. Horvath KA, Smith WJ, Laurence RG, Schoen FJ, Appleyard EF, Cohn LH (1995) Recovery and viability of an acute myocardial infarct after transmyocardial laser. JACC 25:258–263
16. Yano OJ, Bielefeld MR, Jeevanandam V (1993) Prevention of acute regional ischemia with endocardial laser channels. Ann Thorac Surg 56:46–53
17. Whittaker P, Kloner RA, Przyklenk K (1993) Laser-mediated transmural myocardial channels do not salvage acutely ischemic myocardium. JACC 22:302–309
18. Hardy RI, James FW, Millard, RW, Kaplan S (1990) Regional myocardial blood flow and cardiac mechanics in dog hearts with CO_2 laser-induced intramyocardial revascularization. Basic Res Cardiol 85:179–197
19. Whitakker P, Kloner RA Myocardial preconditioning by laser irradiation.
20. Krabatsch T, Tülsner J, Hempel B, et al (1996) Die transmyokardiale Laserrevaskularisation in der Therapie der diffusen koronaren Herzerkrankung. HTG 10:19–26
21. Horvath KA, Mannting F, Cohn LH (1994) Improved myocardial perfusion and relief of angina after transmyocardial laser revascularization. Circulation 90, part 2:I-640
22. Frazier OH, Cooley DA, Kadipasaoglu K, Pehlivanoglu S (1994) Transmyocardial laser revascularization: initial clinical results. Circulation 90, part 2:I-640

CHAPTER 16

Transmyocardial Laser Revascularisation in Edinburgh

I.S. Morgan · C. Campanella

16.1 Introduction

A small proportion of angina sufferers have coronary vascular disease that precludes any attempt at grafting. Of those patients referred for coronary artery bypass grafting (CABG), it is estimated that up to 20% are not suitable for full anatomic revascularisation. Many of them will develop recurrent angina following surgery, and face an increased mortality due to fatal and non-fatal myocardial events.

These bleak figures have stimulated an interest in alternative methods of coronary revascularisation. The development of transmyocardial laser revascularisation (TMLR) has provided an additional tool with which the cardiac surgeon can improve the outcome in patients unsuitable for complete anatomic revascularisation. A number of devices exist at present, including the xenon-chloride excimer, the Holmium:yttrium-aluminum-garnet (YAG) and the carbon-dioxide (CO_2) lasers. Each varies in its energy delivery and ease of operation. The results of a large, randomised, trial comparing TMLR with medical therapy has demonstrated a clear benefit in terms of symptom relief and event-free survival [1, 2]. However, the effect of TMLR on patients undergoing conventional CABG remains unclear.

The primary purpose of this study was to evaluate the effect of the excimer laser as an adjunct to conventional CABG on those patients not suitable for complete anatomic revascularisation.

16.2 Materials and Methods

16.2.1 Patients

In this prospective evaluation study, 30 adults present for elective coronary revascularisation at a single institution were enrolled. Ideally, these patients fulfilled the following criteria: elective CABG, with angiographic evidence of unfavourable anatomy for complete revascularisation; moderate to good left ventricular function; and severe angina despite maximal medical therapy. Patients with any of the following conditions were excluded from participation in the trial : urgent and emergency cases, unstable angina, poor left ventricular function, and those who were candidates for complete anatomic revascularisation. Informed consent was obtained. The local and hospital ethics committees granted permission for this work.

16.2.2
Anaesthesia and Monitoring

Standardised anaesthetic technique was employed. A Servo 900 (Siemens-Elema) was utilised for ventilation, set on intermittent positive pressure. Cefuroxime was used for antibiotic prophylaxis. Monitoring involved continuous measurement of inspired oxygen, arterial oxygen saturation, end-tidal CO_2, electrocardiogram, invasive arterial pressure, non-invasive blood pressure, central venous pressure, urine output with indwelling catheter, oesophageal and skin temperature, and, at 20-min intervals, regular blood gas analysis. Following surgery, all patients were transferred to the intensive care unit.

16.2.3
Cardiopulmonary Bypass

Prior to arterial and venous cannulation, systemic heparin (Heparin Leo, Leo Pharmaceutical Products, Weesp, The Netherlands) was administered at a dose of 300 IU/kg to achieve an activated coagulation time (ACT) of greater than 400 s on a Hemochron analyser (Hemochron 400, International Technidyne, Edison, NJ). The bypass circuit components included a flexible venous reservoir, a cardiotomy reservoir, a membrane oxygenator (Avecor Cardiovascular, Bellshill, Scotland), and a roller pump (Stockert Instruments, Munich, Germany). Standard pump prime comprised: 2000 ml lactated Ringer's solution, 50 ml 8.4% bicarbonate, 8000 IU heparin. Surgery was performed on all patients by the same surgeon using, as far as feasible, standardised techniques. Once bypass had been established, target flow rates of 2.4 l min per square meter were maintained at normothermia, with reduction in flow dependent on temperature. In all cases the flow was linear and non-pulsatile. Moderate hypothermia of 30°C was usual. Aortic cross-clamping was utilised in those patients receiving grafts with antegrade crystalloid cardioplegia (St Thomas' Hospital Solution) cooled to 4°C, and myocardial temperature was monitored. Whenever possible, patients underwent conventional CABG to graftable vessels prior to TMLR. Heparinisation was maintained for the duration of bypass by addition of further heparin if the ACT fell below 400 s. Bypass was weaned in the usual fashion after which heparin was reversed with 3 mg/kg protamine as a slow IV infusion. For the laser procedure, the heart was fibrillated and channels were created in ungraftable areas of myocardium with the excimer laser (Max 20, Auto Suture Deutschland, formerly Medolas). The channels were spaced at 5 mm intervals. Laser settings were at a maximum energy of 30–40 mJ, and a repetition rate of 40 Hz. The technique was later modified adopting anterior left mini-thoracotomy without rib resection. Centrifugal venous assist (Biomedicus BP80, Medtronic, Minneapolis, MN) was used with femoral arterial and venous cannulation. Warfarin was started on day 1 and continued for 3 months for the first 20 patients. We subsequently gave no anticoagulant other than heparin prophylaxis (5000 IU t.i.d.). Functional assessment was made at 3, 6 and 12 months, and graded on the New York Heart Association (NYHA) scale. Pre- and post-operative thallium scanning (pre- and post-exercise), and dobutamine stress tests were performed in selected cases.

16.2.4
Statistical Analysis

After tabulating the data, statistical analysis was performed using Microsoft Excel 97 SR-1. Wilcoxon's rank sum test was used to compare NYHA grades at different time points.

16.3
Results

16.3.1
Patient Characteristics

Characteristics of the patients enrolled in this study and operative details are summarised in Table 16.1. The mean age was 61.6 years, with a male:female ratio of 4:1. Almost half of the patients (46.7%) had undergone CABG previously, and another two had received coronary angioplasty. Twelve patients received only TMLR as therapy. All but one of these were redo cases, and these included nine cases of left anterior mini-thoracotomy. Cardiopulmonary bypass (CPB) time averaged 66.8 min, with the TMLR procedure adding 5–10 min to the usual bypass time for grafts. The number of laser channels created varied, depending on the number of myocardial territories requiring revascularisation.

16.3.2
Anginal Status

16.3.2.1
NYHA Scale

Anginal status as assessed on the NYHA scale is illustrated graphically in Fig. 16.1. Pre-operatively, 50% of patients were in class IV, with a shift down-

Table 16.1. Patient characteristics and operative details

Age (range)±SD	61.6 (39–80)±9.9 years
Sex (M:F)	24:6
Redo operations	14/30 (46.7%)
Thoracotomy	9/30 (30%)
No. of patients receiving	
0 grafts	12
1 graft	12
2 grafts	6
Total	24 (in 18 patients)
TMLR channels created	
Mean (±SD)	45.6 (±20.7)
Range	6–100
CPB time	
Mean (±SD)	66.8 (±21.2) min
Range	1–104 min

CPB, cardiopulmonary bypass.

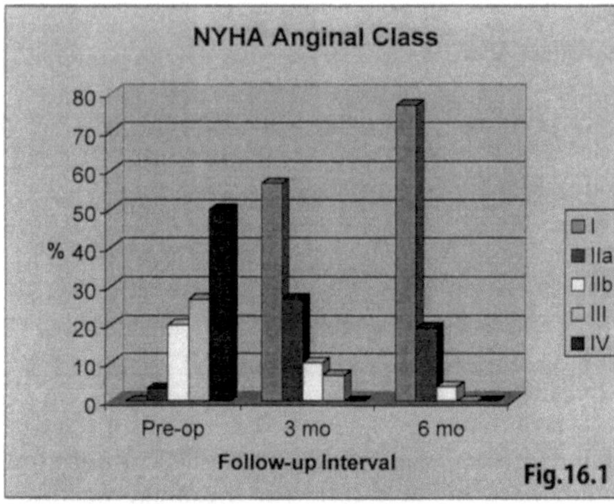

Fig. 16.1. NYHA anginal status for all patients

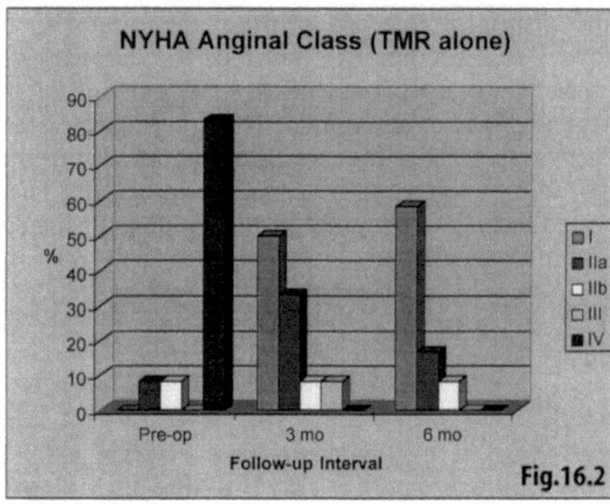

Fig. 16.2. NYHA anginal status for TMLR-only patients

wards at 3 months (average 2.6), and further improvement at 6 months (average 2.8).

When analysed separately, the data for those patients who received only TMLR were even more significant (Fig. 16.2). The average improvement was 2.8 at 3 months, and 3.1 at 6 months.

16.3.2.2
Canadian Cardiovascular Society Scale

When expressed according to the Canadian Cardiovascular Society (CCS) anginal class scale, the findings are similar to those of the NYHA scale (Figs. 16.3–16.4).

The average CCS anginal class is illustrated in Fig. 16.5, where TMLR-only patients are compared with all patients. In the TMLR group, the pre-operative anginal class was 3.75, falling to 1.67 at 3 months, and to 1.4 at

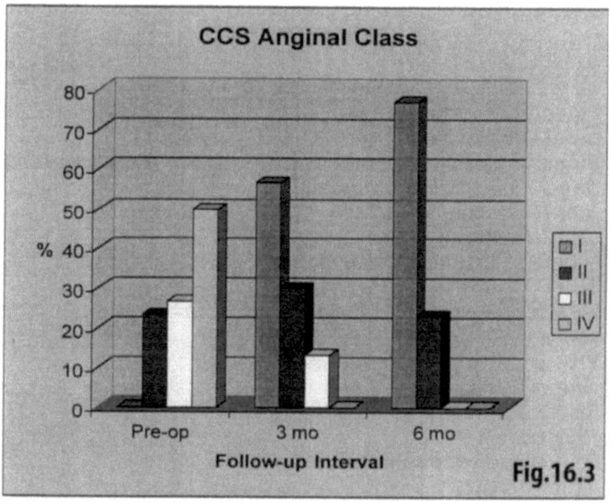

Fig. 16.3. CCS anginal status for all patients

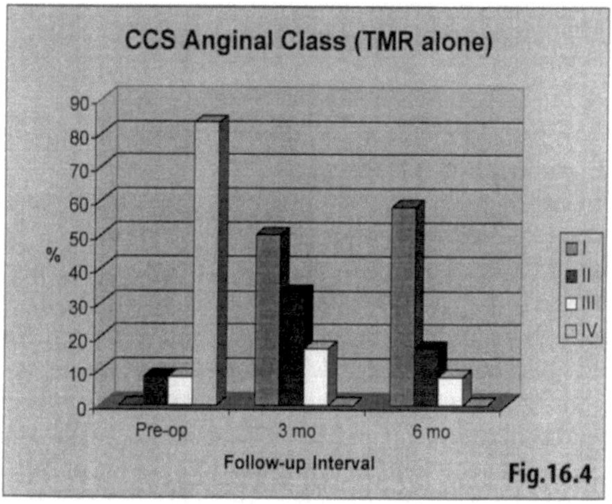

Fig. 16.4. CCS anginal status for TMLR-only patients

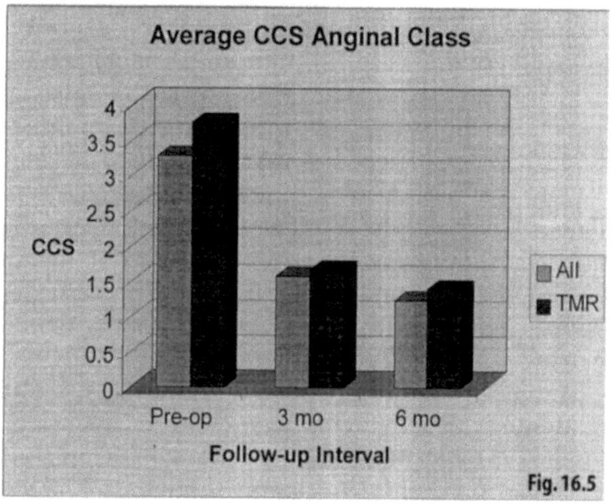

Fig. 16.5. Average CCS anginal class

Table 16.2. Postoperative data

	All patients	TMLR-only patients
Blood drain losses in first 24 h, mean (range) ±SD	850 (210–3740)±778 ml	458 (210–850)±210 ml
Blood transfusion requirements, mean (range) ±SD	2.2 (0–9)±2.3 units	1.5 (0–6)±2.1 units
Inotropic usage	63%	67%
Ventilation time, mean (range) ±SD	15.6 (0.25–96)±23.3 h	9.7 (0.25–43)±12.0 h
Length of ITU stay, mean (range) ±SD	2.3 (1–11)±2.3 d	2.6 (1–10)±3.0 d
Length ofhospital stay, mean (range) ±SD	9 (6–20)±3.3 d	8.5 (6–19)±3.6 d
Pre-operative hospital admissions within 1 year	58	33
Range of times of admission prior to operation	0–11	0–11
Post-operative hospital admissions within 1 year	7	5
Range of times of admission following operation	0–2	0–2

6 months following treatment. The findings for the whole group were similar, although less striking.

Clinical data are presented in Table 16.2. Total drain blood loss was acceptable and comparable with typical bypass patients. Significantly lower blood loss was observed in the 12 patients undergoing only TMLR (458±210 ml vs 850±778 ml, $p<0.01$), although nine of these received a left mini-thoracotomy. Blood transfusion requirements were low (2.2±2.3 units red cell concentrate), with only three patients receiving blood products (platelet concentrate, fresh frozen plasma, cryoprecipitate). Inotrope was marginally higher than usual (63% vs 55%), with 2 patients requiring mechanical assistance from an intra-aortic balloon pump. However, ventilation times (15.6±23.3 h), and length of ITU (2.3±2.3 days), and hospital stays (9±3.3 days) were reasonably short. The majority of the patients (70%) had required admission to hospital for unstable angina in the year preceding surgery, representing a total of 58 admission episodes (1.93±2.5 per patient per year). In the year following surgery, only 16.7% required admission (0.23±0.57 per patient per year).

Objective measures of clinical improvement were obtained for selected patients. A technetium tetrafosmin stress myocardial perfusion scan was performed on four patients, while two had dobutamine stress echocardiography, and another six underwent treadmill exercise testing. All patients demonstrated significant improvement in comparison with pre-operative performance.

The mean duration of follow-up was 11.4 months, and in the longest case, 24 months. Most patients were able to achieve a reduction in number and dose of cardiac medications, although the majority of TMLR-only patients continued on their pre-operative medication for a 3 month period. Two patients died following surgery – one of cardiac failure after 3 months following a prolonged convalescence. His anginal status improved briefly, although poor case selection was undoubtedly a contributory factor. The second patient made an excellent recovery, but died suddenly at 10 months without any preceding illness. Presumably, this was due to dysrhythmia. No postmortem assessment was obtained in either case. Complications directly attributable to the TMLR were uncommon - one patient developed complete heart block immediately following TMLR with 100 channels, requiring the insertion of a permanent pacemaker.

16.4 Discussion

The basis for laser revascularisation began with the observation of myocardial sinusoids in 1933 by Wearn et al. [3]. This was later exploited by Vineberg [4], who implanted the mammary artery directly into the myocardium with some notable long term success [5]. It is likely that these efforts were stimulated by observation of the coronary vasculature of reptilian hearts, which have a rudimentary epicardial coronary system. Their blood flows directly through endomyocardial channels from the ventricular cavity. In an attempt to emulate this type of circulation, many investigators experimented with a variety of devices to create these channels [6–8]. However, it was not until the development of laser technology in the late 1960s that the channels could be created without the accompanying problems of early thrombosis or late fibrosis. Unfortunately, the equipment was too bulky for clinical use in the operating theatre. Much of the early work was pioneered by Mirhoseini in Wisconsin [9–14].

Despite much investigation, the exact mechanism whereby the laser improves myocardial blood flow is not yet clearly understood. Many investigators have demonstrated patent channels by histologic analysis following TMLR [15], whilst others have shown early channel closure [16]. Animal experimental studies give inconclusive results, and do not provide any further clarification [17, 18]. This may be due in part to the different techniques utilised. There are at least three lasers currently available, each with different properties. We chose the excimer laser because we felt that due to its cold beam, it offered the best combination of handling and safety.

Our study demonstrates the effectiveness of the excimer laser in relieving the symptoms of angina in a group of patients unsuitable for conventional coronary revascularisation. The selection of patients for this procedure was based on their unresponsiveness to full medical treatment, as well as on the inadequacy of their anatomy for CABG. We decided at this stage of our investigation to exclude patients with unstable angina, in order to decrease the number of variables inevitably associated with this category of patient. All patients survived the procedure and the immediate postoperative period, and the procedure proved entirely safe. Technically, the switch from median sternotomy to left mini-thoracotomy and femoral cannulation proved extremely satisfactory with respect to blood loss, as well as to pain control and length of hospital stay. The decision to undertake the left thoracotomy and femoral cannulation was made prior to surgery, based on the coronary vasculature. If the angiogram suggested a complete absence of graftable vessels, the left mini-thoracotomy was performed, and if the angiographic findings were confirmed after close inspection of the heart, total transmyocardial revascularisation was undertaken. On the other hand, if angiography showed at least one graftable vessel, then median sternotomy proved to be a more suitable approach. In the immediate postoperative period, due to the underlying pathology of the coronary artery, it was not surprising that the inotropic usage was somewhat higher than standard. Similarly, in a small number of patients, mechanical assistance was required to support haemodynamic parameters in the first few hours.

The objective measurements of clinical improvement were obtained only for a small number of patients due to a variety of logistic problems. However, all demonstrated a significant improvement in comparison with pre-operative performance. This is comparable to findings in other studies [19, 20]. One of the most striking outcomes was the shift in anginal class of patients subjected to TMLR only, as well as of those who received TMLR in association with grafts. The continued improvement at three and six months suggests the development or enrichment of collateral circulation in chronically ischaemic areas. In addition to the improvement of anginal class status, another important outcome is the persistence of that improvement, even up to 24 months following the procedure. It is, nevertheless, difficult to determine from our data the contribution of the coronary revascularisation in association with TMLR, and the role played by the graft itself in improving anginal status. Currently, we must accept the technical limitations which allow identification of the perfusion on a segmental basis only. We hope that in the future, more detailed evaluation might answer this question. From the viewpoint of clinical efficiency, the procedure successfully, reproducibly and predictably relieves angina in a number of patients, but more basic experimental clinical work is required to understand the precise mechanism by which this improvement is brought about.

References

1. Frazier OH, Cooley DA, Kadipasaoglu KA, Pehlivanoglu S, Lindenmeir M, Barasch E, Conger JL, Wilansky S, Moore WH (1995) Myocardial revascularization with laser. Preliminary findings. Circulation 92 [9 Suppl]:II58–II65
2. Cooley DA, Frazier OH, Kadipasaoglu KA, Lindenmeir MH, Pehlivanoglu S, Kolff JW, Wilansky S, Moore WH (1996) Transmyocardial laser revascularization: clinical experience with twelve-month follow-up. J Thorac Cardiovasc Surg 111:791–797, 797–799 (discussion)
3. Wearn JT, Mettier SR, Klump TG, Zschiesche AB (1933) The nature of the vascular communications between the coronary arteries and the chambers of the heart. Am Heart J 9:143–170
4. Vineberg AM (1946) Development of an anastomosis between the coronary vessels and a transplanted internal mammary artery Can Med Assoc J 55:117–119
5. Vineberg AM (1975) Evidence that revascularization by ventricular-internal mammary artery implants increases longevity: twenty-four year, nine month follow-up. J Thorac Cardiovasc Surg 70:381–397
6. Sen PK, Udwadia TE, Kinare SG, Parulkar GB (1965) Transmyocardial acupuncture. J Thorac Cardiovasc Surg 50:181–189
7. Massimo C, Boffi L (1957) Myocardial revascularization by a new method of carrying blood directly from the left ventricular cavity into the coronary circulation. J Thorac Cardiovasc Surg. 34:257–264

8. Hershey JE, White M (1969) Transmyocardial puncture revascularization: a possible emergency adjunct to arterial implant surgery. Geriatrics 24:101–108
9. Mirhoseini M, Cayton MM (1981) Revascularization of the heart by laser. J Microsurg 2:253–60
10. Mirhoseini M, Muckerheide M, Cayton MM (1982) Transventricular revascularization by laser. Lasers Surg Med 2:187–198
11. Mirhoseini M, Fisher JC, Cayton M (1983) Myocardial revascularization by laser: a clinical report. Lasers Surg Med 3:241–245
12. Mirhoseini M (1983) Laser applications in thoracic and cardiovascular surgery. Med Instrum 17:401–403
13. Mirhoseini M, Cayton MM, Shelgikar S, Fisher JC (1986) Laser myocardial revascularization. Lasers Surg Med 6:459–461
14. Mirhoseini M, Shelgikar S, Cayton MM (1988) New concepts in revascularization of the myocardium. Ann Thorac Surg 45:415–420
15. Burkhoff D, Fisher PR, Apfelbaum M, et al (1996) Histologic appearance of transmyocardial channels after 4 1/2 weeks. Ann Thorac Surg 61:1532–1534
16. Cooley DA, Frazier OH, Kadipasaoglu KA, Pehlivanoglu S, Shannon RL, Angelini P (1994) Transmyocardial laser revascularization. Anatomic evidence of long-term channel patency. Tex Heart Inst J 21:220–224
17. Guo JX, Pan J, Ma L, Chen MZ, Xu H, Shi AY (1993) Experimental studies of laser myocardial revascularization in rats. Chin Med J (Engl) 106:665–667
18. Hardy RI, James FW, Millard RW, Kaplan S (1990) Regional myocardial blood flow and cardiac mechanics in dog hearts with CO_2 laser-induced intramyocardial revascularization. Basic Res Cardiol 85:179–197
19. March RJ, Aranki S, Boyce S, Cohn LH, Cooley DA, Crew JR, et al (1997) Improved event free survival following transmyocardial laser revascularisation versus medical management in patients with unreconstructed coronary artery disease. Presented at the 77th Annual Meeting of the American Association for Thoracic Surgery, Washington, DC, 4–7 May 1997
20. PLC Newsletter. Transmyocardial revascularisation – the heart laser (interim report). Simacon, Stanmore, Middlesex. 11 March 1996

CHAPTER 17

Transmyocardial Laser Revascularisation

R. Moosdorf · L. Rybinski · H. Höffken · R. Funck · B. Maisch

17.1 Introduction

Despite the advances made in direct myocardial revascularisation by surgical as well as interventional techniques, there is an increasing number of highly symptomatic patients for whom for none of these methods are suited. This has led to a renewed interest in techniques of indirect myocardial revascularisation, which were abandoned years ago because of the success achieved with bypass grafting and PTCA. Transmyocardial laser revascularisation has picked up the idea of transmural channels, filling with blood from the left ventricle, as first described by Sen et al. in 1965 [4]. Primarily used in combination with coronary bypass grafting, it has now become a sole therapy for end-stage coronary artery disease. While the mechanism of action of this new indirect procedure is still not quite clear, clinical improvements have been demonstrated in numerous studies.

17.2 Transmyocardial Laser Revascularisation

The principle of transmyocardial revascularisation was introduced more than 30 years ago by Sen et al. [4], who performed the first experimental studies before they applied it to patients with ischaemic heart disease, nearly at the same time as Cooley, White and Hershey [5] in the United States. At that time, the left ventricle was punctured by needles, creating transmural channels which were intended to supply the ischaemic myocardium with blood from the left ventricular cavity.

With the introduction of direct myocardial revascularisation, this concept was no longer pursued until the beginning of the 1980s, when Mirhoseini [3] performed his first successful in vivo experiments with a CO_2 laser. He also reintroduced this method into clinical practice, combined with bypass grafting, in patients with diffuse coronary artery disease. Due to the low power of the CO_2 laser at that time, the procedure could only be performed on the arrested heart. With the development of high-powered CO_2 lasers, it was Crew [2] who, in 1991, reported on the first transmyocardial laser revascularisation on the beating heart without cardiopulmonary bypass. The currently used CO_2 laser offers nearly 1000 watts of power, enabling penetration of the left ventricular wall in only a few milliseconds. Triggered by an R-wave, the laser beam is aimed at the myocardium in end diastole, avoiding damage to intracardiac structures and proarrhythmic effects.

The laser beam is totally absorbed by the blood and produces only microbubbles, which can be detected by transoesophageal echocardiography, indicating a successful penetration of the ventricular wall. Usually, one laser channel is drilled per square centimeter of ischaemic myocardium. The concept underlying this new therapy has often been described as a 'reptilisation of the human heart'. The reptilian heart consists of a compact outer myocardial layer, which is supplied by coronary arteries. The inner layer shows deep sinusoids which contribute to myocardial oxygen supply by diffusion and convection. It can easily be appreciated that the small laser channels that are drilled into the human myocardium at a distance of approximately 1 cm from one another can hardly be compared with the large surface area of the reptilian sinusoids with only small islands of myocardium in between. Thus, the underlying mechanism of this new therapy remains to be determined. One possible explanation might be a connection between patent channels and intramyocardial vessels. There might also be an inflammatory response to the laser trauma, which would lead to a neocapillarisation within the ischaemic myocardium. Both theories have to be tested in clinical and especially experimental investigations demonstrating the long-term perfusion of the channels and the surrounding myocardium.

17.3 Clinical Experience

At the department for cardiovascular surgery of the University in Marburg, transmyocardial laser revascularisation has been offered since November 1994 as an additional therapeutic option to patients with intractable end-stage coronary artery disease. A total of 134 patients (117 men, 17 women) have now been treated with this new technique, in 67 cases additional to coronary bypass grafting and in the other 67 cases as the sole therapy. There was an evidently high number of second and third interventions, ranging up to 93% in the laser-only group and 55% in the combined group, which is characteristic for patients with end-stage coronary artery disease. This, together with severity of the disease, explains the hospital mortality of 11.4%, including four patients who were operated on under emergency conditions and with concomitant heart diseases. Preoperatively as well as prior to hospital discharge and after 3, 6 and 12 months, all patients are submitted to intensive investigations including stress-ECG, -echocardiography and -scintigraphy, as well as an intensive clinical investigation and a questionnaire concerning life quality. Coronary angiography is of course mandatory before surgery and is offered to the patients again after 6 months. At present, the complete data of 57 patients after 1 year of follow-up are available, demonstrating a significant improvement in angina. According to the CCS classification, 63% of the patients are in angina class I, 45% in class II and 19% in class III, while 56% were in class III and 44% in class IV preoperatively (see Fig. 17.1). Based on the NYHA classification, 14% are in class I, 54% in class II and 32% in class III, compared with approximately 50% each in class III and class IV preoperatively. Even looking at the group with only laser therapy, 76% of the patients are in angina classes I and II and only 24% in class

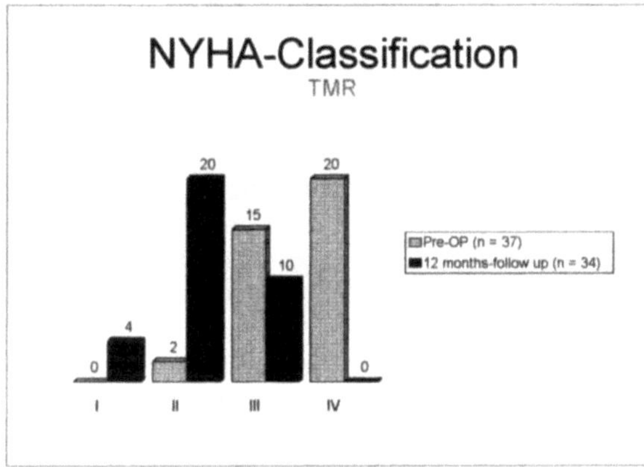

Fig. 17.1. Angina classification (NYHA) preoperatively and after TMLR (12 months)

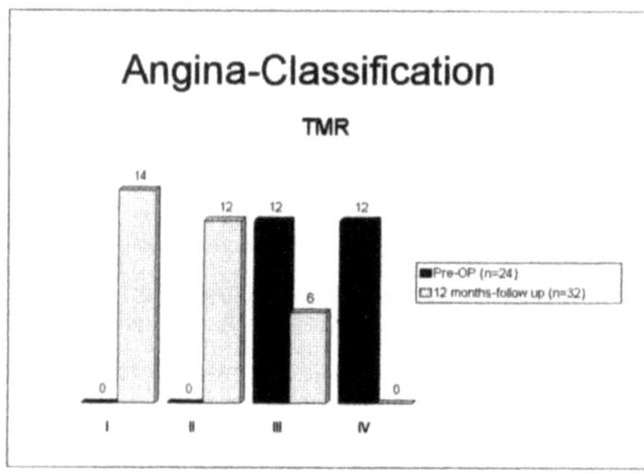

Fig. 17.2. Angina classification (CCS) preoperatively and after TMLR (12 months)

III, compared with 50% in class III and 50% in class IV preoperatively. Again, 60% of them are in NYHA class I and II and only 40% in class III (see Fig. 17.2). The ischaemic tolerance under stress-ECG with St-segment analysis increased from a mean of 25 to 70 watt among the patients who received only laser therapy and from 50 to 85 watt after combined procedures. Nuclear scans showed a significant improvement of perfusion in 40.5% of the patients, who were examined by an independent specialist. After a mean follow-up of 20.1 months, the total mortality was 23.5% – excluding hospital mortality, 14.5%.

This statistic shows a trend towards improved mortality compared with a similar group of patients receiving maximal medical therapy presented by Califf et al. [1]. This trend has to be followed statistically over a longer period to determine whether this new therapy has an impact not only on life quality and hospitalisation rate, but also on life expectancy.

Discussion

Transmyocardial laser revascularization represents a relatively new therapeutic option for patients with endstage coronary artery disease. While the exact pathophysiological mechanism of this treatment still remains to be determined, whether it is a connection of the laser channels to intramyocardial vessels or an induction of neo-angiogenesis or even both, preliminary clinical investigations show a significant improvement in angina and stress tolerance in about two thirds of those patients in whom other treatments were not effective.

Scintigraphy has demonstrated an improvement in myocardial perfusion but not normalization as after direct myocardial revascularization. Further investigations and also new techniques such as positron emission tomography or high resolution echocardiography will be necessary to determine the definitive role of transmyocardial laser revascularization in the surgical armamentarium. It will not be an alternative to direct methods such as coronary bypass surgery or PTCA, but it may be an option for those patients who are no longer amenable to those therapies.

References

1. Califf RM, Daniel BM, Harrell FE, Hlatky MA, Kerry LL, Rosati RA (1988) Importance of clinical measure of ischemia in the prognosis of patients with documented coronary artery disease. JACC 11:20–26
2. Crew JR (1991) Transmyocardial revascularization by CO_2 laser. Surg Technol Int 1:236–238
3. Mirhoseini M, Cayton MM (1981) Revascularization of the heart by laser. J Microsurg 2:253–260
4. Sen PK, Udwadia TE, Kinare SG, Parulkar GB (1965) Transmyocardial acupuncture: a new approach to myocardial revascularization. J Thorac Cardiovasc Surg 50:181–189
5. White M, Hershey JE (1968) Multiple transmyocardial puncture revascularization in refractory ventricular fibrillation due to myocardial ischemia. Ann Thorac Surg 6:557–563

CHAPTER 18

Transmyocardial Laser Revascularisation: Clinical Observations Concerning the Use of an Excimer Laser System

M. Klein · H.P. Dauben · H.D. Schulte · E. Gams

18.1 Introduction

Drug therapy, percutaneous transluminal coronary angioplasty (PTCA) and bypass surgery form the basic strategies for treating coronary heart disease (CAD). Currently, a number of scaled therapeutic approaches are available which, when adjusted to the patient's individual condition, allow for improvements in terms of symptomatology and prognosis and consequently also ensure a long-term improvement of the patient's quality of life.

As an effective therapy for usually primary arteriosclerosis has not yet been found, the progress of the primary disease may require a flexible application of different therapy concepts at any point in time. However, each therapeutic approach has principal limitations.

Whilst diseases involving up to three vessels without expected interventional complications have meanwhile become the domain of cardiological therapy, morphologically severe disorders are treated mainly by heart surgeons. In recent years, heart surgery has increasingly been influenced by demographic and medical developments: the number of difficult second and third operations is continuously rising and, due to the population's increased life expectancy, the number of older patients suffering from complex concomitant diseases which, until a few years ago, were considered contraidications to surgery involving the utilisation of extracorporeal circulation (ECC) is also growing.

The experience gained and innovative technologies developed in the fields of cardioanaesthesia, intensive care, cardiotechnology and new-heart surgical techniques have enabled us to offer these patients a heart operation at an increased but nevertheless justifiable risk. At the same time, the number of patients who show progressive arteriosclerotic alterations of the coronary arterial system that prevent direct revascularisation, even after initially successful interventions, is constantly rising. Here, even maximum medication does not offer patients relief from their complaints. Only a few such patients are eligible for heart transplantation; the majority do not meet the inclusion criteria for this measure.

The majority of these patients do not suffer from manifest heart failure. However, their angina pectoris limits their endurance to the extent that even daily routine activities can be performed only with difficulty, if at all. Frequent hospitalisation is the consequence, and recurrent infarctions finally lead to death.

This clinical problem poses an enormous medical challenge and has prompted a demand not only to extend the therapeutic focus to proximal lesions of the coronary arteries but also to include disorders of smaller and the smallest vessels. This requires techniques that allow for revascularisation of the ischaemic myocardium from an area which is not directly connected to the vessel concerned. In this context, indirect revascularisation techniques - the first surgical option when treating coronary heart diseases - have taken on more and more importance during recent years. Thus, experimental and clinical studies are focusing on techniques of transmyocardial revascularisation, as other methods are nowadays of only historical interest.

18.2 Transmyocardial Revascularisation

Transmyocardial revascularisation (TMR) is based on the idea that by drilling transmyocardial channels through the wall of an ischaemic ventricle a connection between the myocardium and its afferent vessels can be established, so that more arterial blood is supplied directly from the left ventricle to the myocardium. Such networks triggered by a chronic ischaemia can develop in the myocardium to such an extent that in some rare cases survival is possible even when both coronary ostia are occluded.

The most well-known vascular system of this kind are the so-called thebesian veins, which were discovered some 300 years ago (1708, Thebesius). When occluded coronary arteries end in a widely branched capillary net, direct connections to the left ventricle via sinusoid openings can be also found. In the same way, collaterals can be developed between the arterial and venous myocardial network on the one hand and the left ventricle-cavum on the other [1]. However, a sufficient blood supply to the heart, particularly when under stress, is normally impossible.

The heart can accommodate itself to chronic hypoperfusion by developing a so-called hibernating myocardium. Performance decreases, and all possible transitions from hypokinesia to complete akinesia can develop. The extent of such regulating alterations depends on the particular vascular morphology and determines not only - at fluent transitions - the consequently reduced left ventricular ejection fraction (EF) but also the angina pectoris symptomatology and may lead in parallel to the development of a dysrhythmia. If the residual perfusion is also insufficient for structural rescucitation, this condition will finally lead to an infarction.

Of all transmyocardial revascularisation techniques, from simple needle aspiration to the Vineberg operation [2-7], only transmyocardial laser revascularisation (TMLR), which was first introduced experimentally by Mirhoseini in the early 1980s and has been applied clinically since 1986, is of importance. At the beginning, Mirhoseini used a low-energy CO_2 laser, which permitted intervention only on the nonbeating heart. Later, an ECG-triggered, pulsed high-energy CO_2 laser was used for TMLR in order to be able to drill channels also in the beating heart without requiring the use of ECC [8-11]. To control the complete penetration of the left ventricular wall this laser system requires simultaneous transoesophageal echocardiography (TEE). However, as the exact dosing and precise positioning of the laser beam are apparently difficult, damage to the intramyocardial structures can therefore not be completely excluded.

With respect to their technical properties and the specific effect of the light emitted, other laser systems would also have been suited for transmyocardial revascularisation but were not considered at the beginning. One of these is the excimer laser system, which was first used for laser angioplasty. This laser drills transmyocardial channels with the lowest possible energy and causes the smallest necrotic zone within the myocardium. The high-energy UV radiation of the XeCl - excimer laser (wavelength 308 nm) is very efficiently absorbed by the tissue's molecular bindings. A considerable number of these bindings are thereby directly cracked, so that penetration of the excimer laser into the biological material and the thermal damage caused by its radiation is very low. The radiation emitted by the infrared laser (CO_2 laser and holmium:YAG laser) traditionally used for TMLR is absorbed by the tissue water. Depending on the irradiation intensity, the water will only be warmed up, leading to either a thermal load on the tissue or possibly its direct evaporation. The penetration depths as well as the thermal effects vary depending on the wavelengths applied. The thermal side effects of the laser beam are closely related to the penetration depth: the deeper the penetration, the greater the thermal damage that can be expected. Thermal load or damage develops if either the molecular bindings have not been directly cracked or the intensity is insufficient to directly vaporise the tissue water; i.e. the intensity of the laser beam was below the evaporation point.

The predominant effect of the excimer laser is photoablation. This effect can be seen at medium energy and power densities and is caused by the bursting of the molecular bindings, which in turn leads to a layerwise ablation (1–10 μm) of the tissue. The necrotic marginal zones of 30–50 μm created around the excimer laser channel are the smallest, compared with those caused by the other laser systems employed for TMLR. At an adapted chart speed mechanical effects can be almost completely excluded. Transmyocardial channels can also be safely drilled in the beating heart. In addition, the currently available excimer laser systems offer the advantage of easy transportation and can therefore be used in various surgical contexts without requiring time-consuming preparation. A flexible light fibre equipped with a special handle allows for precise and easy dosing of the laser in contact application with the tissue. Its application in transthoracic interventions not involving the use of ECC and carried out by means of a mini-thoracotomy or an endoscopic approach poses no difficulties and requires no additional applicators, as the operating length of the light fibre is more than 4 m. ECG triggering and TEE to control the drilling of channels are not necessary.

18.3 Material and Methods

In Düsseldorf an excimer laser system is used. At the beginning, a Max 10, manufactured by Medolas and initially intended for application in intracoronary arterial laser angioplasty, was used. Since May 1995, the laser type Max 20 TMLR produced by USSC has been employed.

In the period from February 1995 to February 1997, 128 patients underwent transmyocardial laser revascularisation at the Department for Thoracic and Cardiovascular Surgery, Düsseldorf. For the first 18 patients a 600-µm quartz light fibre was used. With an output at the fibre end of 15–20 mJ at a frequency of 25–30 Hz, the operational intensity was rather low. On the average, 1–2 channels/cm^2 were drilled.

The results of this first series were not convincing. At 38.9%, mortality was very high. On histological examination of the hearts of two patients who died 3 and 5 days postoperatively, no open channels were seen.

Furthermore, these patients had been scheduled for TMLR without prior nuclear medical assessment of the myocardium's perfusion and viability; 13 of these 18 patients had an EF below 20% and/or ventricular dysrhythmia that was uncontrollable preoperatively with medication.

Since May 1995, the Max 20 unit, especially configured to TMLR applications, has been employed with a 960-µm fibre. The operating energy has been increased to a maximum of 40 mJ and 40 Hz. In total, 110 patients underwent surgery with this new system up to February 1997. An average of 1–3 channels/cm^2 were drilled.

The following criteria were considered indications for TMLR:

1. Existence of a strong diffuse coronary 2- or 3-vessel disorder
2. Angina pectoris symptoms with significant reduction of life quality
3. Optimised drug therapies that do not lead to a reduction in angina-related complaints
4. Option of bypass operation and/or PTCA significantly limited or nonexistent due to the coronary morphology assessed preoperatively
5. Coincidence of vital myocardial tissue and hypoperfusion – (mismatch) demonstrated by nuclear medicine – in myocardial areas deprived of bypassable coronary arteries and intended for TMLR treatment

The following were considered to be contraindications:

1. Ventricular dysrhythmia untreatable with medication
2. Preoperatively incorrectable haemostatic disorders
3. Left ventricular EF below 20%, if more scarred than hibernating myocardial tissue is identified

The treatment objective was complete or nearly complete revascularisation with all patients, whereby even a critical afferentia via bypass was generally preferred.

The majority of patients suffered from one or more serious additional diseases and most of them had already undergone interconventional angioplastic measures or surgical revascularisation. Under maximum drug therapy, all patients had angina pectoris symptoms grade III–IV according to the classification criteria of the Canadian Cardiovascular Society (CCS). The anamnestic infarct frequency was more than one per patient. Details are included in Table 18.1. The surgical risk was evaluated for all patients by preoperatively preparing a risk profile using the Risk Master (Data Health Research, Oregon, USA), which had been proven valid in a prospective randomised study comprising 1000 patients [12]. Hereby, the calculated mortality risk was assigned to one of the following three categories:

Table 18.1. Demographic and medical data

Time period: June 1995–February 1997	Total	TMLR+ CABG	TMLR	TMLR (Mini-thoracotomy)
No. of patients	110	98	10	2
Sex M:F	94:16	87:11	6:4	1:1
Age mean in years (range)	67.8 (41–86)	67.9 (41–85)	64.3 (52–78)	82 (78–86)
NYHA classification (mean)	2.7	2.7	3.0	3.5
CCS classification (mean)	3.6	3.6	3.6	4.0
LV ejection fraction (*n*)				
>40%	26	22	4	0
20–40%	64	58	4	2
<20%	20	18	2	0
Calculated mortality risk (%)	19.6	16.2	18.9	24.3

Low-risk group: 0–<2.5%
Moderate-risk group: 2.5%–10%
High-risk group: >10%

The patient distribution is seen in Table 18.6.

18.4 Surgical Procedure

In interventions involving the application of ECC the creation of peripherial anastomoses with intermittent clamping of the aorta ascendens was done at a systemic hypothermia of 30°C blood temperature and under artificially induced ventricular fibrillation; 1–3 channels/cm^2 were drilled in the corresponding myocardial areas. Thus the TMLR did not lengthen the intervention time in the combined approach of bypass operation and TMLR. The drilling of one channel took 8–12 s. Heparin/protamine management was carried out as usual.

In interventions not involving ECC a mini-thoracotomy was made in the 5th intercostal space (ICS). After opening the pericardium 1 cm above the n. phrenicus also 1–3 channels/cm^2 were drilled in the beating heart. By means of a special "heart lifter" which can be mounted to the retractor for stability, all free left ventricular wall areas were easily accessed. Postoperatively, patients received 150–250 IU heparin/kg body weight.

The common adjuvant perioperative therapy for both surgical procedures did not differ from the one applied in other comparable routine interventions. For none of our patients was concomitant transoesophageal echocardiography employed.

18.5 Results

The surgical results of 110 patients treated using the excimer laser were evaluated. With 98 patients a combined intervention – bypass operation and TMLR – was carried out. Ten patients underwent TMLR exclusively. As no

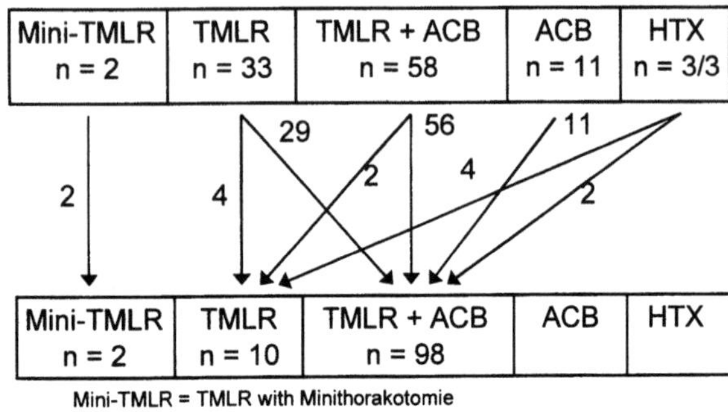

Fig. 18.1. Scheduled vs. actual TMLR procedures

Table 18.2. Laser-specific and intraoperative data

Time period: June 1995–February 1997	Total	TMLR+ CABG	TMLR	TMLR (Mini-thoracotomy)
No. of grafts (mean)	1.25	1.4	–	–
No. of channels (mean)	29	27.5	32.2	34
Mean total energy (J)	124.7	118.25	142.8	146.1
No. of units of RBC (mean)	0.48	0.51	0.50	0
Median drainage volume (ml)	390	420	390	255

Table 18.3. Complications

Time period: June 1995–February 1997	Total	TMLR+ CABG	TMLR	TMLR (Mini-thoracotomy)
Infarctions definite (probable)	2 (4)	2 (1)	0 (2)	0 (1)
Rhythm disturbances	6	5	1	0
Rethoracotomy	2	2	0	0
IABP/assist devices	1	1	0	0
Pneumonia (sepsis)	0	0	0	0
SIRS	2	1	1	0
Wound infections	0	0	0	0
Total	13 (17)	11 (12)	2 (4)	0 (1)

target vessels were detectable on angiography without ECC, two multimorbid patients were first subjected to a left-sided mini-thoracotomy on the beating heart. The demographic and medical data are included in Table 18.1.

Regarding possible bypass operation, there was a considerable discrepancy between the preoperative assessment of the coronary angiography and the coronary morphology found intraoperatively for 42 patients. Twenty-nine patients had been judged falsely negative. Preoperatively, none of these patients seemed suited for a bypass operation, whilst intraoperatively a chance was seen for direct revascularisation of at least one coronary vessel, providing for satisfactory discharge via a peripheral anastomosis. The coronary angiography of 13 patients had been judged falsely positive. In these cases, no or only a limited chance for direct revascularisation was found intraoperatively, so that either a combined approach (TMLR+ACBG: $n=11$) was taken or TMLR exclusively ($n=2$) was performed.

In 62 cases the preoperative assessment was confirmed by the intraoperative findings. Six patients were treated exclusively by TMLR; for two of these patients surgical therapy involving ECC was considered to be too risky. Therefore, TMLR was performed by means of a left-sided mini-thoracotomy. Fifty-six patients underwent a combined surgical intervention (TMLR+ACB) (cf. Fig. 18.1).

The surgical data regarding the laser applications are summarized in Table 18.2. Laser-specific complications, damage to intracardial structures or incessant bleeding from the drilled channels was not observed in any case. In one case, a postoperative circulatory syndrome of low output required the application of an intra-aortic balloon pump. High-dose drug support became necessary for six patients, whilst 19 required low-dose drug support; 84 patients required no circulatory assistance postoperatively.

Definite postoperative myocardial infarcts were found in four patients. In the group of patients who were treated only by TMLR no postoperative infarctions have been observed.

In two cases, a rethoracotomy became necessary at an early postoperative stage. In both cases this was due to bleeding from the pedicle of the inner left internal thoracic artery. The intra- and postoperative complications are summarised in Table 18.3.

The mean drainage volume was 397 ml. A value of 0.48 packed red cells has been calculated as mean transfusion requirement. On average, patients remained 1.4 days in the intensive care unit. The drainage and transfusion volumes are shown in Table 18.2.

The results of the preoperative assessments and the follow-up examinations carried out postoperatively with respect to NYHA and CCS classification are shown in Table 18.4 and Figs. 18.2 and 18.3. After 30 days, a signifi-

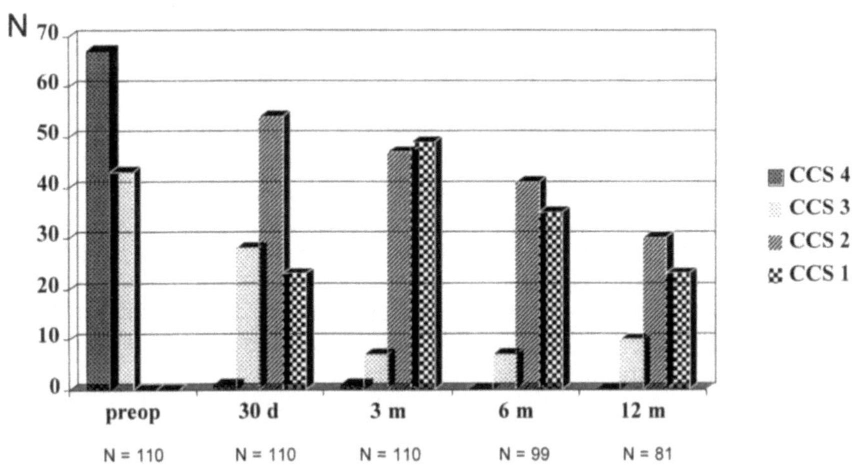

Fig. 18.2. CCS classification, preop and at follow-up

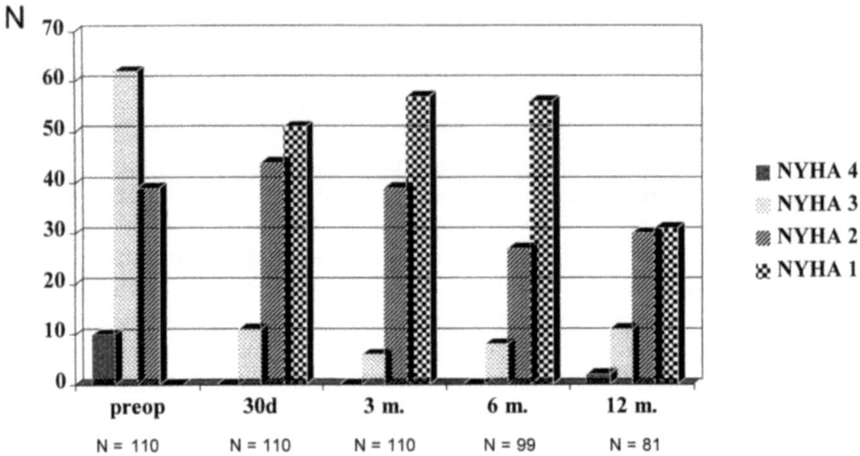

Fig. 18.3. NYHA classification, preop and at follow-up

Table 18.4. NYHA and CCS classifications

Time period: June 1995–February 1997	Total	TMLR+ CABG	TMLR	TMLR (Mini-thoracotomy)
NYHA				
preop MW (*n*)	2.7 (110)	2.7 (98)	3.0 (10)	3.5 (2)
30 days MW (*n*)	1.6 (106)	1.6 (94)	2.1 (10)	2.5 (2)
3 months MW (*n*)	1.5 (103)	1.5 (92)	1.8 (10)	2 (1)
6 months MW (*n*)	1.5 (91)	1.4 (81)	2.0 (10)	–
12 months MW (*n*)	1.8 (72)	1.7 (64)	2.6 (8)	–
CCS				
preop MW (*n*)	3.6 (110)	3.6 (98)	3.6 (10)	4 (2)
30 days MW (*n*)	2.1 (106)	2.2 (94)	1.6 (10)	1.5 (2)
3 months MW (*n*)	1.6 (103)	1.6 (92)	1.5 (10)	1 (1)
6 months MW (*n*)	1.7 (91)	1.7 (81)	1.7 (10)	–
12 months MW (*n*)	1.8 (72)	1.7 (64)	2.3 (8)	–

cant improvement (i.e. by one NYHA and CCS class on the average) was already seen. Further improvement was observed within the first 3 months.

The following checkups initially showed a stabilised endurance and an absence of complaints. Currently, the results of the reexamination carried out after 12 months show a statistically insignificant trend towards slightly deteriorated findings. This trend is observed mainly in the group of patients treated exclusively with TMLR.

The patients described the immediate postoperative decrease in their angina symptomatology as a considerable improvement in their quality of life. An increase in endurance was generally realised somewhat later.

The calculated mortality risk and the actual mortality of the three therapy groups are compared in Table 18.5. According to which "mortality score" is used, the patients are exclusively in either the "moderate-" or the "high-risk" group. When the actual and calculated mortality are compared, the differ-

Table 18.5. Mortality

Time period: June 1995–February 1997	Total	TMLR+ CABG	TMLR	TMLR (Mini-thoracotomy)
Mortality risk (calculated, %)	19.6	16.2	18.9	24.3
Mortality (actual, %)	3.1	4.1	0	0

Table 18.6. Risk stratification

Time period: June 1995–February 1997	Total	TMLR+ CABG	TMLR	TMLR (Mini-thoracotomy)
'Low-risk' patients %-MW (*n*)	2.1 (1)	2.1 (1)	(–)	(–)
'Moderate-risk' patients %-MW (*n*)	6.9 (28)	6.9 (26)	7.4 (2)	(–)
'High-risk' patients %-MW (*n*)	20.1 (81)	19.8 (71)	21.8 (8)	24.3 (2)

Table 18.7. Mortality according to risk group

Time period: June 1995–February 1997 Therapeutic group	Mortality 'Low-risk'	'Moderate-risk'	'High-risk'
Total % (*n*)	0 (0/1)	3.6 (1/28)	3.7 (3/81)
TMLR+CABG % (*n*)	0 (0/1)	3.8 (1/26)	4.2 (3/71)
TMLR % (*n*)	-	0 (0/2)	0 (0/8)
TMLR (Mini-thoracotomy) % (*n*)	-	-	0 (0/2)
Comparable group (CABG patients) % (*n*)	1.2 (2/172)	4.4 (15/341)	10.5 (23/219)

ence found in the "high-risk" group of those patients who underwent a combined intervention is particularly impressive (Tables 18.6 and 18.7). At 4.1%, the actual mortality was 12.1% lower than calculated. Given a preoperatively calculated mortality of 12.3%, the actual mortality amongst a statistically comparable group of patients who were only incompletely treated, without TMLR (due to an unfavourably diffuse coronary heart disease), amounted to 10.7%.

18.6 Discussion

Transmyocardial laser revascularisation is a relatively new indirect approach to myocardial revascularisation. Ideally, laser-drilled transmyocardial channels should provide the preconditions not only for connecting these channels to an intramyocardial network of developed collaterals, but also, particularly, for ensuring that these channels remain open, endothelialise and serve as a long-term vessel replacement in order to reduce the prevailing myocardial ischaemia. However, this method of revascularisation is not actually fully understood with regard to its principle of function [13]. In about two thirds of the cases, clinical follow-up examinations showed an identical improvement in patients' angina pectoris symptomatology and endurance [14–17]. However, there was no clear evidence of improved perfusion in the myocardial areas treated [18]. Experimental data concerning TMLR are very contradictory in part and have been gathered under differing experimental conditions. Whilst some research teams reported a positive effect after laser revascularisation in the acutely ischaemic model [19, 20], this result was not confirmed by other studies [21, 22]. The fact that sufficiently secured data evidencing improved perfusion after TMLR interventions are not currently available has given rise to general doubts concerning the procedure and particularly to varying hypotheses and speculations stimulating the discussion about this issue. The hypothesis of a placebo effect, however, is becoming less and less important against the background of scientifically substantiated findings.

The assumption that myocardial denervation would lead to reduced angina due to the small number of laser channels drilled is also apparently unjustified. The same applies to the hypothesis that TMLR could significantly reduce the amount of ischaemic myocardial tissue and thereby explain the absence of complaints. Improved lymphatic drainage via the laser channels might be conceivable but has not yet been established. This also pertains to the lack of clinical and experimental evidence for a proliferative influence via heat-shock proteins [23, 24], as well as to the hypothesis of laser-induced neoangiogenesis in the context of a reparative process initiated by proliferative granulation tissue. The histological evidence of multivessel granulation tissue (neoangiogenesis) developing with a delay of 3–4 weeks after damage to the myocardium via endocardial biopsy may have been given by Hoffmann et al. [25] and Burkhoff with application of the holmium-laser technique (D. Burkhoff 1997, personal communication), but a reduction in preoperatively documented angina symptomatology was demonstrated for 75% of all patients who had undergone TMLR. These findings can be generally explained by an increased perfusion of the myocardium concerned.

Braunwald [26] defines angina as a missensation in the chest or adjacent area caused by myocardial ischaemia and accompanied by myocardial dysfunction – however, without necrosis. The typical angina pain is directly correlated to an increase in myocardial oxygen requirement under conditions of fixed or limited oxygen provision. If the myocardial ischaemia can be reduced or even relieved, the angina symptoms are also diminished or completely eliminated.

Thus if a reduction in angina-related complaints can be explained only by improved perfusion, the question arises as to which morphological conditions have to prevail in the ischaemic myocardium for the drilling of laser channels to have the intended effect. Unambiguous experimental or clinical data are currently not available. However, proceeding on the assumption that an ischaemic but nevertheless almost functioning myocardium does not provide the ideal preconditions for successful TMLR, indirect revascularisation techniques such as TMLR are no alternative to PTCA and/or bypass surgery. Morphologically preconditions are, more favourable – given the current state of the art – with a hibernating myocardium. If the myocardium remains vital despite being chronically hypoperfused, severe morphological alterations may develop in the course of time. These structural myocardial alterations are expressive of a degenerative process which is, however, reversible up to a certain degree of severity [27]. "Hibernation" is the clinically defined condition of patients suffering from coronary heart diseases who have a chronic dysfunction which may improve following reperfusion [28]. A hibernating myocardium may be manifest both in patients suffering from instable angina and in those with a chronically stable coronary heart disease (CHD). Even under conditions of manifest heart failure the finding of extensive hibernating myocardial areas offers, on principle, the option of successful revascularisation [29–31]. At this stage, however, direct revascularisation techniques are not applicable for an increasing number of patients who present with severe alterations of the coronary arteries subsequent to several prior interventional and/or surgical revascularisation procedures. Indirect revascularisation techniques such as TMLR are often the only surgical therapy which can currently be offered to those patients. In our experience, an afferentia via a bypass must be excluded on rare occasions on the basis of intraoperative findings. These patients should preferably undergo complete revascularisation; i.e. whenever possible critical vessels are bypassed as well. Areas not suited to this option and preoperatively assessed as having a hibernating myocardium are treated by means of TMLR. To diagnose hibernating myocardial areas we prefer using nuclear medical examination techniques. By means of a myocardial scan with ^{99m}Tc-Myoview (or Tc-99-MIBI) carried out at rest and under load, as well as FDG-PET of the myocardium using F-18-FDG, quantitative and qualitative assignments of hibernating areas are possible. However, the evaluation of these findings rarely shows a homogeneous distribution of hibernating myocardium. Correlated to the intraoperatively observed coronary morphology, we generally found bypassable coronary vessels in those areas that were hardly or only slightly hypoperfused. According to previous experience, coronary angiography often allows only a restricted judgement – particularly with respect to these patients. Bearing this in mind, we consider only a few patients to be eligible for TMLR exclusively and consequently strive, whenever possible, for complete revascularisation by combining direct and indirect approaches. For this reason, only 12 of 110 patients underwent an TMLR exclusively, two of them without ECC. None of these patients died postoperatively, and none of them experienced severe postoperative complications. With respect to the angina-related complaints and the patients' endurance capacity, the findings were significantly improved.

The postoperative checkups concerning improved perfusion of the myocardium indicated a positive trend, which was not uniformly documented for all patients, however. The small number of these patients might have allowed for statistical evaluation, which we nevertheless considered to be insignificant.

The 98 patients who received both a coronary bypass and TMLR also showed an immediate postoperative reduction of the preoperatively assessed angina-related complaints. The patients' endurance capacity increased with a delay of approximately 3 months. With these patients, no significant difference from the results established for those patients who had undergone TMLR exclusively was found with respect to myocardial perfusion. Also, this group of patients only showed a trend towards an increased perfusion. Furthermore, it was impossible to differentiate between the effect of a bypass afferentia and the one created by TMLR. However, the fact that an objectively improved perfusion was not unambiguously demonstrated does not necessarily imply that this therapy is ineffective. False indications or insufficiently sensitive measurement techniques may likewise be the reason for this circumstance.

The low total rate of postoperative complications and the low postoperative mortality of 4.1% are, in our view, attributable mainly to improved cardiac function. As previous experience has shown, postoperative cardiac failure is the major cause of postoperative complications which lead either primarily or consecutively to the patient's death [32]. Patients who had statistically absolutely comparable risk profiles and had been evaluated in a prospectively randomised study carried out in our institution [12] showed a mortality of 10.5%. Except for one additional TMLR, these patients received the identical surgical treatment. In principle, we question the significance of retrospective analyses, but we consider these results to be indicative of the efficiency of TMLR as an additional measure applicable in the surgical therapy of severe diffuse coronary heart disease. Even though the physiological mechanism of this procedure is not yet completely understood, we regard the impressively good symptomatologic and endurance results seen in a group of formerly therapeutically refractive patients as being more than a good reason for applying this therapeutic concept to patients suffering from symptomatologically progressive coronary heart disease. In our experience, TMLR with an excimer laser can be offered to patients suffering from end stage coronary heart disease at a justifiable risk. The Excimer Laser system provides optimal flexibility and a high degree of safety during drilling of the TMLR laser channels. Laser-related complications or damage to intracardial structures have not been observed in any case.

Motivated by these initially unexpected positive data, we have prepared a prospective, randomised multicentre study which is intended to evaluate the value of additional excimer laser TMLR in patients who pose a high surgical risk due to their coronary heart disease and offer limited opportunities for direct revascularisation.

References

1. Hoffmann E, Gebhardt C, Kisseler B (1971) Morphologie der ventrikulo-coronaren Anastomosen bei Herzen mit intaktem und pathologisch verändertem Coronargefäßsystem. Langenbecks Arch Chir 328:180–200
2. Goldmann A (1956) Experimental methods for producing a collateral circulation to the heart directly from the left ventricle. Thorac Surg 31:364–374
3. Massimo C, Boffi L (1957) Myocardial revascularization by a new method of carrying blood directly from the left ventricular cavity into the coronary circulation. J Thorac Surg 34:257–258
4. Pifarre R, Jasuja ML, Lynch RD, Neville WE (1969) Myocardial revascularization by transmyocardial acupuncture. J Thorac Cardiovasc Surg 58:424–431
5. Sen PK (1968) Studies in myocardial revascularization. Indian J Med Res 57:415–433
6. Walter P, Hundeshagen HH, Borst HG (1971) Treatment of acute myocardial infarction by transmural blood supply from the ventricular cavity. Eur Surg Res 3:130–138

7. Vineberg A (1954) Clinical and experimental studies in the treatment of coronary artery insufficiency by internal mammary implant. J Int Coll Surg 22:503–518
8. Mirhoseini M, Cayton MM (1981) Revascularization of the heart by laser. J Microsurg 15:315–341
9. Mirhoseini M (1982) Transventricular revascularization by laser. Laser Surg Med 2:187–198
10. Mirhoseini M (1983) Myocardial revascularization by laser: a clinical report. Laser Surg Med 3:241–245
11. Mirhoseini M (1986) Laser myocardial revascularization. Laser Surg Med 6:459–461
12. Klein M, Dauben HP, Schulte HD, Gams E (1998) Centrifugal Pumping During Routine Open Heart Surgery Improves Clinical Outcome. Artif Organs (Accepted for publication)
13. Moosdorf R, Schoebel FC, Hort W (1997) Transmyocardial laser revascularization – morphology, pathophysiology and historical background of indirect myocardial revascularization. Z Kardiol 86:149–164
14. Nägele H, Kalmar P, Lübeck M, Marcsek P, Nienaber CA, Rödiger W, Stiel GM, Stubbe HM (1997) Transmyocardial laser revascularization – treatment option for coronary artery disease? Z Kardiol 86:171–178
15. Cooley DA, Frazier OH, Kadipasaoglu KA, Lindenmeir MH, Pehlivanoglu S, Kolff JW, Wilansky S, Moore WH (1996) Transmycardial laser revascularization: clinical experience with twelve-month follow-up. J Thorac Cardiovasc Surg 111:791–799
16. Horvarth KA, Mannting F, Cummings N, Shernan SK, Cohn LH (1996) Transmyocadial laser revascularization: operative technique and clinical results at two years. J Thorac Cardiovasc Surg 111:1047–1053
17. Klein M, Dauben HP, Schulte HD (1996) Transmyocardial laser revascularization in patients with end-stage coronary artery disease (abstract). Cardiovasc Surg 1:15
18. Frazier OH, Cooley DA, Kadipasaoglu KA, Pehlivanoglu S, Lindenmeir M, Barasch E, Conger JL, Wilansky S, Moore WH (1995) Myocardial revascularization with laser. Preliminary findings. Circulation [Suppl II]:II 58–65
19. Horvarth KA, Smith WJ, Laurence RG, Schoen FJ, Appleyard EF, Cohn LH (1995) Recovery and viability of an acute myocardial infarct after transmycardial laser. J Am Coll Cardiol 25:258–263
20. Yano OJ, Bielefeld MR, Jeevanandam V (1993) Prevention of acute regional ischemia with endocardial laser channels. Ann Thorc Surg 56:46–53
21. Whittaker P, Kloner RA, Przyklenk K (1993) Laser-mediated transmural myocardial channels do not salvage acutely ischemic myocardium. J Am Coll Cardiol 22:302–309
22. Hardy RI, James FW, Millard RW, Kaplan S (1990) Regional myocardial blood flow and cardiac mechanics in dog hearts with CO_2 laser induces intramyocardial revascularization. Basic Res Cardiol 85:179–197
23. Das DK, Engelmann RM, Kimura Y (1993) Molecular adaptation of cellular defences following preconditioning of the heart by repeated ischaemia. Cardiovasc Res 27:578–584
24. Morimoto R, Tissières A, Georgopoulous C (eds) (1994) The biology of heat shock proteins and mollecular chaperones. Cold Spring Harbor Laboratory Press, Cold Spring Harbor
25. Hoffmann E, Gebhardt C, Prückner J, Oppermann C, Purschke R (1971) Die Revaskularisation des Herzmuskels durch Myokardioterebration im Tierexperiment. Arch Kreislaufforsch 66:130–142
26. Braunwald E (ed) (1992) Heart disease: a textbook of cardiovascular medicine, vol 2, 4th edn. Saunders, Philadelphia, pp 1293–1294
27. Elsässer A, Schaper J (1995) Hibernating myocardium: adaption or degeneration? Basic Res Cardiol 90:47–48
28. Rahimtoola SH (1989) The hibernating myocardium. Am Heart J 117:211–221
29. Rahimtoola SH (1991) Clinical overview of management of chronic ischemic heart disease. Circulation 84 [Suppl I]:I 81–84
30. Erdmann E, Kirsch CM (1993) "Stunned" und "hibernating myocardium" – Diagnostik und klinische Implikationen. Z Kardiol 82 [Suppl 5]:143–147
31. Heusch G, Schulz R (1996) Hibernating myocardium: a review. J Mol Cell Cardiol 28:2359–2372
32. Deng MC, Dasch B, Erren M, Möllhoff T, Scheld HH (1996) Impact of left ventricular dysfunction on cytokines, hemodynamics, and outcome in bypass grafting Ann Thorac Surg 62:184–190

Transmyocardial Laser Revascularisation with a Holmium:YAG Laser: Initial Clinical Experience

R. Seitelberger · Th. Wild · J. Wolfram

19.1 Introduction

Transmyocardial laser revascularisation (TMR) is a novel therapeutic approach to ischaemic heart disease. It was originally based on investigations carried out in the 1950s and 1960s aimed at simulating the reptilian concept of sinusoidal myocardial perfusion by needle acupuncture [1–3]. With TMR, finely focused lasers perforate areas of ischaemic myocardium, creating transmyocardial channels [4, 5]. Experimental data suggest that within months, these transmyocardial channels may stimulate new vessel growth in the previously ischaemic region [6, 7]. Encouraging clinical effects have been seen in various multicenter studies: relief from angina, increased myocardial perfusion, and reduced frequency of costly hospitalisation for recurrent angina [8–10].

Currently, three different types of lasers are used clinically for TMR: the 800-watt CO_2 laser, the Excimer laser and, most recently, the 6-watt holmium:YAG laser. Most of the more than 4000 TMR procedures performed worldwide have been done with the CO_2 laser. However, its huge size and the stiff handling of the laser probes will probably lead to its replacement by the newly developed excimer and holmium:YAG TMR systems in the near future. In addition, the holmium:YAG laser even provides the option of drilling laser channels from the endocardial surface part way through the myocardium following percutaneous insertion of highly flexible probes and fibre optics. As part of a worldwide multicentre feasibility study, we have performed TMR with a holmium:YAG laser in 16 patients; this included the first TMR procedure ever to be done with a holmium:YAG laser in late 1995.

19.2 Patient Selection, Methods

Patients classified as having class III or class IV angina according to the Canadian Cardiovascular Angina Score (CCS) were selected for enrollment into the study if PTCA or CABG procedures were considered unfeasible. In addition, patients were required to have either a positive exercise or dipyridamole stress test or respective ECG changes during episodes of angina. Patients with an ejection fraction of <35% or severe chronic obstructive pulmonary disease were excluded from the study.

All procedures were performed with a holmium:YAG laser (CardioGenesis Corporation, USA). In ten patients, TMR was performed via an anterolateral minithoracotomy in the 4th or 5th intercostal space without cardiopulmonary bypass; in six patients it was performed as an adjunct to routine coronary artery bypass grafting via a median sternotomy immediately preceding cessation of cardiopulmonary bypass. In the first four patients with only TMR on the beating heart, an intra-aortic baloon pump was administered preoperatively and removed on the first postoperative day in all cases. The preoperative antianginal drug regimen was continued for at least 3 months postoperatively in all patients.

Patient follow-up included clinical evaluation, exercise stress test and transthoracic echocardiography at discharge and at 3, 6 and 9 months postoperatively. Follow-up data on thallium-persantin and technetium scans at 6 and 12 months postoperatively have not yet been completely analysed. Transthoracic echocardiography images were recorded on videotape. The assessment of ejection fraction was done offline in a split-screen format using sine loops.

19.3 Results

Patients' demographic characteristics, surgical data and perioperative complications are summarised in Table 19.1. Ten patients had had at least one previous coronary bypass operation and only two patients had had no previous revascularisation procedures. One patient died at 2 weeks postoperatively due to multiorgan failure following postoperative myocardial infarction. A second patient committed suicide 4 months postoperatively after receiving diagnostic proof of rectal cancer. Other perioperative complications included pneumonia in two cases and conservatively treated wound infection in one case.

Table 19.1. Pre- and postoperative data on 16 patients who underwent TMR

Preoperative data	
Sex (male/female)	11/5
Age (years)	67.5 (38–74)
Previous CABG (%)	10 (63)
Previous PTCA (%)	6 (37)
CCS class III (%)	12 (75)
CCS class IV (%)	4 (25)
Previous MI (%)	7 (44)
Surgical data	
TMR only (%)	10 (63)
TMR+CABG (%)	6 (37)
No. of channels (range)	19 (10–35)
Intra-aortic balloon pump (%)	4 (25)
Complications	
30-day mortality (%)	1 (6)
Postoperative MI (%)	1 (6)
Wound infection (%)	1 (6)
Pneumonia (%)	2 (13)

CCS, Canadian Cardiovascular angina score; *MI*, myocardial infarction

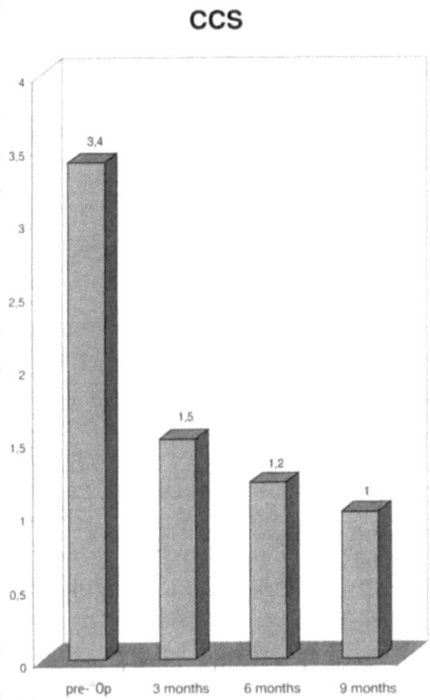

19.1

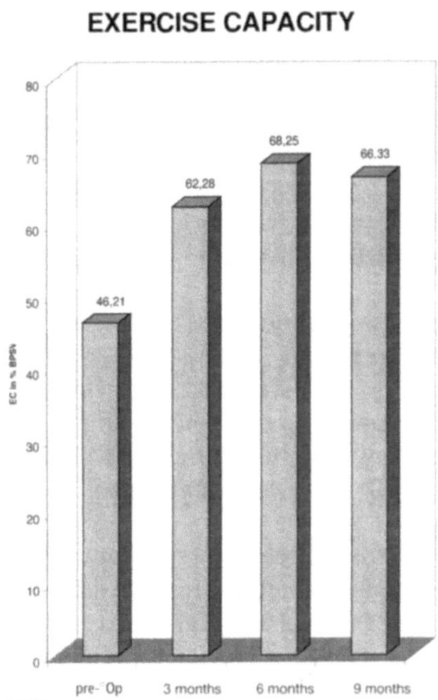

19.2

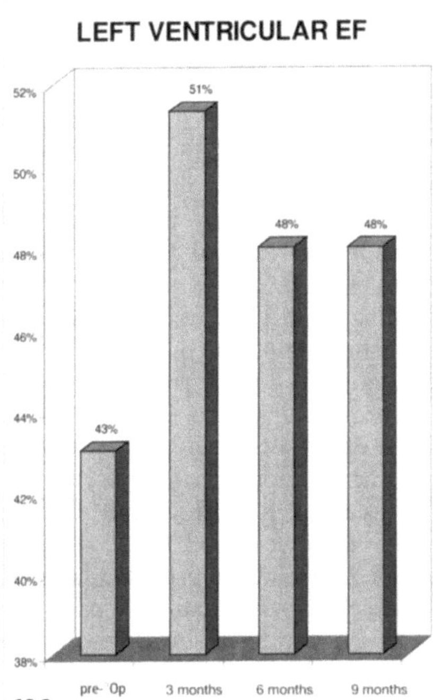

19.3

Fig. 19.1. Changes in angina score for all patients throughout the follow-up period. Data are given as absolute values. *CCS*, Canadian Cardiovascular Angina Score

Fig. 19.2. Changes in exercise capacity (*EC*) for all patients throughout the follow-up period. Data are given as percent EC from Bruce protocol standard values (*BPSV*)

Fig. 19.3. Changes in percent left ventricular ejection fraction (*EF*) for all patients throughout the follow-up period

Postoperative follow-up data are presented in Figs. 19.1–19.3. Data are shown for all 16 patients, since comparison of results between TMR only and combined procedures did not demonstrate any relevant differences. In addition to a significant improvement in angina class (Fig. 19.1), patients demonstrated markedly improved exercise capacity (Fig. 19.2) and, in contrast to all previous publications, an increase in postoperative ejection fraction (Fig. 19.3) during follow-up.

19.4 Conclusion

In spite of continuous advances and considerable efforts aimed at prevention and treatment, coronary artery disease is not only the leading cause of death in most industrialised countries but also a leading cause of severe disability. Conventional treatment regimens for coronary artery disease such as medical therapy, coronary angioplasty (PTCA) or coronary artery bypass grafting (CABG) are well established and effective options for controlling anginal pain.

Unfortunately, however, both PTCA and CABG are indicated only for the treatment of more proximal lesions and may provide incomplete anginal relief if there is surgically inaccessible distal or small vessel disease. In many cases, multiple previous PTCA or CABG procedures prevent further reintervention for various technical reasons. In general, conventional coronary artery disease therapy has little to offer for angina patients with failed or incomplete revascularisation or symptomatic diffuse distal disease.

Transmyocardial laser revascularisation (TMR) represents a novel and promising treatment approach for these patients. Clinical studies completed thus far suggest that TMR may be of immediate use in those patients with severe angina who currently have no treatment options, providing anginal pain relief and improved quality of life.

The most compelling data on the efficacy of TMR comes from a study at eight centres which included 200 patients with severe angina who were not candidates for other procedures [10]. Prior to TMR, these patients had a mean angina class of 3.8. At 3, 6 and 12 months following the procedure, the mean angina class had dropped to 1.5 or lower. In addition, in the 12 months prior to receiving TMR, these patients averaged 2.5 hospital admissions for angina as compared with only 0.3 admissions for angina during the 12 months following the procedure.

The results of our initial experience with a new holmium:YAG laser for TMR clearly demonstrate that this new device is safe and easy to handle and appears to provide effective relief of angina throughout the first postoperative year. Perioperative mortality and morbidity are in line with those in other TMR series. Exercise capacity is substantially increased, translating into significantly improved quality of life for almost all patients.

The relatively small but consistent increase in postoperative ejection fraction in our study is in contrast to all previous experience with TMR. In this respect, we speculate about whether the larger size of the channel core and the area of tissue thermally damaged by the holmium:YAG laser as compared with the CO_2 or excimer laser also amounts to a faster and/or more pronounced stimulation of angiogenetic activity in the underperfused myocardium [11, 12]. However, due to the small number of patients in our series, this initial observation has yet to be substantiated.

In conclusion, our initial experience demonstrates that TMR can be effectively performed with laser systems other than the CO_2 laser. Clinical and functional follow-up in ongoing multicentre trials will enable us to answer more detailed questions about patient selection and long-term clinical outcome.

References

1. Lary BG (1963) Effect of endocardial incisions on myocardial blood flow. Arch Surg: 87:424–427
2. Sen PK, Daulatram J, Kinare SG, Udwadia TE, Parulkar GB (1968) Further studies in multiple transmyocardial acupuncture as a method of myocardial revascularization. Surgery 64:861–870
3. Vineberg AM, Munro DD, Cohen H, Buller W (1955) Four years' clinical experience with internal mammary artery implantation in the treatment of human coronary artery insufficiency including additional experimental studies. J Thorac Surg 29:1–32
4. Mirhoseini M, Fisher JC, Cayton MM (1983) Myocardial revascularization by laser. Laser Surg Med 3:241–245
5. Mirhoseini M, Shelgikar S, Cayton MM (1988) New concepts in revascularization of the myocardium. Ann Thorac Surg 45:415–420
6. Whittaker P, Rakusan K, Kloner RA (1996) Transmural channels can protect ischemic tissue. Assessment of long-term myocardial response to laser- and needle-made channels. Circulation 93:143–152
7. Kohmoto T, Fisher PE, DeRosa C, Smith CR, Burkhoff D (1996) Evidence of angiogenesis in regions treated with transmyocardial laser revascularisation. Circulation 94 [Suppl 1]:294
8. Cooley DA, Frazier OH, Kadipasaoglu KA, et al (1996) Transmyocardial laser revascularization: clinical experience with twelve-month follow-up. J Thorac Cardiovasc Surg 111:791–799
9. Frazier OH, Cooley DA, Kadipasaoglu KA, Pehlivanoglu S, Barasch E, Conger JL, Lindenmeir MH, Gould KL, Wilansky S, Moore WH (1995) Myocardial revascularization with laser: preliminary findings. Circulation 92:1158–1165
10. Horvath KA, Mannting F, Cummings N, Shernan SK, Cohn LH (1996) Transmyocardial laser revascularization: operative techniques and clinical results at two years. J Thorac Cardiovasc Surg 111:1047–1053
11. Burkhoff D, Fisher PE, Apfelbaum M, Kohmoto T, DeRosa CM, Smith CR (1996) Histologic appearance of transmyocardial laser channels after 4 weeks. Ann Thorac Surg 61:1532–1535
12. Fisher PE, Kohmoto T, DeRosa CM, Spotnitz HM, Smith CR, Burkhoff D (1997) Histologic analysis of transmyocardial channels: comparison of CO_2 and holmium: YAG lasers. Ann Thorac Surg 64:466–472

PART V

Imaging Techniques

CHAPTER 20

Assessment of Myocardial Perfusion and Metabolism: Promises and Limitations

H. R. VOSBERG

20.1 Introduction

Coronary artery disease is characterised by progressive sclerosis of the coronary arteries accompanied by loss of myocardial motility and function. In this process increasing coronary artery stenosis leads to a progressive reduction in regional perfusion and thus to regional substrate and oxygen deficiencies. In coronary artery stenosis of up to 70% the perfusion is still sufficient for a normal myocardial performance at rest. However, during exercise the necessary enhancement of perfusion can not always be maintained, leading to a substrate and oxygen deficiency and to clinical presentation of stress induced angina. Severe repeated or longer lasting ischaemia may induce serious metabolic disturbances that lead to deficiency of energy production and consequently to a loss of myocardial motility. This situation is called "stunned myocardium" and can last for hours to weeks despite of sufficient reperfusion.

In stenosis of more than 80% perfusion is already impaired at rest leading to a loss of myocardial motility and function. At this stage of the disease regional hypo- and akinesia occur already at rest despite of maintained myocardial viability. The energy production of these cells is just sufficient to survive but not to achieve contraction work. This condition is referred to as "hibernating myocardium" [4].

An even more severe reduction of perfusion leads to progredient or sudden death of myocardial cells with the development of smaller or greater myocardial scars.

Surgical revascularisation or PTCA is necessary in patients with perfusion deficiencies at stress. In patients with myocardial hypo- or akinesia, viability of the myocardium in hypoperfused areas has to be confirmed preoperatively to avoid ineffective therapy [15].

For preoperative assessment of regional myocardial perfusion, metabolism, and function several well established methods are available.

20.2 Available Methods of Investigation

The investigation of *myocardial perfusion* is based on two quite different approaches:

1. **Coronary arteriography** demonstrates the anatomy of the coronary arteries down to a diameter of about 1 mm, but yields no information on the perfusion at the cellular level. Coronary angiography is essential for

Table 20.1. Radioactive tracers

Radioactive tracers for investigation of myocardial perfusion
^{15}O-water
^{13}N-Ammonia
^{201}Tl-Thallium
^{82}Rb-Rubidium
^{99m}Tc-Sestamibi
^{99m}Tc-Tetrafosmin

planing of bypass surgery and PTCA, however the extent of coronary artery stenosis and its impact on regional perfusion is difficult to estimate [10].

2. **Myocardial scintigraphy** supplies information on myocardial perfusion at the cellular level. There are different techniques of investigation and several radioactive tracers as **perfusion markers** available (Tab. 20.1). All of these are accumulated in the myocardium after i.v. injection, but the intracellular uptake is based on different cellular mechanisms. The resulting regional activity distribution reflects mainly regional myocardial perfusion, but as intracellular accumulation is to some extent energy dependent in most of the used substances, the information on perfusion may be blurred in hypoxic tissues [15].

Only **15-O-water** is diffusing purely passively into the cells, thus regional distribution depends exclusively on regional perfusion. It is an ideal perfusion marker as the diffusion into the cells is rapid and thus independent of blood flow velocity [11].

13-N-Ammonia too diffuses passively into the cells, but it is fixed there by entering into the glutamate metabolism. Thus the accumulation is not only depending on perfusion but also on cell viability and metabolism [17].

The perfusion markers **201-Thallium**, and **82-Rubidium** are potassium analoga and are actively transported from plasma into the cells by the Na^+/K^+-pump. Therefore regional tracer distribution is not only influenced by perfusion but also by an energy depending uptake mechanism [10, 15].

The process of intracellular accumulation of **99^m-Tc-Sestamibi** and **99^{m}Tc-Tetrofosmin** is not yet completely understood, but an intact transmembrane potential seems to be essential. Cell ischaemia with failure of the Na^+/K^+-pump leads to a loss of intracellular potassium and by this to a disturbance of the transmembrane potential. Thus the accumulation of the 99m-Tc-tracers too depends to some extent on the energy demanding Na^+/K^+-pump. Therefore the uptake reduction of both, the anions (201 Tl^+ and 82 Rb^+) and the technetium complexes in hibernating myocardium is more severe than would be expected from the perfusion deficit alone [6, 16, 19].

Using these tracers one has to take into account the different biological and physical properties of these substances, leading to different technical requirements and investigation protocols.

As 15-O and 13-N are cyclotron produced positron emitting radioactive isotopes with very short half lives of 2 and 10 minutes respectively, they can only be used at PET (positron emission tomography) centres with a cyclotron. They can serve as "gold standard" in scientific investigations, but are hardly available for use in routine diagnostic.

82-Rb is a positron emitting isotope, and requires registration with a PET-scanner too. However, no cyclotron is needed because the 82-Rb with a very short half life of 1.3 min is produced in a radioactive generator by desintegration of 82-Strontium. The "mother nuclide" 82-Sr in the generator has a half life of 25.5 days and thus can be delivered to every PET-scanner. The short half life of the "daughter nuclide" 82-Rb allows for repeated investigations of the same patient at short time intervals. Admittedly, physical stress testing by tread mill exercise is difficult inside a PET scanner, as the registration has to be started at the moment of the injection, i.e. during continued stress when the patient actually has to rest on the scanner table. The main draw back for this approach, however, is the price of the generator.

201-Thallium is not fixed intracellularly, but rather diffuses back into the circulation. This myocardial "wash out" is again depending on perfusion, e.g. a high perfusion leads to a high 201-Tl accumulation initially, but to a fast wash out later on, while low perfusion results in a low accumulation and a slow wash out. This behaviour can be utilised for a special investigation protocol: when 201-Tl is injected at maximal stimulated coronary perfusion (work load at a tread mill or pharmacological coronary dilatation – referred to as "physical/pharmacological *stress*") a scintigraphy registered within the first 15 minutes represents the regional distribution of maximal perfusion, while a second scintigraphy after 3–5 hours rest shows a redistribution of the 201-Tl corresponding to perfusion at rest.

In this technique myocardium supplied by an artery with a haemodynamically significant stenosis shows a relative perfusion deficit at "stress" registration. In the "rest" registration this area seems to be "filled in", due to faster "wash out "in the higher perfused areas. In areas with sufficient perfusion at rest and a good cell performance an additional "new fill in" can be observed [10].

As 99m-Tc-Sestamibi and -tetrofosmin are substantially fixed intracellularly, probably in the mitochondria, registration can be delayed to one or two hours after injection of the tracer, when the activity has cleared already from lungs and liver. However, there is also a disadvantage: as there is no "redistribution" of these tracers, stress and rest conditions have to be examined separately. One- or two-days-protocols have been suggested with these substances [10, 12].

Because of limited spatial resolution of the scintigraphic techniques, reduced regional tracer accumulation can be related to both, a reduced perfusion in a myocardial wall of normal thickness or to a normal perfusion in a region of thinned myocardium, e.g. a non transmural scar. As the first mentioned situation needs coronary intervention while the second one is an irreversible and stable state a further differentiation of this finding is necessary. For this purpose investigation of the *myocardial metabolism* is needed.

Several radioactive tracers have been developed to investigate free fatty acid and carbohydrate metabolism, and oxygen consumption [Tab. 20.2].

The metabolism of **free fatty acids** (FFA) is one of the main energy producing processes of myocardial cells, especially in the fasting state. Thus, in-

Table 20.2. Radioactive tracers

Radioactive tracers for investigation of myocardial metabolism		
Fatty acids	Glucose	Oxygen
^{11}C-Palmitate	^{18}F-Fluorodeoxyglucose (FDG)	^{15}O-Oxygen
^{11}C-methylated fatty acids		^{11}C-Acetate
^{123}J-decanoic acid		
^{123}J-oPPA and -pPPA		

vestigation of FFA metabolism is of major interest. 11-C-palmitate was the first radioactive fatty acid to be used as a marker of myocardial FFA metabolism. The regional accumulation of the 11-C-palmitate is strongly related to regional perfusion, as the extraction fraction is high. The 11-C-activity disappears from the myocardium in a biphasic mode. The first high disappearance rate is probably related to beta-oxidation, while the second lower rate constant may reflect the triglyceride or lipoprotein metabolism.

Unfortunately, quantitative data on regional energy production due to FFA metabolism can not be derived from this investigation as there are more FFA than only palmitate metabolised simultaneously. Furthermore the FFA utilisation is different at all in the fasted and the fed state and in areas with sufficient and deficient oxygen supply [9, 14, 18].

Other tracers for FFA metabolism like 11-C-methylated fatty acids or 123-J-iodinated decanoic acids share very similar draw backs, as they follow the same biochemical regulations. Until now the information supplied by these tracers does not seem to differ from that derived with perfusion markers, as the first step regulating regional distribution is regional perfusion. Thus, routine investigation of FFA metabolism in the heart muscle is still an aim, not a reality [7, 13, 15].

18-F-Fluorodeoxyglucose (FDG) is a glucose analogon that is used as a metabolic marker for carbohydrate metabolism and myocardial viability. It is transported from the blood into the cell by the same transporter as glucose and is phosphorylated intracellularly by the same enzyme system as glucose, the hexokinase. However, as it is a deoxyglucose, it is not further metabolised, but is rather trapped intracellularly, where it accumulates. By continuously measuring 18-F-FDG uptake in the myocardium, the 18-F-FDG concentration in the blood, and the actual blood glucose level it is possible to derive quantitative information on the regional glucose metabolism in terms of mmol glucose per gram tissue per minute.

This quantitative approach, how promising it may be, is questionable in scientific investigations because of two major problems: 1. The cellular handling of FDG and glucose is not quite identical. Especially the membrane transporter "glut-4" and the hexokinase obviously have different affinities for FDG and glucose. Only recently investigations have shown evidence of an about 2-fold preference of the glut-4 transporter for FDG over glucose, while the hexokinase system showed an opposite preference for glucose over FDG. These and some more not yet exactly defined differences between glucose and FDG are compensated for by the so called "lumped constant", which is mostly set to 0.67 to convert FDG metabolism data to estimates of glucose consumption. An identical value for the lumped constant is mostly used for all metabolic states of the myocardium, even though this has never been validated for the heart. In fact, recent investigations have shown, that this may be wrong for the fasting state with preferential FFA metabolism, for hyperinsulinaemia with preferential glucose metabolism, and especially not for hypoxia. In these clinically common metabolic states, variations of the lumped constant between 0.4 and 1.3 have been estimated. The second problem is, that at different metabolic states like fasting, after glucose load, or during euglycaemic hyperinsulinaemic clamp the regional glucose metabolism changes differently in normoxic and hypoxic regions respectively. A hypoxic region with a preferably anoxic glycolysis will show an isolated FDG uptake in the fasted state, as the normoxic myocardium is utilising FFA at the same time. After glucose load or in hyperinsulinaemic clamp all of the myocardium will metabolise glucose, leading to a homogeneous FDG uptake in the heart. Thus, FDG investigations have to be done under standardised, controlled metabolic conditions. Without knowledge of the actual regional lumped constant, the calculation of quantitative turnover rates for glucose from FDG data can be very erroneous. Using FDG uptake values without calculation of glucose consumption per time has shown to be a very valuable and reliable approach to investigate myocardial metabolism. It is the "gold standard" to assess myocardial viability in clinical settings [2, 3, 9, 14].

Measuring **oxygen consumption** using 15-O_2 inhalation would be optimal to identify regional hypoxia. Unfortunately, it is not a routine method as it requires a PET centre with a cyclotron running on-line (half life of 15-O: 2 min!). Furthermore, the investigation is complicated by count spillover from the high oxygen activity in lungs and cardiac ventricles into the myocardial region, obscuring the information of interest.

A more satisfying approach to investigate oxygen supply is the calculation of regional oxygen consumption from measurements of **11-C-acetate** turnover. 11-C-acetate is metabolised in the last step of the Krebs cycle and its turnover is thus strongly correlated to oxygen consumption. The application of this method for clinical investigations again is limited, because of the short half life of 11-C of 20 min, and the requirement for a PET centre with a cyclotron [5, 8].

The activity registration should be done with SPET (single photon emission tomography) or PET (positron emission tomography) technique respectively, depending on the mode of radioactive desintegration: with or without emission of positrons. The advantage of the PET-technique over the SPET-registration is a better spatial resolution and the possibility of correction for gamma quants absorbed in the body, resulting in terms of: activity per volume of tissue (Bq/ml). Using appropriate mathematical models it is even possible to calculate quantitative values for perfusion in ml/g tissue/min. Unfortunately, PET centres with cyclotrons are still rare.

State of the art is the reprojection of the measured data into a 3-D-model of the activity distribution in the body. From this data set three perpendicular slice orientations are commonly reconstructed: 1. perpendicularly to the long heart axis (so called "short axis" slices) and 2. vertically and horizontally parallel to the long axis ("long axis vertically/horizontally"). Using the heart axis for orientation of the slices helps to overcome anatomical variability of the position of the heart. On these slices all regions of the myocardium can be identified. Areas with reduced or abolished perfusion/metabolism show reduced or missing radioactivity (Fig. 20.1).

For the investigation of regional *myocardial motility and function* different techniques are applied:

1. X ray cardiocinematography of the myocardial cavum in two perpendicular planes is usually performed in combination with coronary angiography. Unfortunately, as usual in planar radiography only the contour building parts of the myocardium can be assessed. Furthermore, investigation under work load stress is not possible. Thus this method yields mostly incomplete information about myocardial function only at rest.
2. Cardiac ultrasound (CUS) is widely used to demonstrate regional wall motion disturbances. In contrast to x-ray cardiocinematography this method allows to depict the heart dynamically in arbitrary planes and thus en-

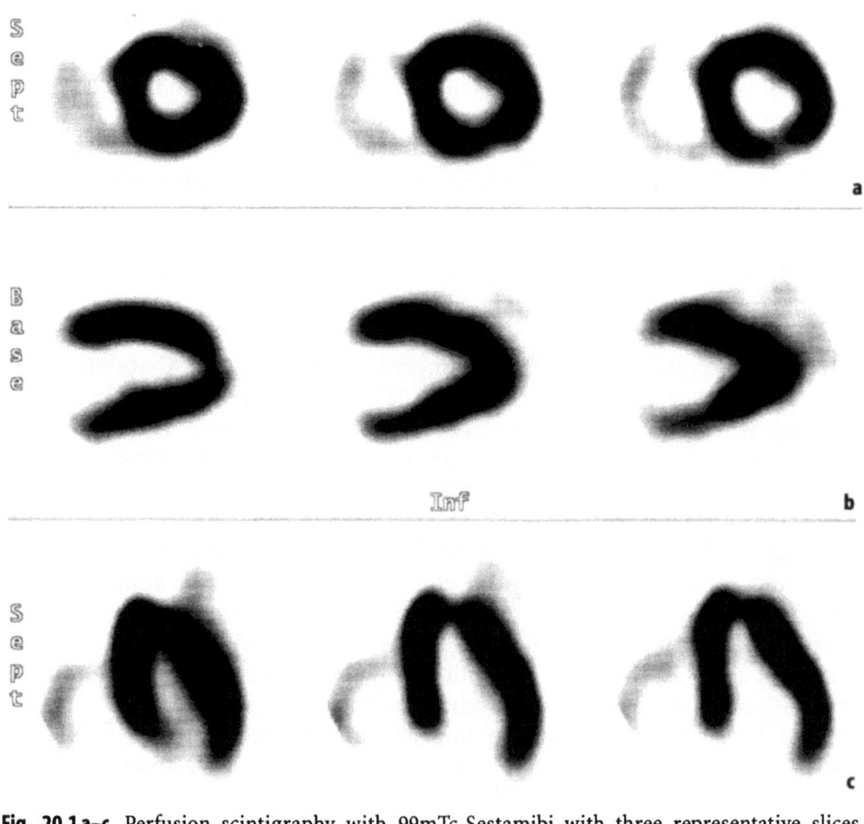

Fig. 20.1 a–c. Perfusion scintigraphy with 99mTc-Sestamibi with three representative slices (thickness: 8mm) of the three perpendicular planes:
a short axis slices; **b** vertical long axis slices; **c** horizontal long axis slices.
Using high attenuation the thin right ventricular wall can faintly be seen. Usually, only the strong, thick left ventricular myocardium is depicted.

ables to assess regional wall motion as well as valvular function. Finally this method allows also to measure changes of cardiac emptying and wall motion during physical and pharmacological stress. But omitting standardisation of documentation can impede the fusion of information on regional wall motion assessed with CUS and regional perfusion/metabolism measured with PET or SPECT.

3. ECG gated blood pool (GBP) scintigraphy allows for registration of the inner ventricle contour as the border of an intracardiac radioactive blood pool. Registration can be done in several projections and under different stress modalities. GBP scintigraphy allows to quantify enddiastolic emptying regionally as well as for the ventricle as a whole. Regional and global information on the performance of the mechanical heart cycle can be drawn and documented.
4. ECG-gated SPECT or PET registrations of the myocardium depicted with a perfusion or metabolism marker are at the stage of validation. With these techniques it is possible to show a beating myocardium as a computer animation with the regional perfusion/metabolism colour coded. By this the correlation of regional perfusion/metabolism and regional wall motion is perfect at a glance. Quantification of the wall motion as regional amplitudes or regional ejection fractions is also possible.
5. MRI and CT investigations especially of myocardial wall thickening are on the way but still have to be validated.

20.3 Recommended Investigations

For planning a surgical revascularisation, with or without TMLR (trans myocardial laser revascularisation), preoperative diagnostic has to supply sufficient information on the coronary status, regional myocardial perfusion and metabolism, and regional wall motion. Areas at risk of perfusion deficiency, even if only occurring at stress, have to be identified. In areas which are already hypo-, dis-, or akinetic one has to distinguish between myocardium with reduced perfusion but persistent myocardial viability, and areas that are already completed scars [1, 8, 20].

To cover this for routine diagnostic the combination of coronary angiography with an investigation of regional perfusion (using 201-Tl or a 99m-Tc-Tracer and SPET), and regional metabolism (using F-18-FDG) is mostly used [1]. To get meaningful FDG data, the metabolic state during the investigation has to be controlled and stable. The following patterns of regional perfusion, metabolism and function can be found:

1. Normal regional perfusion, glucose metabolism, and function: Normally supplied myocardium.
2. Normal regional perfusion and glucose metabolism but hypo- or akinesia: So called "stunned myocardium". This occurs after severe longer lasting ischaemia (e.g. an infarction with early reperfusion) and recovers to normal function within days to several weeks.
3. Identical ("matching") reduction (but not complete loss) of perfusion, glucose metabolism and function: Non transmural scar.

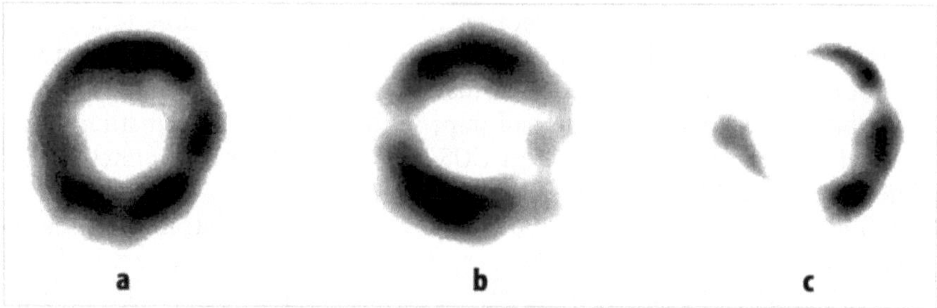

Fig. 20.2. a Short axis slice of a FDG study showing homogeneous FDG uptake in all wall regions.
b slice of the same heart and same position but from a 99mTc-Sestamibi study with a severe perfusion deficit in the lateral wall reaching from anterolateral to dorsolateral. Small perfusion deficit in the septal wall.
c Demonstration of areas with significant perfusion/metabolism discrepancies: mismatch areas, "hibernating myocardium".

4. Reduced or nearly abolished perfusion and function but normal or even elevated glucose metabolism (a so called perfusion-metabolism "mismatch"): "Hibernating myocardium" with partly anaerobic glycolysis. This constellation requires urgently revascularisation to salvage myocardial function (Fig. 20.2).
5. Totally omitting regional perfusion and metabolism: myocardial necrosis or scar. Revascularisation will not lead to recovery.

TMLR is an approach to improve regional myocardial blood supply independent from the coronary artery system. To demonstrate effects of this intervention on myocardial perfusion or metabolism, only the described scintigraphic investigations, that give information at the cellular level, may be the appropriate means. The combination of perfusion and metabolism investigations before and after TMLR should be adequate to show improvement of regional perfusion and/or metabolism due to treatment.

Investigations with radioactive isotopes lead to exposure to ionising radiation of the subject examined. The burden of this is relatively small compared to coronary arteriography and x-ray cinematography. The single investigation leads to a dose of about 10–20 mSv, which causes only a neglectable stochastic risk compared to the high and live threatening risk involved with coronary heart disease.

References

1. Altehoefer C, Kaiser HJ, Doerr R, Feinendegen C, Beilin I, Uebis R, Buell U (1992) Fluorine-18 deoxyglucose PET for assessment of viable myocardium in perfusion defects in Tc-99m MIBI SPET: a comparative study in patients with coronary artery disease. Eur J Nucl Med 19:334–342
2. Bax JJ, Veening MA, Visser FC, van Lingen A, Heine RJ, Cornel JH, Visser CA (1997) Optimal metabolic conditions during fluorine-18 fluorodeoxyglucose imaging; a comparative study using different protocols. Eur J Nucl Med 24:35–41
3. Botker HE, Böttcher M, Schmitz O, Gee A, Hansen SB, Cold GE, Nielsen TT, Gjedde A (1997) Glucose uptake and lumped constant variability in normal human hearts determined with (18F)fluorodeoxyglucose. J Nucl Cardiol 4:125–132

4. Braunwald E, Rutherford EJD (1986) Reversible ischaemic left ventricular dysfunction: evidence for the hibernating myocardium. J Am Coll Cardiol 8:1467–1470
5. Buxton DB, Nienaber CA, Luxen A, Ratib O, Hansen H, Phelbs ME, Schelbert HR (1988) Non-invasive quantitation of regional myocardial oxygen consumption in vivo with (1-C-11) acetate and dynamic positron emission tomography. Circulation 79:134–142
6. Carvalho PA, Chiu MI, Kronauge JF, Kawamura M, Jones AG, Holman BL, Piwnica-Worms D (1992) Subcellular distribution and analysis of technetium-99m-MIBI in isolated perfused rat hearts. J Nucl Med 33:1516–1521
7. Freundlieb CH, Höck A, Vyska K, Feinendegen LE, Machulla HJ, Stöcklin G (1980) Myocardial imaging and metabolic studies with 17-(123-J)iodoheptadecanoic acid. J Nucl Med 21:1043–1050
8. Gropler R, Geltmann E, Kondapuram S (1992) Functional recovery after coronary revascularisation for chronic vascular disease is dependent on maintenance of oxidative metabolism. J Am Coll Cardiol 20:569–577
9. Hariharan R, Bray M, Ganim R, Doenst T, Goodwin GW, Taegtmeyer H (1995) Fundamental limitations of (18F)2-deoxy-fluoro-D-glucose for assessing myocardial glucose uptake. Circulation 91:2435–2444
10. Hör G, Baum RP, Maul FD (1992) Myocardial perfusion. In: Pabst HW, Adam WE, Ell P, Hör G, Kriegel H (ed) Handbook of Nuclear Medicine, Vol 2, Fischer, Stuttgart
11. Iida H, Kanno I, Takahashi A. et al. (1988) Measurement of absolute myocardial blood flow with H_2-15-O and dynamic positron emission tomography. Strategy for quantification in relation to the partial-volume effect. Circulation 78:104–115
12. Iskandrian AS, Verani MS, Heo J (1994) Pharmacological stress testing: mechanism of action, haemodynaemic response, and results in detection of coronary artery disease. J Nucl Cardiol 1:94–111
13. Kaiser KP, Geuting B, Grossmann K, Vester E, Lösse B, Antar MA, Macchulla HJ, Feinendegen LE (1990) Tracer kinetics of 15-(ortho123,131-J-phenyl)pentadecanoic acid (oPPA) and 15-(para123,131-J-phenyl)pentadecanoic acid (pPPA) in animals and man. J Nucl Med 31:1608–1616
14. Kalff V, Schwaiger M, Nguyen N, McClanahan TB, Gallagher K (1992) The relationship between myocardial blood flow and glucose uptake in ischaemic canine myocardium determined with F-18 deoxyglucose. J Nucl Med 33:1346–1353
15. Opie LH, Hesse B (1997) Radionuclide tracers in the evaluation of resting myocardial ischaemia and viability. Eur J Nucl Med 24:1183–1193
16. Piwnica-Worms D, Kronauge JF, Chiu ML (1990) Uptake and retention of hexakis(2-methoxyisobutylisonitrile)technetium (I) in cultured chick myocardial cells: mitochondrial and plasma membrane potential dependence. Circulation 82:1826–1838
17. Schelbert HR, Phelps ME, Huang SC, MacDonald NS, Hansen H, Selin C, Kuhl DE (1981) N-13-ammonia as an indicator of myocardial blood flow. Circulation 63:1259–1272
18. Schön H, Schelbert HR, Najafi A et al. (1982) C-11 labelled palmitic acid for the noninvasive evaluation of regional myocardial fatty acid metabolism with positron emission tomography. II. Kinetics of C-11 palmitic acid in acutely ischaemic myocardium. Am Heart J 1103:548–561
19. Sinusas AJ, Shi QX, Saltzberg MT, Vitols P, Jain D, Wackers FJT, Zaret BL (1994) Technetium-99m-tetrofosmin to assess myocardial blood flow: Experimental validation in an intact canine model. J Nucl Med 35:664–671
20. vom Dahl J, Eitzman DT, Al-Aouar ZR, Kanter HL, Hicks RJ, Deeb GM, Kirsh MM, Schwaiger M (1994) Relation of regional function, perfusion, and metabolism in patients with advanced coronary artery disease undergoing surgical revascularisation. Circulation 90:2356–2366

Intraoperative Perfusion Measurements in MIDCAB and TMLR Surgery by Thermal Imaging: A New Clinical Software

M. ZUCKER · R. IVRON

21.1 Introduction

Thermography was first applied in cardiac surgery as a method for analysing the static temperature distribution in the myocardium to reveal general pathological information [1–4]. Nevertheless, the use of this information for the diagnosis of a disease was controversial because steady-state thermal imaging was not able to follow the dynamic physiological characteristics of the vascular system [5, 6]. For example, poorly perfused or ischaemic regions of the myocardium were hard to detect because blood from small collaterals and capillaries around a defective area caused it to warm. The same phenomenon occurred with artery occlusion; the atherosclerosis reached an equilibrium temperature with the blood flow and even severe stenosis was not revealed.

Therefore, in order to follow and measure dynamic myocardial performance by thermal imaging, it was necessary to develop a way to analyse transitional temperature processes in the myocardium in real-time [7]. By analogy, no significant evidence may be shown on the ECG when a patient is tested for CAD in a steady-state resting condition; however by following the ECG waves in the dynamic condition – during a stress test, for example – a CAD can be detected.

In the following we present a new approach to the measurement of intraoperative regional perfusion based on dynamic thermography and application of the method to MIDCAB and TMLR surgery.

21.2 Method

The principles of perfusion measurement are illustrated in Fig. 21.1. The idea is to create a transitional temperature change in a region of interest in the myocardium and to analyse the thermal response in real-time. A transitional thermodynamic response is elicited by splashing approximately 20 ml saline at room temperature over the region of interest in the myocardium (Fig. 21.1).

The thermodynamic response is shown in Fig. 21.2. The temperature which represents the steady-state condition of the tissue is $T_1(t<0)$. $T_1(t=0)$ represents the temperature of the tissue at the end of the cooling process. We found that the rewarming rate of the tissue (the slope, dT_1/dt $(t>0)$) to the original temperature is correlated to the perfusion of the tissue. Practically speaking, the better the perfusion, higher is the slope of the rewarming

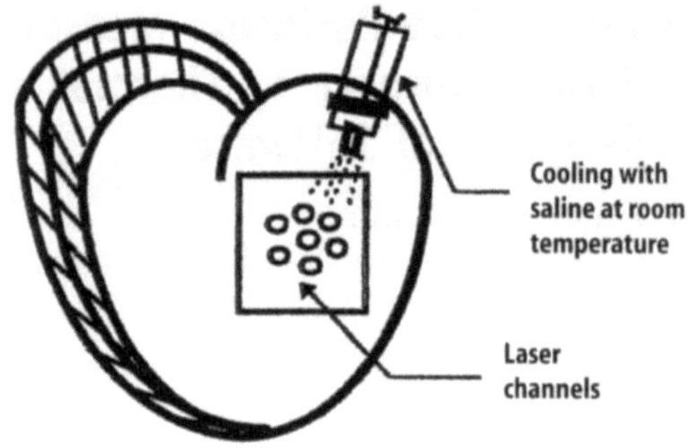

Fig. 21.1. Perfusion measurement: a defined region of interest in the myocardium is cooled with saline at room temperature and the thermodynamic response is analysed

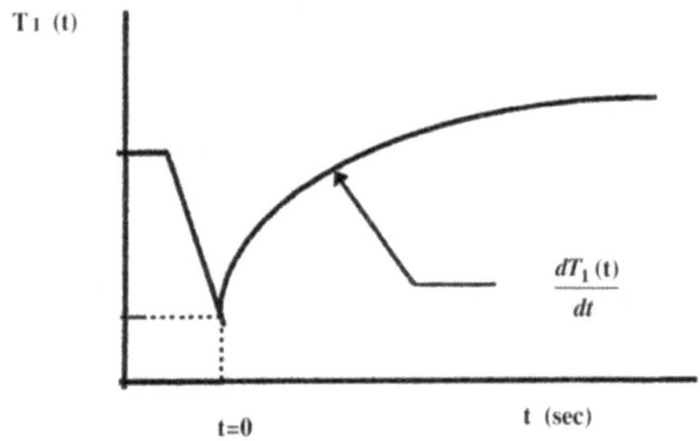

Fig. 21.2. Physical model of perfusion measurement

curve. In order to eliminate sensitivity to the amount of saline splashed and the saline temperature, the perfusion value is normalised to the difference between $T_1(t<0)$ and $T_1(t=0)$ (Fig. 21.2). Computer software detects the minimum temperature in the cooling process and fits an exponential approximation to the measured curve. The perfusion value is extracted and represented in arbitrary units.

21.3 Applications

One of the important applications of perfusion measurement is in MIDCAB surgery. In order to assess the improvement of LAD perfusion during surgery, it is necessary to measure the perfusion of the LAD when the LIMA is clamped and released. An example of this procedure is given in Figs. 21.3–21.5. Figure 21.3 shows a thermal angiogram of the LAD and its diagonal after a LIMA graft is anastomosed to the LAD. Figure 21.4 shows measurement of the LAD perfusion distal to the anastomosis when the LIMA is clamped. Even though the LIMA is clamped, the LAD can still be observed in the steady-state angiogram because it is perfused by collateral flow (Fig. 21.4). The perfusion value of the LAD in this condition is 147 (arbitrary units). In Fig. 21.5, a measurement of the LAD perfusion when the

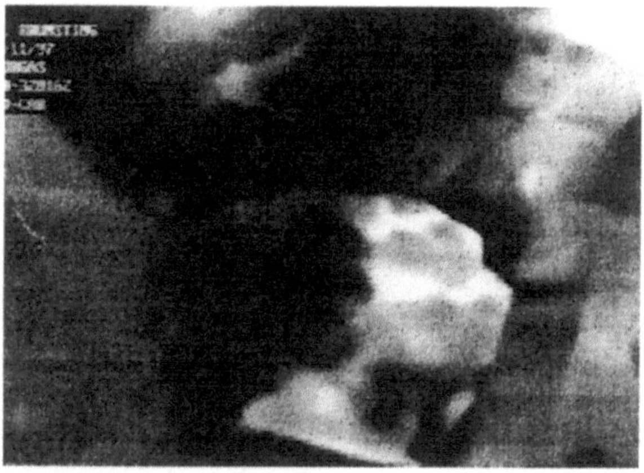

Fig. 21.3. Thermal angiogram of the LAD and its diagonal

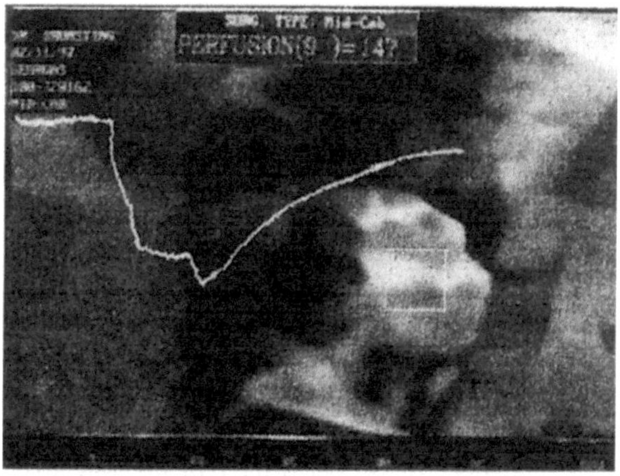

Fig. 21.4. Perfusion measurement of the LAD when the LIMA was clamped. Measurement was performed by splashing saline at room temperature over the region of interest. The perfusion value is represented in arbitrary units in the figure

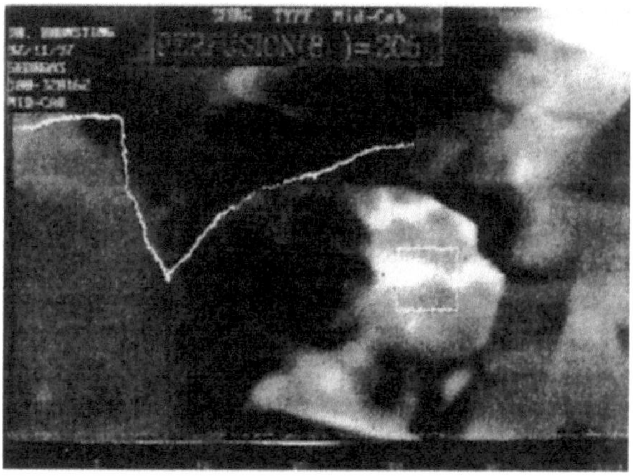

Fig. 21.5

LIMA was released is shown. The perfusion value is 205 (arbitrary units). Therefore, the improvement (P.I.) of LAD perfusion during surgery was 38%. According to our experience with 30 MIDCAB cases, the improvement of

Fig. 21.6

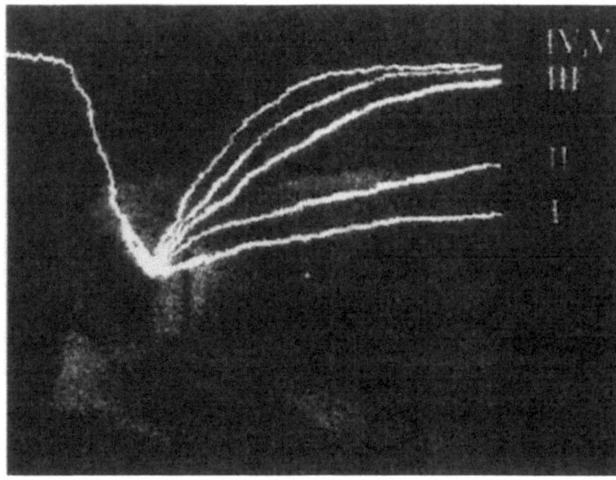

LAD perfusion in this type of surgery is more than 40%. In cases where P.I. values are less than 20% another surgical procedure (for example, adding of laser channels) should be considered.

Intraoperative perfusion measurement has a major significance in TMLR surgery as well. Application of the laser in surgery raises two questions: the first is how to identify optimal regions for lasing in the myocardium and the second is how to assess the optimal number of channels that should be drilled in the selected myocardial region during surgery.

A partial solution to the first of these issues can be suggested by assuming that neighbouring regions in a healthy heart should possess an equal perfusion value if they have the same myocardial wall thickness. By dividing and marking the myocardial tissue into six to ten regions, regional perfusion measurements can be performed in the way that was described previously. Regions which have relatively low perfusion values are to be selected for lasing.

Figure 21.6 shows perfusion results in a myocardial region treated by the laser. The size of the region is 2×2 cm^2. Perfusion improvement evaluations were performed when the region stopped bleeding after two, four, five and six channels had been drilled. It can be seen (Fig. 21.6) that the slope of the rewarming curves increases until a saturation value is reached. The total number of channels drilled in this operation, providing maximal perfusion increase, was 30.

21.4 Summary and Conclusions

The ability to follow transitional temperature processes in the myocardium enables us, for the first time, to perform intraoperative perfusion measurements by thermal imaging. The idea is to create a forced temperature change in a region of interest in the myocardium and to analyse the response in real-time. We found that the rewarming rate of myocardial tissue to the original temperature after cooling is correlated to its perfusion.

Perfusion measurement is useful in CABG, MIDCAB and TMLR surgery in order to assess and verify the functioning of the surgical procedure. In CABG and MIDCAB the perfusion of the LAD is expected to rise following grafting of an internal mammary artery. In TMLR surgery, the perfusion function makes it possible to select optimal regions for lasing and helps to estimate the optimal number of channels to be drilled in order to achieve maximal perfusion improvement.

In general, thermal angiography has a unique advantage over alternative methods in that it reveals, intraoperatively, technical imperfections and therefore allows improvement of the surgical procedure without delay [8-10]. The imaging equipment is flexible and simple to operate and there are no procedure-related complications.

References

1. Seynk S, Malm A, Bornmyr S (1971) Intraoperative cardiothermography. A new method for detecting ischemic areas in the heart muscle and for investigating the results of revascularization procedure in coronary surgery. Eur Surg Res 3:1-12
2. Eckroth R, Berggrer H, Sudow G, et al. (1980) Thermographic demonstration of uneven myocardial cooling in patients with coronary lesions. Ann Thorac Surg 29:341-345
3. Tzivoni D, Cribier A, Ganz W, et al. (1982) Evaluation of changes in epicardial blood flow in experimental animals by cardiothermography. Eur Heart J 3:382-338
4. Pantaleo D, Rocco P, Marchese AR (1984) Thermographic evaluation of myocardial cooling and intraoperative control of graft patency in patients with coronary disease. J Cardiovasc Surg 25:554-559
5. Godik EE, Gulyaev YV (1991) Functional imaging of the human body. IEEE Eng Med Biol
6. Gulgaev YV, Markov AG, Koreneva LG, Zakharov PV (1995) Dynamical infrared thermography in humans. IEEE Eng Med Biol
7. Adachi H, Johnson DL, Baumgartner WA, et al. (1986) Real-time infrared imaging for perfusion assessment in heart surgery: an experimental model. Thermology 2:7-12
8. Mohr FW, Matloff J, Grundfest W, Chaux A, et al. (1989) Thermal coronary angiography: a method for assessing graft patency and coronary anatomy in coronary bypass surgery. Ann Thorac Surg 47:441-449
9. Falk V, Walther T, Philipppi A, Autschbach R, et al. (1995) Thermal coronary angiography for intraoperative patency control of arterial and saphenous vein coronary artery bypass grafts. Cardiovasc Surg 10:147-160
10. Merin G, Elami A, Zucker M (1995) Intraoperative detection of unsuspected distal coronary obstruction by thermal coronary angiography. Cardiovasc Surg 3:599-601

PART VI

Experimental Finding

TMLR With and Without Additional Single Grafting: Differences in Postoperative Outcome?

M. Misfeld · E.-G. Kraatz · C. Schmidtke · F. Führmeyer · H.H. Sievers

22.1 Introduction

In the past few years transmyocardial laser revascularisation (TMLR) has been introduced into clinical practice as a new operative technique. It constitutes a new therapeutic concept for those patients who suffer angina despite maximal anti-ischaemic medication and who are not suitable for conventional interventional procedures like coronary artery bypass grafting (CABG) or percutaneous transluminal angioplasty (PTCA) due to severe diffuse coronary artery disease (CAD). TMLR has been accepted as a procedure for myocardial revascularisation because postoperative results reveal an improvement of clinical symptoms and myocardial perfusion [3, 5, 6, 9, 16]. However, TMLR is still the subject of controversy, since the exact mechanism of action has not been unequivocally clarified to date. The basic principles of myocardial laser treatment are the techniques to achieve improved myocardial perfusion as delineated by Beck [1] and Vineberg [25], as well as by Massimo and Boffi [13] and later by Sen et al. [22]. Alligator hearts serve as an anatomic model because, of all amphibians, they possess a complete interventricular septum, and therefore a parallel to the human heart can be drawn. On the other hand, in alligators left ventricular myocardial perfusion is – to a large extent – supplied directly by channels originating from the left ventricle [11]. Following further development of laser therapy, the first clinical TMLR trials with an 800-watt carbon dioxide laser were conducted by Mirhoseini and co-workers [17]. In this first series of investigations 16 patients had improved with regard to their clinical symptoms at follow-up 6 years after the operation.

TMLR is performed either as the only procedure [3, 5, 9, 20] or in combination with CABG [23]. Both techniques result in an improvement of clinical symptoms. Nevertheless, the rather high early mortality of up to 10% with laser procedures alone should not be disregarded [5, 9]. Might one possible explanation for this finding be myocardial oedema caused by TMLR intraoperatively? This oedema seems to compromise left ventricular function.

To examine in how far an additional bypass operation affects the early and late postoperative course after TMLR and whether the additional graft serves as a "protecting graft", the data of patients who underwent TMLR only were compared with those of patients treated with TMLR in combination with additional single bypass grafting.

22.2
Methods

22.2.1
Patients

After approval by the ethics committee of the Medical University of Lübeck had been obtained, TMLR only was performed in 34 patients (group I) between October 1995 and February 1997. Within the same period a combined procedure of TMLR and single coronary artery bypass grafting was conducted in 14 patients (group II). The following criteria served as indications for laser treatment:

1. Angina class III or IV (Canadian Cardiovascular Society Classification) despite maximal antianginal medication
2. The impracticability of conventional revascularisation via CABG or PTCA as agreed on with the treating cardiologist
3. Positive evidence of myocardial vitality documented by thallium-201 single-photon-emission computer tomography (^{201}Tl-SPECT)

Patients with an ejection fraction (EF) below 25% were excluded from this study. The indication for an additional bypass was given whenever coronary angiography demonstrated that one of the three main coronary branches could possibly be revascularised via CABG despite diffuse CAD.

The mean age of the 28 men and six women in group I was 64±8.6 years. For the 11 men and three women in group II the mean age was 65±8 years. The mean preoperative angina class (CCS-Classification) was 3.5±0.5 in group I and 3.4±0.5 in group II. In group I the mean preoperative EF was 55±14%; in group II it was 58±16%. The mean number of hospital stays within the preceding year was 2.9±1.9 for group I and 2.6±2.2 for group II. The relevant anamnestic data of both groups are listed in Table 22.1.

Table 22.1. Patient demographics

	Group I (n=34) No. (%)	Group II (n=14) No. (%)
Previous MI	27 (79)	9 (64)
Previous CABG	19 (56)	3 (21)
Previous PTCA	6 (18)	None
Cardiovascular risk factors		
- Diabetes mellitus	9 (26)	5 (36)
- Arterial hypertension	22 (65)	10 (71)
- Nicotine	27 (79)	9 (64)
- Hyperlipoproteinaemia	16 (47)	7 (50)
- Familiary disposition	5 (15)	2 (14)

Group I, TMLR alone; *Group II*, TMLR plus single bypass; *MI*, myocardial infarction; *CABG*, coronary artery bypass grafting; *PTCA*, percutaneous transluminal coronary angioplasty

22.2.2
Surgical Technique

In all patients an arterial and a central venous line were placed for perioperative monitoring. Intraoperatively, transoesophageal echocardiography (TEE) was performed in order to register the laser shot by means of an intraventricular vaporisation cloud. Furthermore, TEE following the procedure helped to exclude mitral valve damage, which is occasionally reported after TMLR. On the basis of preoperative myocardial scintigraphy findings, TMLR was conducted with an 800-watt CO_2 laser (PLC Medical Systems, Inc., Milford, Mass.). A helium-neon laser served as a localiser beam. The energy applied was 40 J with an impulse range of 50 ms. Lasering of the beating heart was triggered electrocardiographically and was conducted in the nonvulnerable phase of the cardiac cycle in a density of approximately one channel/cm^2. Myocardial areas appearing akinetic or aneurysmatic macroscopically were spared from TMLR. Spontaneous squirting bleeding from a laser channel and evidence of vaporisation bubbles in intraoperative TEE were considered criteria of successful lasering. An intra-aortic balloon pump (IABP) was inserted prophylactically with an EF<40% and intraoperatively consecutive to symptoms of left ventricular decompensation under moderate catecholamine support.

TMLR Alone. Following 45° right lateral positioning and intubation with a double-lumen tube for isolated right-sided ventilation, an anterolateral thoracotomy was performed in the fourth or fifth intercostal space. Under preservation of the phrenic nerve, the pericardium was opened. The mean number of laser channels was 30±8. In all patients a mediastinal drain, a pleural drain and a pleural catheter for topical analgesia were placed.

TMLR and Single CABG. In group II bypass grafting applying extracorporeal circulation (ECC) was performed prior to TMLR. Shortly before ECC was terminated, laser treatment was conducted in the beating heart using the technique described above. Also, the myocardial regions supplied with a single bypass were additionally lasered. In 64% of the patients a venous graft was used as a bypass (three patients received an LAD graft, two patients an RCX graft and four patients an RCA graft). In 36% of this group the internal mammary artery (IMA) was used as a bypass onto the LAD (in two patients without ECC). The mean number of laser channels was 19±4. All patients were equipped with two mediastinal and – consecutive to IMA preparation – with a pleural drain.

22.2.3
Postoperative Patient Management

For at least 24 h the patients were monitored in the intensive care unit. Intravenous heparinisation was started 6 h following TMLR, the aim being to achieve a partial thromboplastin time of 45 s. On the third postoperative day treatment with phenprocoumon was initiated. The internationalised normal ratio (INR) aspired to was 2.5. Anticoagulation was continued up to 6 months postoperatively. All patients were started on 100 mg of acetylsalicylic acid daily as a permanent medication on the first postoperative day. Anti-ischaemic medication taken prior to surgery was continued for at least another 6 months following the operation in order to ensure comparability of the results.

22.2.4 Follow-up

Postoperative follow-up investigations were carried out after 3, 6 and 12 months. These investigations included repeat myocardial scintigraphy. The analysis comprised the number of segments with normal myocardial perfusion, scars, reversible impairment of perfusion, and segments with a combination of permanent and reversible impairment of perfusion. Improvement of perfusion in more than one segment was considered significant. The results of the postoperative myocardial scintigraphy were compared with the preoperative findings. Further, the findings in group II were evaluated with regard to the myocardial region that was revascularised by bypass grafting or TMLR. For the purposes of follow-up ergometry was also carried out. An amelioration of symptoms was defined as an increase of ergometric capacity by two or more exertional levels (one exertional level being equivalent to 25 watt, 2 min). Using to a standardised questionnaire, each patient was interviewed with reference to intensity and frequency of angina, physical activity, present medication and number of further hospital stays.

22.2.5 Statistical Analysis

If not stated otherwise, all results are given as mean±standard deviation of the mean. For statistical evaluation a Student's *t*-test was applied. Differences were considered significant at a level of $p \leq 0.05$.

22.3 Results

22.3.1 Perioperative Results

No patient suffered mitral valve dysfunction as a result of TMLR. Bleeding from a laser channel required rethoracotomy in one patient of group I. The mean duration of surgery was 219±93 min in group I and 237±52 min in group II. The time to extubation was 13±10 h in group I and 12±5 h in group II. Thorax drains were removed after 24 h in all patients. An IABP was inserted prophylactically in four patients of group I; intraoperatively, IABP insertion was required in eight patients. The mean EF of these patients was 47±14%. In group II an IABP was inserted intraoperatively in one patient who had an EF of 60%. Table 22.2 lists perioperative complications.

Table 22.2. Perioperative complications

	Group I ($n = 34$) No. (%)	Group II ($n = 14$) No. (%)
Death	3 (8.8)	None
Bleeding	6 (18)	3 (21)
Infection	1 (3)	None
Supraventricular/ventricular arrhythmia	6 (18)	1 (7)
Left ventricular failure	12 (35)	1 (7)
MI	3 (9)	1 (7)
Others	2 (6)	None

Group I, TMLR alone; *Group II*, TMLR plus single bypass; *MI*, myocardial infarction [definition: a new Q in ECG and creatine kinase (*CK*) more than eight times the normal value with a CK-MB more than 10% of CK]; *Others*, renal failure

Table 22.3. Clinical status preoperatively and at 3, 6 and 12 months follow-up

	Angina class [a]			
	Preoperatively	3 months	6 months	12 months
Group I	3.5±0.5	1.2±1.0[b]	1.1±0.7[b]	0.9±0.9[b]
Group II	3.4±0.5	1.2±1.0[b]	1.2±1.1[b]	0.7±0.8[b]

Group I, TMLR alone; *Group II*, TMLR plus single bypass
[a] Canadian Cardiovascular Society classification.
[b] $p<0.001$.

Hospital mortality of group I was 8.8% (three patients). One patient died during surgery because of an acute myocardial infarction with persisting low output syndrome. Two other patients died within the first 30 postoperative days. One of these patients suffered an acute myocardial infarction, the other died of septic shock. None of the patients in group II died within the first 30 postoperative days.

22.3.2 Follow-up

In group I, 76% of the patients had improved clinically by two or more angina classes (CCS-Classification) after 3 months. After 6 months this was true for 83%, after 12 months for 93%. After 3 months, 78% of the patients in group II showed an amelioration of clinical symptoms; 78% had improved after 6 months and 86% after 12 months. In comparison to the mean preoperative angina score (group I: 3.5±0.5, group II: 3.4±0.5), the mean postoperative angina score was significantly lower at each follow-up ($p<0.05$). Table 22.3 illustrates the postoperative improvement of clinical symptoms compared with preoperative status.

Improved myocardial perfusion was documented in 88% of the patients in group I after 3 months. Nevertheless, 57% of these patients had residual areas of ischaemia. Compared with this, 79% of the patients in group II had a better myocardial perfusion after 3 months, whereas in 36% of these patients residual

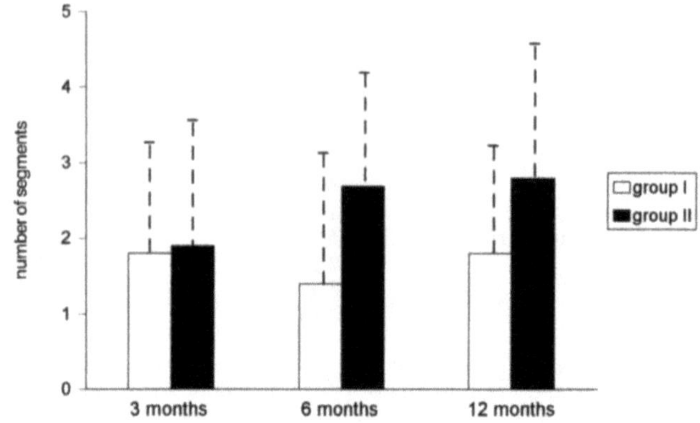

Fig. 22.1. Myocardial perfusion compared with preoperatively as the mean number of segments which showed increased perfusion in ^{201}Tl-SPECT analysis at 3 months (group I = TMLR alone, n = 27; group II = TMLR plus single bypass, n = 14), 6 months (group I: n =22, group II: n = 7) and 12 months (group I: n = 12, group II: n=5) follow-up; segments: septal (not lasered), anterior, apical, lateral and inferior. p = not significant for group I versus group II

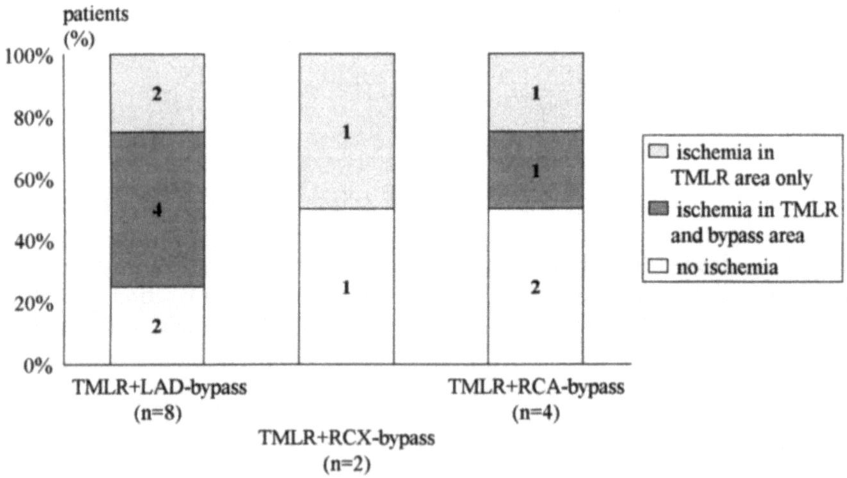

Fig. 22.2. Last available ^{201}Tl-SPECT analysis of group II (TMLR plus single bypass). Correlation between myocardial perfusion and revascularisation procedure (TMLR or bypass)

ischaemia was verifiable. Myocardial scintigraphy demonstrated that perfusion had improved in 94% of group I after 6 months (residual ischaemia in 72%) and in 88% after 12 months (residual ischaemia in 86%). In group II an improvement of myocardial perfusion was substantiated by scintigraphy in 71% (residual ischaemia in 60%) after 6 months and in all patients (residual ischaemia in 80%) after 12 months. Five-segment analysis (septal = not lasered, anterior, apical, lateral and inferior) of the ^{201}Tl-SPECT findings – in comparison to preoperative status – showed that myocardial perfusion was better in 1.8±1.5 segments after 3 months, in 1.4±1.7 segments after 6 months and in

1.8±1.4 segments after 12 months in group I. In group II, myocardial perfusion had improved in 1.9±1.7 segments after 3 months, in 2.7±1.5 segments after 6 months and in 2.8±1.9 segments after 12 months (Fig. 22.1).

Further evaluation of myocardial scintigraphic findings in group II revealed that – in the last available analysis – four patients (29%) had residual ischaemia in the region that had been revascularised by an LAD bypass. In none of the two patients with a bypass to the circumflex distributory was residual ischaemia demonstrated in the bypass region. One patient (25%) supplied with an RCA bypass still had ischaemia in the bypassed region. Figure 22.2 illustrates the myocardial scintigraphic findings in relation to the revascularisation procedure (bypass and TMLR).

Improved ergometric capacity was substantiated in 66% of the patients in group I compared with 64% in group II.

Total mortality of group I was 11.8% in the follow-up period of 11.6±4.6 months. None of the patients in group II died during follow-up.

22.4 Discussion

On the basis of the initial publications of Beck [1], Vineberg [25], Massimo and Boffi [13] and Sen et al. [22], TMLR was introduced into clinical practice by Mirhoseini et al. [15, 18] as a new procedure for the therapy of severe diffuse CAD not suitable for conventional revascularisation in patients who, because of persisting clinical symptoms, require further treatment. Although the exact mechanism of action of TMLR is still not clear [19], its clinical effect is evident. There is still some speculation about whether the laser channels remain open. In histological investigations Mirhoseini showed that channels were open and endothelialised even 2 years after TMLR [4, 14, 15]. Other research groups demonstrated the various stages of wound healing and found occluded, nonendothelialised laser channels in deceased patients at various times after TMLR [2, 7, 8, 12, 14].

Our data analysis of 34 TMLR procedures alone and 14 combined procedures (TMLR and single CABG) revealed rather similar medical histories of the patients. With regard to postoperative clinical symptomatology, a comparable improvement was found up to 12 months postoperatively, as has been described by other authors with regard to TMLR alone [3, 6, 9, 16, 19–21]. Similar clinical improvement after combined procedures has also been documented previously [23]. According to follow-up investigations, the following aspects need to be considered in the evaluation of clinical symptomatology: Immediately after TMLR, patients are free of complaints, and symptoms of angina pectoris are reduced in the further postoperative course as well. Considering this, one possible explanation for the mode of action of TMLR might be the induction of angioneogenesis, as shown by Unger et al. [24] in an animal model after implantation of the internal mammary artery into the left ventricular myocardium. However, this theory would not sufficiently account for the immediate relief of clinical symptoms in the postoperative phase. To what extent this early effect of laser therapy is attributable to a form of partial sympathectomy remains to be established.

It seems certain that TMLR results in an improvement of myocardial perfusion [3, 5, 9, 10]. Despite this, however, left ventricular function will not be improved TMLR [5, 20]. According to our own experience with 70 laser operations conducted so far, patients are – on the contrary – intraoperatively compromised by cardiac oedema. This is reflected by the rather large number of 12 patients (35%) who suffered complications perioperatively in the form of left ventricular failure, necessitating the insertion of an IABP. In the literature this is substantiated by a relatively high perioperative mortality [5, 9]. Under the assumption that an additive bypass revascularisation of one of the three main coronary vessels in spite of severe diffuse CAD is favourable to early postoperative recovery, providing a certain amount of myocardial protection and a possible enhancement of neocapillarisation in the postoperative course, the results of 34 TMLR procedures only and 14 combined procedures (TMLR and single CABG) were analysed retrospectively. In the evaluation of long-term results, no significant differences were found with regard to clinical status or ergometric capacity. There was a tendency to better myocardial perfusion in patients with TMLR and additional single bypass, although the analysis of scintigraphic findings revealed that impairment of perfusion was present also in the areas revascularised via bypass grafting as an expression of the severity of diffuse CAD. Thus, enhancement of neocapillarisation does not appear to be promoted by additional bypass grafting.

In contrast to group I, with a total mortality of 11.7%, no patient in group II died. Furthermore, an IABP was inserted in only one patient (7%) of group II perioperatively compared with 12 patients (35%) in group I. The preoperative risk profile and ejection fractions were similar in both groups. Patients in group II had a smaller number of previous myocardial infarctions, which limits the value of these results. However, the addition of bypass revascularisation seems to be favourable to the perioperative course.

This study is also restricted by the fact that our patient collective was not randomised. The reason for this is that, in our clinic, a combined procedure is indicated whenever a coronary artery is still suitable for conventional revascularisation via bypass grafting. In all other cases only TMLR was performed. Furthermore, it must be stated that our clinical results are subject to a 'learning curve' as also shown in the investigations of other research groups [20]. Thus, none of the last 30 patients treated with TMLR in our department died, while the total mortality was 7.1% (five patients). The number of combined procedures did not increase in this context.

Based on the results of this study, there is evidence that patients who undergo CABG in addition to TMLR whenever possible have a better perioperative course than patients who receive TMLR treatment alone. In this respect, a certain protective function can be ascribed to the bypass vessel ('protection graft'). In our investigation, however, long-term clinical results were not affected by the addition of single bypass revascularisation. Nevertheless, bypass grafting of one of the three main coronary arteries supplementary to TMLR should be aspired to whenever possible. Longer follow-up periods within the scope of larger randomised clinical trials are required to further clarify the effect of a 'protecting vessel'.

References

1. Beck CS (1935) The development of a new blood supply to the heart by operation. Ann Surg 102:801–813
2. Burkhoff D, Fisher PE, Apfelbaum M, Kohmoto T, DeRosa CM, Smith CR (1996) Histologic appearance of transmyocardial laser channels after 4.5 weeks. Ann Thorac Surg 61:1532–1535
3. Cooley DA, Frazier OH, Kadipasaoglu KA, Lindenmeir MH, Pehlivanoglu S, Kolff JW, Wilansky S, Moore WH (1996) Transmyocardial laser revascularization: clinical experience with twelve months' follow-up. J Thorac Cardiovasc Surg 111:791–799
4. Cooley DA, Frazier OH, Kadipasaoglu KA, Pehlivanoglu S, Shannon RL, Angelini P (1994) Transmyocardial laser revascularization. Anatomic evidence of long-term channel patency. Texas Heart Inst J 21:220–224
5. Frazier OH, Cooley DA, Kadipasaoglu KA, Pehlivanoglu S, Lindenmeir M, Barasch E, Conger JL, Wilansky S, Moore WH (1995) Myocardial revascularization with laser: preliminary findings. Circulation 92 [Suppl II]:II-58–II-65
6. Frazier OH, Kadipasaoglu K (1996) Transmyocardial laser revascularization. Curr Opin Cardiol 11:564–567
7. Gassler N, Wintzer HO, Stubbe HM, Wullbrand A, Helmchen U (1997) Transmyocardial laser revascularization. Histological features in human nonresponder myocardium. Circulation 95:371–375
8. Hardy RI, Bove KE, James FW, Kaplan S, Goldman L (1987) A histologic study of laser-induced transmyocardial channels. Lasers Surg Med 6:563–573
9. Horvarth KA, Mannting F, Cummings N, Shernan SK, Cohn LH (1996) Transmyocardial laser revascularization: operative technique and clinical results at two years. J Thorac Cardiovasc Surg 111:1047–1053
10. Klein M, Dauben HP, Schulte HD (1996) Transmyocardial laser revascularization in patients with end-stage coronary artery disease (abstract). Cardiovasc Surg Sept 1996:15
11. Kohmoto T, Argenziano M, Yamamoto N, Vliet KA, Gu A, DeRosa CM, Fisher PE, Spotniz HM, Burkhoff D, Smith CR (1997) Assessment of transmyocardial perfusion in alligator hearts. Circulation 95:1585–1591
12. Krabatsch T, Schaper F, Leder C, Tulser J, Thalmann U, Hetzer R (1996) Histological findings after transmyocardial laser revascularization. J Cardiovasc Surg 11:326–331
13. Massimo C, Boffi L (1957) Myocardial revascularization by a new method of carrying blood directly from the left ventricular cavity into the coronary circulation. J Thorac Surg 34:257–264
14. Mirhoseini M, Muckerheide M, Cayton MM (1982) Transventricular revascularization by laser. Lasers Surg Med 2:187–198
15. Mirhoseini M, Shegilkar S, Cayton MM (1988) New concepts in revascularization of the myocardium. Ann Thorac Surg 45:415–420
16. Mirhoseini M, Shelgikar S, Cayton MM (1990) Clinical and histological evaluation of laser myocardial ravascularization. J Clin Laser Med Surg 9:73–78
17. Mirhoseini M, Shelgikar S, Cayton MM (1993) Transmyocardial laser revascularization: a review. Lasers Surg Med 11:15–19
18. Mirhoseini M, Cayton MM, Shegilkar S (1994) Transmyocardial laser revascularization J Am Coll Cardiol 1A:484
19. Moosdorf R, Schoebel FC, Hort W (1997) Transmyocardial laser revascularization – morphology, pathophysiology and historical background of indirect myocardial revascularization. Z Kardiol 86:149–164
20. Nägele H, Kalmar P, Lübeck M, Marcsek P, Nienaber CA, Rödiger W, Stiel GM, Stubbe HM (1997) Transmyocardial laser revascularization – treatment option for coronary artery disease?. Z Kardiol 86:171–178
21. PLC Systems Inc. (1996) The heart laser. Clinical data sheet. September
22. Sen PK, Udwadia TE, Kinare SG, Parulkar GB (1965) Transmyocardial acupuncture – a new approach to myocardial revascularization. J Thorac Surg 50:181–189
23. Trehan N, Mishra M, Kohli VM, Mishra A, Jangid DR, Bapna R (1996) Transmyocardial laser revascularization as an adjunct to coronary artery bypass grafting. Indian Heart J 48:381–388
24. Unger EF, Sheffield CD, Epstein SE (1990) Creation of anastomoses between an extracardiac artery and the coronary circulation. Circulation 82:1449–1466
25. Vineberg A (1954) Clinical and experimental studies in the treatment of coronary artery insufficiency by internal mammary artery implant. J Int Coll Surg 22:503–518

CHAPTER 23

Transmyocardial Laser Revascularisation (TMLR): Experimental Studies on Acute Regional Ischaemia

G. Lutter · M. Yoshitake · N. Takahashi · E. Nitzsche · J. Martin · K. Sarai · Ch. Lutz · M. Bürkle · B. v. Specht · F. Beyersdorf

23.1 Introduction

Transmyocardial laser revascularisation (TMLR) is a new surgical technique for patients with symptomatic end-stage coronary artery disease that is untreatable by conventional revascularisation. TMLR creates transmural channels in the myocardium via laser ablation. Hypothetically, this allows direct perfusion from the left ventricular cavity via the channels to the myocardium [1]. The clinical experience gained from single- and multicentre studies with TMLR [2, 3] indicates that angina is relieved significantly, perfusion and treadmill tolerance are improved and hospital admissions are decreased. Other centres report similar results but no significant improvement in regional perfusion and metabolism; results of a long-term follow-up showed no significant improvement of regional myocardial perfusion in the lased areas [4, 5]. Naegele et al. even observed reduced myocardial perfusion and viability after TMLR [5].

However, the exact mechanism by which TMLR facilitates these subjective and objective improvements remains unknown. This study was initiated to evaluate the short-term effectiveness of TMLR in the setting of an acute coronary occlusion in pig hearts.

23.2 Materials and Methods

23.2.1 Animals and Anaesthesia

The study was approved by the Experimental Animal Protection Committee of the University of Freiburg. Pigs of the "German land race" weighing 28–35 kg were premedicated with an intramuscular injection of 0.2 mg/kg flunitrazepam and 7 mg/kg ketamine hydrochloride. An ear vein was cannulated and anaesthesia was induced with 0.1 mg/kg flunitrazepam and 10 mg/kg ketamine hydrochloride by titrated i.v. injection.

After muscular relaxation had been induced with 0.1 mg/kg i.v. vecuronium bromide, an endotracheal tube was inserted and mechanical ventilation was begun. Tidal volume and respiratory rate were adjusted while maintaining oxygen tension at >100 mmHg, carbon dioxide tension at 35–42 mmHg and pH 7.3–7.4. Anaesthesia was maintained by continuous i.v. infusion of

Supported by the Clinical Research Center II of the Albert-Ludwig University Freiburg, grant no. B4.

0.06 mg/kg per hour vecuronium, 0.004 mg/kg per hour fentanyl dihydrogen citrate, 5.2 mg/kg per hour propofol, and 0.04 mg/kg per hour flunitrazepam. At the end of the experiment the animals were killed by means of an intravenous injection of potassium chloride.

23.2.2 Experimental Groups

Following thoracotomy, haemodynamic and perfusion measurements were performed and all animals were randomised into one of four experimental groups:

1. *Control group, no ischaemia:* Four pigs underwent isolation of the LAD without occlusion and were kept anaesthetised for 6 h (after thoracotomy) to determine the effect of thoracotomy and anaesthesia.
2. *Ischaemic group.* In seven pigs myocardial infarctions were created by isolated occlusion of the LAD beyond the first diagonal branch after a 30-min observation period following thoracotomy (time period equal to that with laser groups). The occlusions were left in place for 6 h. No laser treatment was performed in these cases.
3. *Laser group 1.* Nine pigs received the same treatment as the ischaemic group as well as prophylactic treatment by TMLR 0.5 h prior to coronary occlusion. They were treated by creation of *one* laser channel (1 mm diameter) per cm^2 in the ischaemic LAD area. To define this area of risk the LAD was occluded for 10 s prior to laser treatment. After LAD occlusion the animals were monitored for 6 h.
4. *Laser group 2.* Eight pigs were treated with the same regimen as laser group 1. However, in contrast to laser group 1, these animals received *two* laser channels (1 mm diameter) per cm^2.

23.2.3 Monitoring

The right and left external jugular veins were surgically exposed and cannulated with a sheet. An intravenous line (14-gauge) was placed into the left external jugular vein to provide access for fluid and medications. A 7-French Swan-Ganz thermodilution catheter (Baxter Healthcare Corporation, Irvine, Calif.) was inserted through the right external jugular vein into the pulmonary artery in order to record pulmonary artery pressure, cardiac output, pulmonary capillary wedge pressure and central venous pressure. The left carotid artery was cannulated with a 14-gauge polyurethane catheter to monitor systolic and mean arterial pressure (MAP) and to facilitate arterial blood-gas analysis. Both catheters were connected to pressure transducers (SX 509597, Medex Medical GmbH, Ratingen, Germany) which drove an amplifier monitor (Sirecust 404–1, Siemens, Erlangen, Germany). The right femoral artery was cannulated with a 14-gauge polyurethane catheter to take blood samples for measurement of the perfusion. A 7-F polyurethane catheter was inserted into the left atrium through the left atrial appendage to monitor left atrial pressure and to inject the microspheres. Electrocardiographic leads were affixed to the left thorax and extremities and connected to a monitor. Sinus rhythm and any kind of rhythm disturbance were registered.

23.2.4
Experimental Preparation

Following anterolateral thoracotomy, 150 IU/kg heparin and 1 g magnesium were given i.v. to all pigs. Lidocaine was administered at 40–60 μg/kg per minute in a continuous drip. The heart was suspended in a pericardial cradle. A 7-F cannula was placed through the left hemiazygos vein into the sinus coronarius for venous blood-gas analysis and enzyme probes. The LAD was dissected and isolated immediately distal to the bifurcation of the first diagonal branch, and a snare occluder was placed loosely around the LAD for subsequent occlusion to produce an area at risk of about 30%.

Complications such as atrial fibrillations were treated with local administration of 50–100 mg lidocaine hydrochloride, ventricular fibrillations with electrical countershocks (10–20 J) and intervening open-chest cardiac compression.

23.2.5
Laser Procedure

Transmyocardial laser revascularisation was accomplished with an 800-watt (spot size 1 mm, wavelength 10.6 μm) pulsed CO_2 laser coupled to an articulating arm (Laser Engineering, Milford, Mass.). The maximal output is 80 J, and the pulse width can be adjusted from 5 to 99 ms. Laser activation was synchronised with the R-wave of the electrocardiogram to avoid creating arrhythmias by stimulating the heart during the electrically vulnerable ventricular repolarisation period. The CO_2 laser was aimed with a helium-neon laser (5 mW, wavelength 632.8 nm). The articulating arm connected to a focusing probe was placed against the epicardium of the heart within the area of risk and fired, creating a transmyocardial channel. Channels were created in a distribution of one (laser group 1) or two (laser group 2) channels per square centimetre. After each channel was formed, manual pressure with gauze was gently applied to the epicardial surface to secure haemostasis. Drilling took an average of 17 min per animal (laser group 1) and 40 min per animal (laser group 2) to complete (Table 23.2.).

23.2.6
Miscellaneous Measurements

23.2.6.1
Haemodynamics

Baseline haemodynamic measurements were recorded before and shortly after thoracotomy and TMLR (in the laser groups). Further haemodynamic assessments were performed hourly. Cardiac output was measured by the thermodilution technique. Cardiac preload was increased by stepwise volume loading controlling left atrial pressure, and Starling curves were registered in all groups shortly after thoracotomy and at the end of the 6-h observation period. Left ventricular stroke work was calculated and normalised for heart weight as stroke work index in mJ/g:

$$SWI = \frac{(MAP - LAP) \times CO}{HR \times HW} \times 0.133 \times 1000\,,$$

where SWI is the stroke work index (mJ/g), MAP the mean arterial pressure (mmHg), LAP the left atrial pressure (mmHg), CO the cardiac output (l/min), HR the heart rate (beats/min), HW the heart weight (g). For comparison between the experimental groups we used the maximal achieved left ventricular stroke work index ($LVSWI_{max}$).

23.2.6.2
Perfusion

Regional myocardial blood flow of the LAD and RCX territory was measured based upon the microsphere and arterial reference sample technique. Microspheres of 15±3 μm labelled with ^{95}Nb, ^{103}Ru and ^{141}Ce were injected over a 30-s period into the left atrium while a reference sample was withdrawn from the descending aorta for 2 min at a rate of 10 ml/min, starting 5 s before the injection of the spheres as described previously [6, 7]. The spheres were suspended before injection in blood with 0.01% Tween 80 and were vigorously agitated prior to their use. The number of spheres injected was calculated so that a 0.5-g sample of myocardium contained 800 spheres. The microsphere suspensions were injected into the left atrium shortly after thoracotomy in all groups, after the TMLR procedure (only in the laser groups), and at the end of the study (after the 6-h observation period in all groups). The heart was removed after the experiment and samples of endocardial, mid-myocardial, and epicardial muscle were obtained and placed into tared vials. The radioactive content of each nuclide was determined by γ-spectrometry and blood flow was calculated as described previously [6, 7].

23.2.6.3
Histochemical Assessment and Histology

Monastryl blue vital dye (2% solution, 0.25 mg/kg body wt.) was injected via the left atrium in all animals with LAD occlusion to delineate the area at risk. The area of the left ventricle that did not receive monastryl blue vital dye was measured by planimetry and considered to be the area at risk. After 15 s the heart was arrested with a hyperkalemic solution at 4°C, excised and inspected, and the heart weight was assessed. The ventricles were cut into 5-mm-thick transverse sections. The slices were then incubated in a 1% solution of TTC (triphenyl tetrazolium chloride) made up in 8 mmol/l dibasic and 2 mmol/l monobasic phosphate buffer (pH 8.4) for 30 min at 37°C [8, 9]. Thus prepared, the sections underwent planimetric analysis to determine the area at risk (AR of the left ventricle, expressed as the ratio AR/LV) and the area of necrosis in the area at risk (AN, expressed as the ratio AN/AR). Myocardial samples were fixed in 10% formalin, embedded in paraffin, cut and stained with hematoxylin/eosin.

23.2.6.4
Statistical Analysis

Statistical analysis was performed with Student's or Welch's *t*-test or the Wilcoxon test to compare either paired or unpaired data as appropriate. A *p*-value less than 0.05 was considered statistically significant. Results are expressed as mean value±standard deviation. Only data are used of animals who survived the whole 6-h observation period. Myocardial flow heterogeneity occurred in laser group 1 and in the ischaemic group at baseline and at the end of the experiment. The flow ranged from one third to more than three to six times the mean. Consequently, the values of the RMBF which were greater than three times the standard deviation have been excluded from analysis (<3% of the RMBF data) [10, 11].

23.3
Results

The results are shown in Tables 23.1–23.3 and Figs. 23.1 and 23.2.

1. No ischaemia: global haemodynamics (max. LWSVI) and perfusion were minimally changed, and intractable ventricular fibrillation occurred in one case shortly after thoracotomy. Mean arterial blood pressure remained at control levels. Histology did not show any ischaemia.
2. Ischaemia, laser 1 and 2 groups: all seven pigs in the ischaemic group had ventricular fibrillation (100%) during the first hour of LAD occlusion

Table 23.1. Incidence of VF and mortality

		Incidence of VF	Intractable VF	Overall mortality
Control group	($n=4$)	25%	25% ($n=1$)	25% ($n=1$)
Ischaemic group	($n=7$)	100%	14% ($n=1$)	14% ($n=1$)
Laser group 1	($n=9$)	56%*	11% ($n=1$)	11% ($n=1$)
Laser group 2	($n=8$)	38%*	12.5% ($n=1$)	12.5% ($n=1$)

VF, Ventricular fibrillation
* $p<0.05$ versus ischaemic group

Table 23.2. Intraoperative data[a]

	Laser group 1 ($n=9$)	Laser group 2 ($n=8$)	
No. of channels	17.2±2.7 (15–23)	39.2±5.2 (23–49)	$p<0.05$
No. of unconfirmed channels	0.9±0.4 (0–3)	1.3±0.41 (1–2)	n.s.
Pulse energy in joules	23.4±2.1 (20–26)	32.0±4.8 (25–40)	n.s.
Pulse width in ms	29.2±2.4 (25–32)	38.3±4.8 (32–45)	n.s.

[a] All values expressed as mean±standard deviation, with range in parentheses.

Table 23.3. Regional myocardial blood flow (ml/100 g per minute)

	Baseline				Post laser		6 h Ischaemia			
	Control	Ischaemia	Laser 1	Laser 2	Laser 1	Laser 2	Control	Ischaemia	Laser 1	Laser 2
LAD region										
epi	95±41	140±128	143±96	96±47	80±43	99±44	180±177	3±5	5±5	3±3
mid	101±47	154±115	146±88	103±54	92±43	85±40	162±148	1±1	4±12	2±3
endo	162±98	209±129	223±187	108±46	190±106	125±51	184±133	7±13	1±7	1±1
transmural	120±59	187±139	199±141	102±46	120±50	103±38	175±149	4±5	3±10	2±10
endo/epi-ratio	1.67	1.50	1.9	1.18	2.25	1.32	1.54	0.62	0.23	0.34
LCx region										
epi	73±37	175±147	184±96	132±76	120±80	96±50	203±197	148±102	134±92	193±103
mid	96±60	209±152	222±16	147±73	126±67	100±53	157±97	177±150	177±97	199±82
endo	174±72	198±172	215±187	156±82	248±186	147±72	105±81	180±126	173±109	242±137
transmural	114±51	194±69	207±141	145±71	145±92	114±50	155±110	168±96	161±145	211±90
endo/epi-ratio	2.9	1.13	1.16	1.26	2.07	1.76	1.02	1.22	1.28	1.47

Values are mean±standard error of the mean. *Epi*, epicardial; *mid*, midmyocardial; *endo*, endocardial; *LAD*, left anterior descending coronary artery, *LCx*, left circumflex coronary artery; *post laser*, 15 min after TMLR

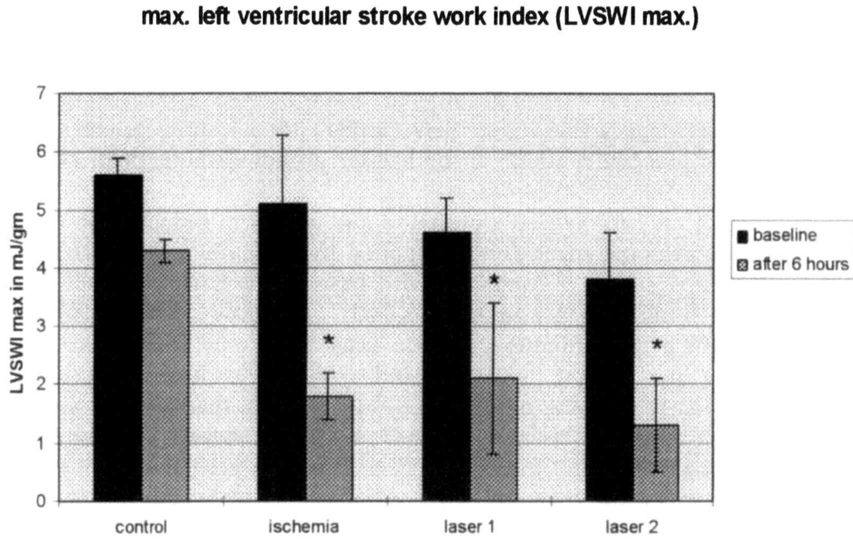

Fig. 23.1. The maximal left ventricular stroke work index ($LVSWI_{max}$.) is demonstrated after a 6-h observation period in all study groups and with 6 h of ischaemia in the ischaemic and laser groups compared with baseline values. In all three ischaemic groups a comparable reduction in LVSWI was found at the end of the experiment, with a significant reduction as compared with the control group, *$p<0.01$. Mean values (*column height*) and standard deviation (*error bars*) are shown

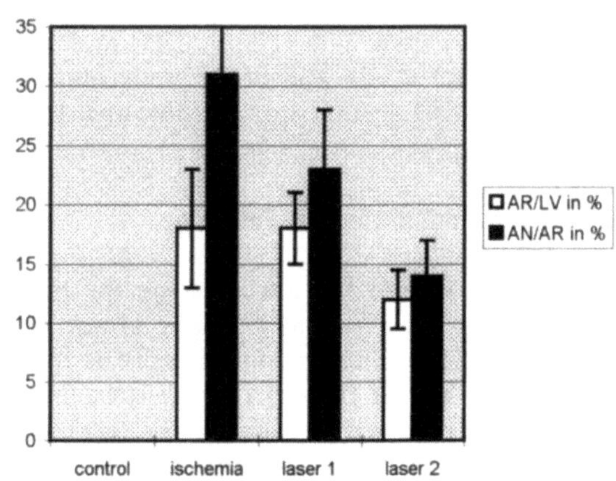

Fig. 23.2. Percent of area of necrosis (*AN*) in the area at risk (*AR*) for control ($n=3$), ischaemic (n=6), laser 1 ($n=8$) and laser 2 ($n=7$) groups. Mean values (*column height*) and standard deviation (*error bars*) are shown. Note: the AR of the ischaemic and laser groups did not differ significantly, but the AN in the AR of laser groups 1 and 2 was reduced compared with the ischaemic group (laser group 1: 23% vs. ischaemic group: 31%, p=n.s.; laser group 2: 14% vs. 31%, * $p<0.01$)

(without TMLR). In contrast, ventricular fibrillation occurred significantly less often in laser group 1 (56% ; 5/9, $p<0.05$) and laser group 2 (38%; 3/8, $p<0.05$) (Table 23.1).

In each of the study groups one pig died of intractable ventricular fibrillation during the 6-h observation period and could not be studied. All pigs in whom ventricular fibrillation occurred required electrical countershocks and intervening open-chest cardiac compression (2–5 min). Intraoperative data are shown in Table 23.2.

23.3.1
Regional Myocardial Blood Flow

Data indicated that (prior to ischaemia) the LAD and LCx territories showed normal regional myocardial blood flow (RMBF) for all study groups. Even after the laser procedure, RMBF in both laser groups demonstrated normal values (Table 23.3).

Occlusion of the LAD caused a profound and persistent reduction in transmural flow to regional myocardium supplied by the LAD in the ischaemic and laser groups after 6 h compared with baseline (ischaemic group: from 187±139 to 4±5 ml/100 g per minute, $p<0.001$; laser group 1: from 199±141 to 3±10 ml/100 g per minute, $p<0.001$; laser group 2: from 102±46 to 2±10 ml/100 g per minute, $p<0.001$) and with the control group (from 120±59 to 175±149 ml/100 g per minute; p=n.s.). Thus, there was no significant difference between laser-treated and ischaemic hearts regarding the amount of blood flow into the infarcted LAD region after 6 h (p=n.s.). In contrast, normal RMBF in remote myocardium supplied by the LCx was assessable in all study groups.

23.3.2
Systemic Haemodynamics

The maximal LVSWI at baseline and end of study are summarised in Fig. 23.1 for all groups. After 6 h, maximal LVSWI in the ischaemic and laser groups 1 and 2 was reduced significantly as compared with the preoperative value (36% vs. 38% and 41%; $p<0.05$) and with the 6-h value of the control group ($p<0.01$). At the end of the study maximal LVSWI in the ischaemic, laser 1 and laser 2 groups did not show any difference.

23.3.3
Macroscopic and Microscopic Pathology

The area at risk of the left ventricle for the ischaemic (18±5%) and laser groups (laser group 1: 18±3%, laser group 2: 12±3%) did not differ significantly (Fig. 23.2). The amount of necrosis in the area at risk in laser groups 1 and 2 was smaller than that in the ischaemic group (23%; 14% versus 31%, $p<0.01$). Longitudinal and transverse sections of myocardium demonstrated typical features of open laser channels [12].

23.4
Discussion

Previous experimental studies tested transmyocardial laser channels in dog hearts [13–16], which have variable native collateral circulations. Therefore, it is impossible to know whether any beneficial, preventive effect against ischaemia was attributable to the channels or whether the treated hearts had intrinsic collateral blood flow. Such limitations also apply to sheep [17] and, to a lesser extent, to rabbit hearts [18]. In contrast, pig and rat hearts [19] have very little native collateral circulation, so that pigs were used to evaluate the short-term effectiveness of TMLR in the setting of an acute myocardial infarction. This model of acute regional ischaemia demonstrates that CO_2-laser revascularisation significantly diminishes the incidence of ventricular fibrillation and necrosis in the area at risk and does not change regional myocardial perfusion and global left ventricular function.

TMLR limits expansion of the myocardial infarction zone after acute coronary occlusion: laser group 2 showed a significantly smaller area of necrosis in the area at risk (laser group 1 did not reach significance) than the ischaemic group (TTC technique: laser group 1: 23%; laser group 2: 14% vs. ischaemic group: 31%, $p<0.01$). In sheep, using the same technique, Horvath et al. [17] demonstrated minimal necrosis in the area at risk (6%) compared with controls (39%). Their smaller area of necrosis cannot be explained by better coronary collateralisation in sheep, because their area at risk was nearly the same as that in this study (14% vs. 16%) and the control animals showed high amounts of necrosis (39%).

The maximal LVSWI in the ischaemic and laser groups 1 and 2 did not show any difference at the end of the experiment. All groups showed an average mean reduction of 39% of their baseline value. It might be speculated that the similarity in measurements of global left ventricular function between the three ischaemic groups after 6 h of oberservation was due to too short a time period (half an hour) between creating CO_2 channels and causing the infarction. The possible new collateralisation by the microchannels (direct blood flow) did not improve myocardial function in the laser groups compared with the ischaemic group. These haemodynamic results mirror those seen in the RMBF measurements. No significant difference was seen between laser-treated (laser group 1: 3±10 ml/100 g per minute and laser group 2: 2±10 ml/100 g per minute) and ischaemic hearts (ischaemia group: 4±5 ml/100 m per minute) with regard to the extremely low blood flow into the infarcted LAD region after 6 h (p=n.s.). Even in laser group 2, with double the number of laser channels compared with laser group 1, a higher blood flow was not observed. A longer time period with existing microchannels might have improved the blood flow through angiogenesis and thus the global contractility of the lased myocardium.

There is little experimental evidence in the literature about whether blood flow through the microchannels is the mechanism of action. In most studies the RMBF was not determined. In contrast, Kohmoto et al. measured regional myocardial blood flow (with coloured microspheres) after using a holmium:YAG laser in ischaemic canine hearts. They found only a very low blood flow (<1 ml/100 g per minute), and, as we have observed in this study, the amount of collateral flow into the channel region was not increased compared with nontreated myocardium [20].

Laser group 2, with twice the number of laser channels, was less prone to ventricular fibrillation and demonstrated a smaller area of necrosis compared with laser group 1. These results may signify that the creation of two channels per square centimetre is preferable in terms of preventing ischaemia.

In their long-term study with pigs, Goda et al. used a CO_2 laser (creating 0.2 mm laser channels) and saw no difference in the amount of the ischaemic and necrotic area between the laser and the control group, but they observed stronger regression of ischaemic ST-elevations in the laser group [21]. In their acute CO_2-laser study, Nagata et al. found a significantly higher stroke work index and RMBF in the laser group compared with controls [22].

Occlusion of the LAD coronary artery distal to the first diagonal branch produced an area at risk of 31±9%, which does not involve sufficient myocardium to cause cardiac shock (i.e., 40% of LV mass) [23]. Therefore, this experimental model did not reflect the natural history of single-vessel disease with more proximal LAD occlusion. This more limited area at risk was chosen to allow evaluation of the ischaemic myocardium. Other influences affecting our results, such as general anaesthesia with barbiturates, thoracotomy, lidocaine to reduce arrhythmias, and coronary dissection, remain unclear. Myocardial flow heterogeneity occurred in the laser 1 and the ischaemic group at baseline and at the end of the experiment. The flow ranged from one third to three to six times the mean in these groups. This is presumably related to inadequate mixing, which can occur with any number of injected spheres or due to the degree of spatial heterogeneity [10, 11]. Consequently, the RMBF values which were greater than three times the standard deviation were excluded from analysis (<3% of the RMBF data).

It has been stated that it is theoretically impossible for blood to flow directly from the ventricle into the myocardium during either systole or diastole [24, 25]. In normal myocardium the endomyocardial pressure approaches left ventricular pressure during systole and diastole [26]. This endocardial pressure permits blood flow into the myocardium, but this flow may be enhanced by diminished tissue pressure due to ischaemia.

Various animal models have provided contradictory results that have led investigators to draw opposing conclusions as to patency and perfusion through laser channels. The reason might be that these models do not accurately reproduce the complex anatomy and pathology of human atherosclerotic heart disease. The only current clinical indication for TMLR is a chronically ischaemic myocardium (myocardial hybernation). Further studies are in progress to quantify perfusion through the CO_2 channels, to monitor regional and global function, and to determine the amount of angiogenesis and metabolic changes in chronic ischaemia.

Acknowledgements. Dr. Lutter is supported by the Clinical Cardiovascular Research Center II at the University of Freiburg, Germany.

References

1. Mirhoseini M, Shelgikar S, Cayton MM (1988) New concepts in revascularization of the myocardium. Ann Thorac Surg 45:415–420
2. Horvath KA, Mannting F, Cummings N, Shernan SK, Cohn LH (1996) Transmyocardial laser revascularization: operative techniques and clinical results at two years. J Thorac Cardiovasc Surg 111:1047–1053

3. Horvath KA, Cohn LH, Cooley DA, Crew JR, Frazier OH, Griffith BP, Kadipasaoglu K, Lansing A, Mannting F, March R, Mirhoseini MR, Smith C (1997) Transmyocardial laser revascularization: results of a multicenter trial with transmyocardial laser revascularization used as sole therapy for end-stage coronary artery disease. J Thorac Cardiovasc Surg 113:645–654
4. Lutter G, Frey M, Saurbier B, Nitzsche E, Kobba J, Martin J, Beyersdorf F (1997) TMLR: clinical results of patients transferred for transmyocardial laser revascularization. J Heart Failure 4:49
5. Naegele H, Kalmar P, Lübeck M, Marcsek P, Nienaber CA, Rödiger W, Stiel GM, Stubbe HM (1997) Transmyocardial laser revascularization – treatment option for coronary artery disease? German J Cardiol 86:171–178
6. Hirzel HO, Nelson GR, Sonnenblick EH, Kirk ES (1976) Redistribution of collateral blood flow from necrotic to surviving myocardium following coronary occlusion in the dog. Circ Res 39:214–222
7. Hirzel HO, Sonnenblick EH, Kirk ES (1977) Absence of a lateral border zone of intermediate creatine phosphokinase depletion surrounding a central infarct 24 hours after acute coronary occlusion in the dog. Circ Res 41:673–683
8. Lie JT, Pairolero PC, Holley KE, Titus JL (1975) Macroscopic enzyme mapping verification of large, homogeneous, experimental myocardial infarcts of predictable size and location in dogs. J Thorac Cardiovasc Surg 69:599–605
9. Kloner RA, Darsee JR, DeBoer LW, Carlson N (1981) Early pathologic detection of acute myocardial infarction. Arch Pathol Lab Med 105:403–406
10. Buckberg GD, Luck JC, Payne B, Hoffman JIE, Archie JP, Fixler DE (1971) Some sources of error in measuring regional blood flow with radioactive microspheres. J Appl Physiol 31:598–604
11. King RB, Bassingthwaighte JB, Hales JRS, Rowell LB (1985) Stability of heterogeneity of myocardial blood flow in normal awake baboons. Circ Res 57:285–295
12. Lutter G, Schwarzkopf J, Schlensak C, Martin J, Kobba J, Beyersdorf F (1997) Transmyocardial laser channels: histologic findings after two hours. J Heart Failure 4:114
13. Whittaker P, Kloner RA, Przyklenk K (1993) Laser-mediated transmural myocardial channels do not salvage acutely ischemic myocardium. J Am Coll Cardiol 22:302–309
14. Hardy RI, James FW, Millard RW, Kaplan S (1990) Regional myocardial blood flow and cardiac mechanics in dogs with CO_2 laser-induced intramyocardial revascularization. Basic Res Cardiol 85:179–197
15. Landreneau R, Nawararong W, Laughlin H, et al. (1991) Direct CO_2 laser revascularization of the myocardium. Lasers Surg Med 11:35–42
16. Jeevanandam V, Auteri JS, Oz MC, Watkins J, Rose EA, Smith CR (1990) Myocardial revascularization by laser-induced channels. Surg Forum 41:225–227
17. Horvath KA, Smith WJ, Cohn LH, et al (1995) Recovery and viability of an acute myocardial infarct after transmyocardial laser revascularization. J Am Coll Cardiol 25:258–263
18. Hale SL, Kloner RA (1992) Effect of ischemic preconditioning on regional myocardial blood flow in the rabbit heart. Coron Artery Dis 3:133–140
19. Whittaker P, Rakusan K, Kloner RA (1996) Transmural channels can protect ischemic tissue. Assessment of long-term myocardial response to laser- and needle-made channels. Circulation 93:143–152
20. Kohmoto T, Fisher PE, Gu A, Zhu SM, Yano OJ, Spotnitz HM, Smith CR, Burkhoff D (1996) Does blood flow through holmium:YAG transmyocardial laser channels? Ann Thorac Surg 61:861–868
21. Goda T, Wierzbicki Z, Gaston A, Leandri J, Vouron J, Loisance D (1987) Myocardial revascularization by CO_2 laser. Eur Surg Res 19:113–117
22 Nagata Y, Aoyama T, Mase T, Shioi K, Nogaki H (1996) Effectiveness of transmyocardial laser revascularization on ischemic heart – experimental study. J Cardiovasc Surg 4 [Suppl 1]:15
23. Page DL, Caulfield JB, Kastor JA, DeSanctis R, Sanders CA (1971) Myocardial changes associated with cardiogenic shock. N Engl J Med 285:133–137
24. Piffare R, Jasuja ML, Lynch RD, Neville WE (1969) Myocardial revascularization by transmyocardial acupuncture. J Thorac Cardiovasc Surg 58:424–431
25. Piffare R (1968) Intramyocardial pressure during systole and diastole. Ann Surg 168:871–875
26. Nematzadeh D, Rose JC, Schryver TH, Huang HK, Kot PA (1984) Analysis of methodology for measuring intramyocardial pressure. Basic Res Cardiol 79:86–97

Subject Index

MIX
Papier aus verantwortungsvollen Quellen
Paper from responsible sources
FSC® C105338

If you have any concerns about our products,
you can contact us on
ProductSafety@springernature.com

In case Publisher is established outside the EU,
the EU authorized representative is:
Springer Nature Customer Service Center GmbH
Europaplatz 3, 69115 Heidelberg, Germany

Printed by Libri Plureos GmbH
in Hamburg, Germany